Creating Urban and Workplace Environments for Recovery and Well-being

This essential book offers suggestions for how cities and spaces can be planned and designed to reduce the impact of stress, provide opportunities for recovery, and promote the resilience of individuals in urban communities.

Connecting research from different scientific disciplines, the book provides a broader perspective of creating healthy lifestyle in society. It focuses on mental health and well being by exploring how urban and workplace environments can be created to enhance and promote recovery. Divided into three parts, the book begins by investigating the multi-dimensional challenges of planning and design for stress reduction and recovery in urban areas. Part 2 concentrates on the design of residential and working environments, including commuting between the two, while Part 3 considers how neighbourhoods and entire cities contribute to or obstruct stress reduction, recovery, and well-being. The book concludes by demonstrating how the insights from the book can be implemented in practice to create restorative and inclusive environments. Bringing together leading experts, the book offers an interdisciplinary perspective for increasing well-being in urban developments.

The book will be of interest to researchers and practitioners in related fields, including environmental psychologists, urban planners, architects and landscape architects, healthcare staff, and policymakers.

Stephan Pauleit is Chair for Strategic Landscape Planning and Management at Technical University of Munich, Germany.

Michael Kellmann is Professor of Sport Psychology at the Faculty of Sport Science at Ruhr University Bochum, Germany. He is also Honorary Professor in the School of Human Movement and Nutrition Sciences at The University of Queensland, Australia.

Jürgen Beckmann is Professor of Sport Psychology, Emeritus of Excellence, at the School of Medicine and Health at Technical University of Munich, Germany. He is also Honorary Professor in the School of Human Movement and Nutrition Sciences at The University of Queensland, Australia.

Advances in Recovery and Stress Research: Multi-Disciplinary Approaches Series

Series Editors

Michael Kellmann, Ruhr University Bochum, Germany, and The University of Queensland, Australia

Jürgen Beckmann, Technical University of Munich, Germany, and The University of Queensland, Australia

Advances in Recovery and Stress Research: Multi-Disciplinary Approaches covers a broad range of areas in which recovery plays a crucial role, providing the current status of research on recovery and stress. In particular, it aims to be unique in addressing fields in which recovery and stress play an important role, but recovery has not received adequate attention, for example, in the areas of health promotion as well as performance promotion in work settings. Another feature of the series is that it contains both up-to-date theoretical and applied perspectives from multi-disciplinary approaches.

Recovery and Well-being in Sport and Exercise
Interdisciplinary Insights
Edited by Michael Kellmann and Jürgen Beckmann

The Importance of Recovery for Physical and Mental Health
Negotiating the Effects of Underrecovery
Edited by Michael Kellmann, Sarah Jakowski, and Jürgen Beckmann

Fostering Recovery and Well-being in a Healthy Lifestyle
Psychological, Somatic, and Organizational Prevention Approaches
Edited by Michael Kellmann and Jürgen Beckmann

The Recovery-Stress Questionnaires
A User Manual
Edited by Michael Kellmann and K. Wolfgang Kallus

Creating Urban and Workplace Environments for Recovery and Well-being
New Perspectives on Urban Design and Mental Health
Edited by Stephan Pauleit, Michael Kellmann, and Jürgen Beckmann

For more information about this series, please visit: www.routledge.com/Advances-in-Recovery-and-Stress-Research/book-series/ARSR

Creating Urban and Workplace Environments for Recovery and Well-being

New Perspectives on Urban Design and Mental Health

Edited by
Stephan Pauleit, Michael Kellmann, and Jürgen Beckmann

Routledge
Taylor & Francis Group
LONDON AND NEW YORK

Designed Cover Image: liuzishan via Getty Images

First published 2025
by Routledge
4 Park Square, Milton Park, Abingdon, Oxon OX14 4RN

and by Routledge
605 Third Avenue, New York, NY 10158

Routledge is an imprint of the Taylor & Francis Group, an informa business

British Library Cataloguing-in-Publication Data
A catalogue record for this book is available from the British Library

ISBN: 978-1-032-56427-2 (hbk)
ISBN: 978-1-032-56424-1 (pbk)
ISBN: 978-1-003-43547-1 (ebk)

DOI: 10.4324/9781003435471

The Open Access version of Chapter 11 was funded by ECR Publication Fund.

Contents

Contributors

Åshage, Anna, Swedish University of Agricultural Sciences, Sweden

Bauer, Amelie, Ludwig-Maximilians-University Munich, Germany

Beckmann, Jürgen, Technical University of Munich, Germany, and The University of Queensland, Australia

Bengtsson, Anna, Swedish University of Agricultural Sciences, Sweden

Ceccato, Vania, KTH Royal Institute of Technology, Sweden

Chalmin-Pui, Lauriane S., University of Sheffield, United Kingdom

de Vries, Sjerp, Wageningen Environmental Research, Netherlands

Egerer, Monika, Technical University of Munich, Germany

Elfering, Achim, University of Bern, Switzerland

Grahn, Patrik, Swedish University of Agricultural Sciences, Sweden

Gu, Lanqing, Technical University of Darmstadt, Germany

Huber, Fabrice, Université de Neuchâtel, Switzerland

Iovița, Claudia, Kopvol architecture and psychology, Germany

Jarvis, Ingrid, University of British Columbia, Canada

Kallus, K. Wolfgang, Karl-Franzens-University Graz, Austria

Kellmann, Michael, Ruhr University Bochum, Germany, and The University of Queensland, Australia

Knöll, Martin, Technical University of Darmstadt, Germany

Koppen, Gemma, Coburg University of Applied Sciences, Germany

Lehmann, Hannah, University Hospital of Munich, Ludwig-Maximilians-University Munich, Germany

Marselle, Melissa, University of Surrey, United Kingdom

Pauleit, Stephan, Technical University of Munich, Germany

Phillips, Mark N., Coburg University of Applied Sciences, Germany

van den Bosch, Matilda, Barcelona Institute for Global Health, Spain, and the European Forest Institute, Biocities Facility, Italy

Vollmer, Tanja C., Technical University of Munich, Germany

Zölch, Teresa, Department for Climate and Environmental Protection, City of Munich, Germany

Series foreword

Advances in Recovery and Stress Research: Multi-Disciplinary Approaches covers a broad range of areas in which recovery plays a crucial role, providing the status of research on recovery and stress. In particular, it aims to broaden the understanding of recovery and be unique in addressing fields in which recovery and stress play an important role but recovery has not received adequate attention. Examples are the areas of health promotion as well as performance promotion in work settings. Another feature of the series is that it contains both up-to-date theoretical and applied perspectives from multidisciplinary approaches.

It is the idea of the series *Advances in Recovery and Stress Research: Multi-Disciplinary Approaches* to publish a volume each year. We started with *Recovery and Well-being in Sport and Exercise* (Volume 1), followed by *The Importance of Recovery for Physical and Mental Health: Negotiating the Effects of Underrecovery* (Volume 2), and with Volume 3, *Fostering Recovery and Well-being in a Healthy Lifestyle: Psychological, Somatic, and Organizational Prevention Approaches. The Recovery-Stress Questionnaires: A user manual* (Volume 4) and *Creating Urban and Workplace Environments for Recovery and Well-being: New Perspectives on Urban Design and Mental Health* (Volume 5) are on the way, and Volume 6 is already organised, but the title is not finalised. Always current information on the series can be found at www.routledge.com/Advances-in-Recovery-and-Stress-Research/book-series/ARSR.

We thank Routledge for the flexibility and engagement for this adventure to develop the series *Advances in Recovery and Stress Research: Multi-Disciplinary Approaches.*

Michael Kellmann
Jürgen Beckmann

Preface

The 21st century experiences unprecedented rates of population increase in urban areas. Already now, over 50% of the human population is living in urban areas, and this share is expected to increase to 68% by 2050 (United Nations, 2019). Together with still strong overall population growth, this trend is likely to add another 2.5 billion inhabitants to urban areas globally, mostly in countries of the Global South, while industrialised countries, such as in Europe and North America, are already highly urbanised.

Cities are centres of social, cultural, and economic innovation and hence provide many opportunities for fulfilling human needs. At the same time, living in cities can be stressful, with negative impact on human health and well-being. Stressors in cities are related to density of living with unsustainable modern lifestyles in connection with environmental pollution, high economic and technological dynamics, and other factors. Moreover, climate change leads to an increasing heat impact and hence loss of thermal comfort, which has a negative impact on not only physical but also mental health. While exposure to harmful levels of stressors for human living must be reduced, increased stress cannot be entirely avoided in dense urban settlements. Moreover, stress must not be considered as being negative for humans, per se, as long as humans can restore from it and build resilience and manage to deal with it. Our concept of recovery not only involves regeneration from stress, or the replenishment of personal resources, but has also expanded into a concept of building resilience. Only recently, positive psychology has begun to address recovery in the field of mental health as a broader concept in a similar way, as a resource that enables individuals not only to recover from stress but also to show resilience to health-threatening stress.

Urban planning and design have a long history of striving for the creation of healthy places for humans. Much emphasis has been placed on a reduction of negative health impacts from environmental pollution, leading to sometimes strong legislation to control air pollution, to control noise, or to provide pure drinking water. Considerably less attention has still been given to mental health and well-being, however, despite an increasing body of scientific evidence that is building up, for example, on the beneficial effects of exposure to urban green for physical and mental health as well as the well-being of the city-dwellers.

This book will address this neglected aspect and connect research from different scientific disciplines to the broader perspective of creating a healthy lifestyle in society. It will explore how urban and workplace environments can be created to enhance/promote recovery as an underestimated factor in creating urban and workplace environment. The book should provide impetus in many areas in which the impact of recovery is important, such as architecture, workplace, and health.

References

United Nations. (2019). *World urbanization prospects: The 2018 revision*. Department of Economic and Social Affairs, Population Division. Retrieved June 27, 2024 from https://www.un.org/en/desa/2018-revision-world-urbanization-prospects#:~:text=Today%2C%2055%25%20of%20the%20world's,increase%20to%2068%25%20by%202050

Stephan Pauleit
Michael Kellmann
Jürgen Beckmann

Part I

Conceptualising the problem

1 Urban flourishing

Human recovery and urban resilience as hubs for the city of the future

Stephan Pauleit, Jürgen Beckmann, and Michael Kellmann

Introduction

Cities have become the most important human habitat in the 21st century. According to the United Nations, more than 50% of the world's population lives in cities (United Nations, 2019), and this share is expected to grow to more than two-thirds by 2050.

Many cities are currently witnessing a phase of rapid social and technological changes that have an impact on urban development. The digital revolution influences all spheres of urban living and the economy. Retail is changing dramatically due to online trade, for example, and department stores are disappearing from city centres as a result. Teleworking from home is gaining influence and reducing the need for office space and mobility. The Covid-19 pandemic has accelerated these processes. In general, digitalisation is fundamentally changing the way humans interact with each other and the social fabric (OECD, 2019). Positive effects include increased individual flexibility, which can positively affect well-being and potentially reduce carbon footprint due to decreased commuting necessities. Increasing digitalisation has accelerated the development of a 'network society' (Castells, 1996) that is organised around networks based on shared interests, values, or activities that are not constrained by geographical proximity. Negative aspects of this development are increased individual isolation (Rainie & Wellman, 2012) and the further promotion of sedentary behaviour instead of a physically active lifestyle (Thivel et al., 2018).

The quest for sustainability and climate change adaptation is becoming ever more important in urban development. The 'ecological footprint' of the City of London alone – the area of land needed to provide its necessary resources and absorb the wastes generated by it – was estimated to exceed 40 times its biological capacity (Lyndhurst, 2003). Consequently, cities are also major contributors to global warming due to their enormous emissions of greenhouse gases (Mukim & Roberts, 2023).

Pauleit, S., Beckmann, J., & Kellmann, M. (2025). Urban flourishing: Human recovery and urban resilience as hubs for the city of the future. In S. Pauleit, M. Kellmann, & J. Beckmann (Eds.), *Creating Urban and Workplace Environments for Recovery and Well-being* (pp. 3–20). Routledge.

DOI: 10.4324/9781003435471-2

At the same time, urban areas are increasingly affected by heatwaves, storms, and floods (Revi et al., 2014). Global and local crises are becoming more frequent and severe. The belief in the complete controllability of these crises through technology in a progressively complex and unpredictable world has dwindled. For the future of the city and its inhabitants, it will be crucial to strengthen the capacity for urban recovery, that is, the ability to recover from acute crises, but even more so to enhance urban resilience as urban systems' capacity to adapt and even to transform in the face of fundamental changes, such as climate change or technological upheavals, without compromising its functions and quality of life (Meerow et al., 2016). Urban recovery and urban resilience, therefore, have become key goals for urban development and need to be considered as imperatives for their sustainability.

Increased focus on health and well-being

How cities are built, how life is organised in them, and how they change have significant consequences for people's health and well-being. Air and water pollution, contaminated soils, noise, and malnutrition constitute persisting major health concerns worldwide.

A major cause of health problems in modern society, the so-called civilisation diseases, is the increasing physical inactivity among people. Already in 1954, Collins coined the notion of a 'sedentary society'. The problem and its consequences have escalated much since then. The prevalence of being sedentary has increased substantially in recent decades. This increase is associated with, for example, higher rates of obesity and type 2 diabetes (Lavie et al., 2019; Owen et al., 2010). Factors that prevent sedentary behaviour are physical activity–related cognitions, a more positive attitude towards physical activity, having greater social support or norms for physical activity, greater self-efficacy or control for physical activity, higher physical activity intentions, and higher intrinsic and identified motivation towards physical activity (Rollo et al., 2016). In general, motivational psychology has demonstrated that environmental stimuli (situational cues) can instigate motivation to become active or trigger habits related to physical activity with positive health impacts (Beckmann et al., 2024). Such environmental stimuli are provided, for instance, by the provision of accessible and attractive green spaces (Biernacka & Kronenberg, 2019). Positive effects of regular visits to green spaces and contact with nature on mental health have been established in many studies (Markevych et al., 2017; Marselle, 2019; White et al., 2021). Visiting green spaces can reduce psychological stress, increase individual resilience to future stress experiences (Grahn & Stigsdotter, 2003), and strengthen social cohesion (Birtchnell et al., 2019; Kaźmierczak, 2013). There is now a large body of further evidence on the positive effects of urban greening on human physical and mental health (van den Berg et al., 2015). Conceptual frameworks have been proposed to establish causal pathways between exposure to and contact with nature and human health and well-being (Markevych et al., 2017; Marselle, 2019) and, recently, between nature contact and community and individual resilience (*Nature-based Biopsychosocial Resilience Theory*; White et al., 2023). In the latter concept, green spaces are considered as an adaptive resource that can be drawn upon in times of stress. It is therefore problematic that green spaces and nature are often lacking in urban areas. Moreover, while green spaces can have positive impacts on health in cities and their loss may be problematic, research suggests that other aspects of cities may be causing additional stress.

In recent decades, especially in post-industrial service societies, issues of chronic stress in the never-resting '24-hour city' have become critical (Lederbogen et al., 2011). For example, a survey in the United Kingdom showed 74% of the respondents to be so stressed that they were overwhelmed or felt unable to cope (Mental Health Foundation, 2018). Meta-studies established significantly higher levels of mental health problems, such as anxiety and mood disorders, as well as schizophrenia, in urban areas (Lederbogen et al., 2011; Peen et al., 2010). Brain imaging studies have recently demonstrated a higher vulnerability to social stress among urban residents (Lederbogen et al., 2011). However, epidemiological evidence was inconclusive in a study for the United States (Breslau et al., 2014), and for low- and middle-income countries (DeVylder et al., 2018; Solmi et al., 2017). Moreover, levels of stress and mental disorders can vary to a large degree within urban areas (Lederbogen et al., 2011; Solmi et al., 2017).

Urban areas can be stressful places and have negative impacts on mental health due to environmental factors, such as air and noise pollution, the predominance of artificial structures, the concurrent lack of green space, the density of population, as well as social and economic factors, such as deprivation (Ventriglio et al., 2020; Xu et al., 2023). Moreover, lifestyles have changed and diversified in recent decades and are characterised by greater flexibility of working hours, less economic security, acceleration, digitalisation, loss of social cohesion and isolation, and generally, the perception of a highly uncertain future (Burton, 1990; Ventriglio et al., 2020). Therefore, a major focus of urban development needs to address how cities can be designed and how living in cities can be organised to reduce stress and its adverse impacts on human health and well-being, as well as to improve human recovery from stress. Moreover, it needs to be asked whether and how increasing the resilience of urban systems can promote human recovery, and vice versa. Both perspectives of human recovery and urban resilience will be explored in the following sections, in turn, while the final section aims to establish the interrelationships between the two.

Human recovery

Human recovery from stress has been defined in different ways in different contexts. In Kellmann and Kallus's (2001) approach, a broader perspective on recovery is advocated that goes beyond regeneration or 'being cured' or 'being normal again'. In this broader perspective, recovery is addressed as a resource that enables an individual not only to recover from stress but also to show resilience to health-threatening stress. Thereby, recovery promotes health and well-being (Beckmann et al., 2023). According to Kallus (2016, p. 42), recovery is defined

Box 1.1 Central characteristics of recovery (modified based on Kallus & Kellmann, 2000, p. 210)

Recovery:

- Is a process in time and is dependent on the type of and duration of stress.
- Depends on a reduction of stress, a change of stress, or a break from stress.
- Is individually specific and depends on individual appraisals.
- Can be passive, active, and pro-active.
- Is closely tied to situational conditions (e.g., sleep, social contact).

as "an inter- and intraindividual multilevel (e.g., psychological, physiological, social) process in time for the re-establishment of personal resources and their full functional capacity". Box 1.1 highlights some of the main characteristics of recovery, which will be briefly outlined.

The recovery process needs time. How much time is needed to recover from stress depends on the type of stress, its intensity, and the duration. Ideally, the recovery process involves a break from stress, or at least a reduction of stress. Sometimes, the recovery process can also consist of a change of stress, switching behavioural systems that involve different types of stress. For example, a person spending the whole day sitting at a desk and doing paperwork may shift to physical activity after work, changing from mental stress to somatic stress. The latter supports replenishing the person's mental resources. Physical activity is an active recovery approach. The office worker could alternatively take a nap, that is, pursue a passive recovery strategy.

Individuals differ regarding which recovery approach suits them best. The individually most adequate recovery strategy needs to be selected and executed for successful recovery. Additionally, a person may be proactive in planning or scheduling self-initiated recovery strategies, including social activities chosen by the individual and catered to the individual's needs (Kellmann, 2002; Kellmann et al., 2018, 2023). Situational conditions play a crucial role in finding recovery. For example, a noisy environment can interfere with good sleep quality. Also, heat can negatively affect recovery, such as hindering physical activity and negatively impacting sleep quality. Especially, in the case of physical activity as the preferred recovery strategy, environmental conditions must be given that make the execution of physical activity possible, and these need to be easily accessible. The affordances (sensu what the environment offers to the individual; Gibson, 1979) will be low if one has to drive 45 minutes to find adequate conditions for one's recovery activities. Adequate conditions that promote positive recovery outcomes are in particular natural settings with trees and water (Donnelly & MacIntyre, 2019).

According to the previously described characteristics of the recovery model, specific prerequisites for adequate recovery must be met. A vicious cycle can be initiated if the necessary conditions are not met, such as a lack of time or adverse situational circumstances. Opportunities for people to recover from stress can be insufficient because demanding and excessive life activities leave little time for recovery. Commuting to work in big cities can be very time-consuming and reduces the time available for recovery (Elfering & Huber, this volume, Chapter 2). With a lack of recovery, people may become chronically stressed to the point that they even fail to become aware of their recovery needs and/or find their best recovery strategy (Beckmann, 2023). If awareness of the need for recovery leads to pro-active strategies, the vicious circle can be avoided. Recovery habits can be developed that can be initiated by situational cues (cf., affordances) provided by the environment, which calls for an interaction of developing individual awareness and environmental design (Beckmann & Heckhausen, 2024).

A central aspect of the recovery model postulated by Kellmann and Kallus (2001) refers to a balance of stress and recovery. The assumption is that with increasing stress an increase in recovery must co occur to maintain a balance between the two, to avoid adverse outcomes and promote positive outcomes in health, well-being, and quality of life (Beckmann et al., 2024). While this model was initially developed for the sport context, it can be much more generalised.

Limited resources (e.g., time) can initiate a vicious cycle: under increased stress and an inability to meet the increased recovery demands, increased levels of stress are experienced. The increased stress level can then interfere with finding time for recovery or finding ways to cope with the situation. In this model, the simplest case is a symmetrical increase in stress and recovery demands: the two axes drift apart with elevated stress levels ('scissors' function). Up to intermediate levels of stress, one can find adequate recovery (solid arrows in Figure 1.1). Beyond, the stress capacity threshold, recovery demands cannot be met or will require additional recovery activities. Humans must be given special opportunities to recover in order to re-establish an optimal level of functionality or performance. If the recovery needs are not met because the stress threshold is exceeded and, at the same time, recovery resources are exhausted or depleted, stress will accumulate and underrecovery symptoms (e.g., burnout, overtraining in athletes) are likely to develop.

The underlying mechanism of Kellmann's *Scissors Model* can be compared to the health-oriented model of *Salutogenesis* developed by Antonovsky (1979, 1987). The salutogenic approach proposes a health ease/disease continuum – also called a breakdown continuum – on which an individual can be located. The question is not whether someone is ill but rather how far away a person is from the end points. The person's position on the breakdown continuum depends on current resistance deficits and the availability of general resistance resources for tension management. Notably, the stress buffer in Kellmann's recovery model has similarities with the function of Antonovsky's general resistance resources.

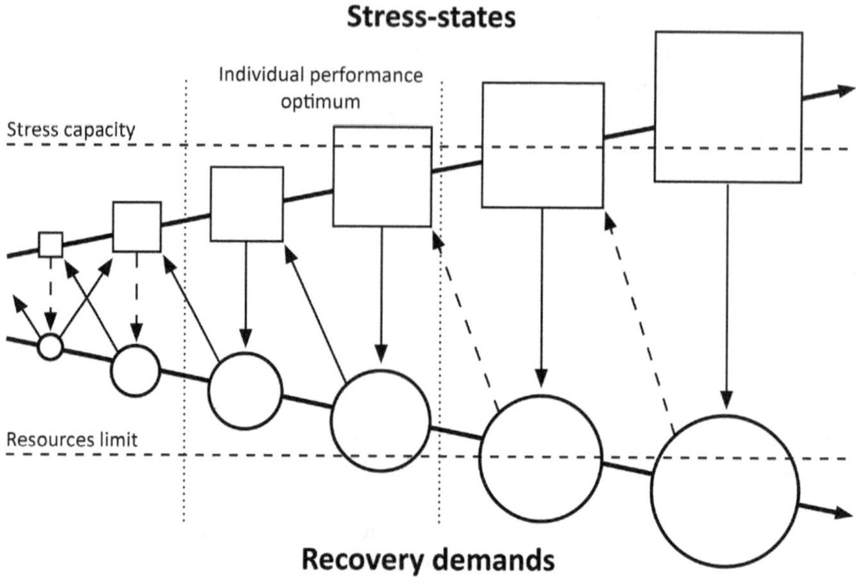

Figure 1.1 The *Scissors Model* of the interrelation of stress states and recovery demands.

Source: Reprinted with permission from Kallus, K. W., & Kellmann, M. (2000). Burnout in athletes and coaches. In Y. Hanin (Ed.), *Emotions in sport* (pp. 209–230). Human Kinetics.

In summary, Kellmann's recovery model suggests it is not harmful to be high on stress, as long as the individual knows how to recover optimally. The model describes the process of readjustment. Recovery as a resource can also be addressed as a result of the recovery process. Rather than merely re-establishing an equilibrium, the recovery process may overcompensate to generate a stress buffer, increasing available recovery resources and raising the threshold for negative stress effects.

Recently, a broader perspective of human recovery was advocated (Beckmann et al., 2023) in which recovery is addressed as a resource that promotes health and well-being. It involves gaining or recapturing meaning and purpose in life, and self-determination, resulting in personal empowerment and resilience. Beckmann and Kellmann (2024, pp. 218–219) emphasise that

> recognizing the systemic nature of stress and recovery is vital for designing effective interventions and policies. By fostering a balance between stress and recovery across physiological, psychological, and social dimensions, individuals and societies can cultivate resilience, promote optimal well-being, and mitigate the negative effects of chronic stress.

Citizens in modern cities need to be resilient to various environmental, social, and lifestyle-related stresses and manage to maintain vital urban and human functions. This involves developing the capacity to provide optimal levels of stimulation, affordances for physical activity, and a perception of security enabling health promotion and well-being not only for the affluent. Affordances 'suggest' or 'invite' action. According to Norman (1988), affordances 'suggest' how an object may be interacted with. Gibson (1979) defined affordance as what the environment provides or furnishes. He points out that individuals need to control their perception of affordances (selective attention) and initiate acts, for example, a one-metre-high step does not permit climbing to a crawling infant. It might provide rest to a tired adult or suggest an opportunity to get an overview of the environment.

Similarly, Lewin (1935) described demand characteristics of the environment. Demand characteristics call for action. They offer need fulfilment or, in Lewin's terms, the discharge of motivational tension. Lewin describes this in an example of a person who intends to post a letter. Forming this intention has created a motivational tension. When walking through town, the person may not intentionally look for a mailbox, but seeing one will automatically trigger posting the letter. Thus, environmental affordances can suggest the execution of a behavioural intention or even trigger behavioural habits. For example, a fitness machine in a park can incite walkers to spontaneously engage in physical activity suggested by the machine (Figure 1.2).

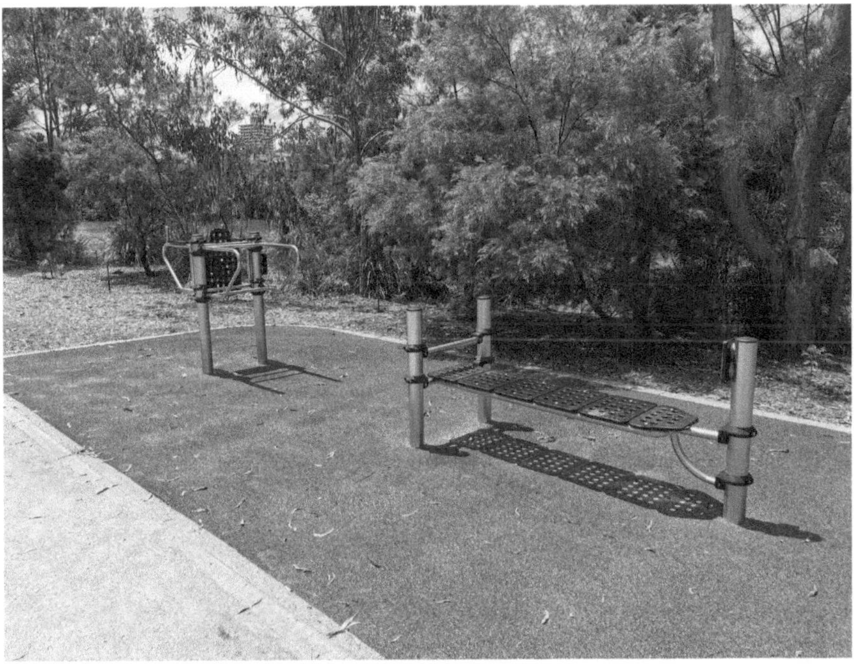

Figure 1.2 Physical activity affordances on the walkway at The University of Queensland, Brisbane, Australia.

Source: Photo by Michael Kellmann.

Gibson (1979) stated that humans tend to alter and modify their environment to change its affordances to better suit them and make living easier. Hammoud et al. (2021) found high population density to be associated with loneliness, but if neighbourhoods produced feelings of social inclusivity, feelings of loneliness were decreased. Also, exposure to nature was linked to reduced odds of loneliness. Furthermore, Fraser et al. (2024) report studies showing that social infrastructure, such as parks, supports the development of social ties, mitigates political polarisation, and improves health. Urban design focusing on the development of social infrastructure could thus pave the way to, for example, healthier lifestyles in terms of physical activity in nature or increased interpersonal encounters and interactions.

This section introduced human recovery from urban stresses as a process that depends on the interplay of individual human recovery demands and stress states. The *Scissors Model* postulates that recovery from increasing severity of stress requires additional recovery activities. The availability of individual, social, and environmental resources (social infrastructure) is crucial to stimulate recovery activities. As will be shown in the following section, the concepts of urban recovery and resilience are closely related to this line of thought, however, with a focus on the entire urban system.

Urban recovery and resilience

Urban recovery can be understood as the response of urban systems to disasters that may have natural and/or human causes, such as earthquakes, hurricanes, wars, or the recent Covid-19 pandemic. Strengthening the capacity for recovery at the urban system scale is about creating social, institutional, political, economic, and infrastructural conditions to be well prepared for disasters, to enable a rapid and targeted response during the disaster, and to effectively support the recovery of affected people after the disaster, as well as to repair the damage. Making efforts to protect urban areas from natural hazards, such as building dikes along a river, are important, but the reduction of urban vulnerabilities before, during, and after the occurrence of the hazard is emphasised in urban recovery. The availability of assets at city, community, and individual levels is critical in this regard (Herslund et al., 2016). These comprise the availability and the state of 1) physical assets, including, for instance, the availability of and access to nature and natural resources, the provision of ecosystem services, and the layout of urban areas; 2) social assets, such as access to sufficient economic resources or health literacy, the existence of social networks, and the sociodemographic composition (e.g., a balanced age structure); 3) institutional assets, like an effective and fair local administration and governance system; and 4) attitudinal assets, such as risk awareness and training. These four broad types of assets and how they interact may increase or reduce the vulnerability of people, communities, and the overall urban system.

'Resilience' expands this perspective further. The term is used in different fields of research and application, such as disease prevention, the management of organisations, (disaster) risk management, economics, and social-technical systems science (Therrien et al., 2015). For urban systems, Meerow et al. (2016, p. 49) defined resilience as the

> ability of an urban system – and all its constituent socio-ecological and socio-technical networks across temporal and spatial scales – to maintain or rapidly return to desired functions in the face of a disturbance, to adapt to change, and to quickly transform systems that limit current or future adaptive capacity.

Therefore, resilience goes beyond the ability to return to a previous state after some disturbance ('bouncing back'; Figure 1.3) but offers a transformative perspective ('bouncing forward'; Figure 1.3). This view emphasises the importance of learning processes within the urban system that enable the transformation of existing urban regimes to respond successfully to future challenges while maintaining qualities and functions essential for the health and well-being of humans and other organisms now and in the future. With *Transformation Theory*, an entire body of research has emerged over the past two decades that explores how such transformations can be achieved by overcoming system lock-ins and path dependencies (Geels, 2004; Loorbach et al., 2017).

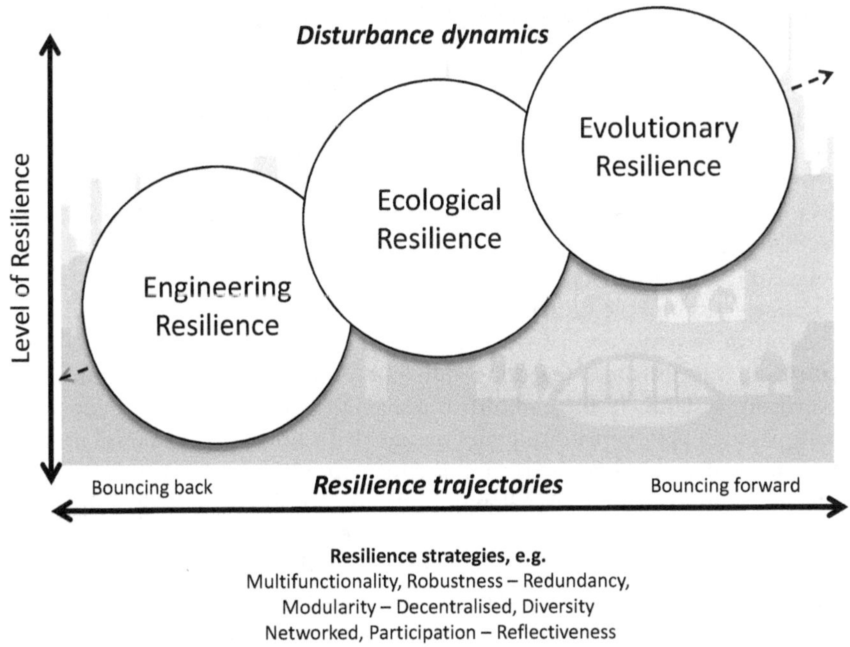

Figure 1.3 Resilience types.

Source: Adapted from Davoudi (2012).

Resilience Theory distinguishes three types of resilience: 1) *engineering resilience*, wherein systems can return to their initial state after disturbances to preserve what already exists ('bouncing back'); 2) *ecological resilience*, wherein ecosystems can shift between different states of stability but maintain basic ecological structures and functions; and 3) *evolutionary resilience*, in which systems can transform into new systems driven by fundamental changes of the environment and/or disruptive innovations within the system ('bouncing forward').

Much of urban 'resilience thinking' has been derived from insights gained in research on socio-ecological systems (Holling, 1973; Walker & Salt, 2006). It has caught the interest of urban planners (Davoudi, 2012) that have to deal with the complexity and, hence, the unpredictability of urban systems' behaviour and are facing global change. Various authors have proposed principles or strategies for strengthening urban resilience, such as the promotion of multifunctionality of urban spaces; redundancy and modularity of urban infrastructures, which are robust, flexible, and decentralised; enhancement of biological, social, and economic diversity and networking; inclusive and participatory approaches to urban governance; the strengthening of natural and social capital; and pilot projects that provide arenas for shared learning and reflection as a basis for adaptive and integrated planning (Ahern, 2011; Ribeiro & Gonçalves, 2019; Wilkinson, 2012).

The role of urban nature, understood here as all areas that contain plants and non-human animals in cities, from street trees, managed parks, and gardens, to remnants of pristine wilderness (Bratman et al., 2012), deserves particular attention in urban resilience strategies. There is strong evidence that urban nature, with its diversity of organisms, plays a crucial role in strengthening the resilience of urban landscapes by maintaining natural processes that provide ecosystem services for the health and well-being of humans (Coutts, 2016; McPhearson et al., 2015). 'Urban green infrastructure' is an approach to promote urban nature by developing networks of green and blue spaces with multiple ecosystem services in urban areas through strategic planning and management (Pauleit, Hansen, et al., 2017; Pauleit, Zölch, et al., 2017).

The selective sample of general principles/strategies for designing and managing urban systems towards resilience requires further definition and contextualisation, for instance, regarding different urban areas, infrastructures, and governance systems. In the end, urban resilience as a policy concept, like other concepts, such as sustainability, defies unique definitions and measures but needs to be adapted to local contexts in a discursive process. It may have its greatest value as a 'boundary' concept, allowing a diverse constituency to develop a joint vision in a systems perspective (Jacobs, 1999; Meerow & Newell, 2016).

Also, monitoring of urban resilience is under debate (Gerges et al., 2023). One example is the City Resilience Index developed by Arup (2014; Cao et al., 2021), with 52 indicators of four categories: leadership and strategy (knowledge), health and well-being (people), economy and society (organisation), as well as infrastructure and ecosystems (place). Thus, the index recognises the important link between urban resilience and human health and well-being yet is mostly concerned with provision of effective life support systems (water and energy supply, etc.), livelihood, and health infrastructures.

Organisations such as the Resilience Alliance, the Resilient Cities Network, UNEP (United Nations Environmental Program), ICLEI – Local Governments for Sustainability, the World Bank, and the 100 Resilient Cities initiative by the Rockefeller Foundation promote the uptake of resilience thinking in municipal practice all over the world through conferences, publications, and networks. One example is the Resilient Melbourne Strategy which proposes 33 strategy actions under four action areas: adapt, survive, thrive, and embed (City of Melbourne, 2016). Some of the actions are a metropolitan urban forest strategy that aims to increase urban tree cover, a metropolitan cycling network, a community resilience framework, resilience research at local universities, a smart city initiative, and resilience training for local government. Another action aims to improve the mental well-being of young people in Melbourne (VicHealth, 2019).

Relating human recovery and urban resilience

Urban resilience shares similarities with and is related to human recovery (Figure 1.3). This is not surprising, as the roots of the concept of resilience can be found, among others, in psychology (Brown & Westaway, 2011). Yet urban resilience thinking has been more informed by insights gained from social-ecological systems research but has given little attention to aspects of human recovery. Both human recovery and urban resilience are grounded in a non-equilibrium worldview where stress/disturbances are a part of the system and may be even necessary for human health and well-being and urban sustainability, respectively, if they do not exceed certain thresholds ('tipping points' and 'stress capacity', respectively). As the *Scissors Model* for human recovery suggests, an individual's capacity to tolerate stress is not fixed but can increase or decrease, depending on the availability of resources to fulfil recovery demands. Similarly, the strengthening of urban resources/assets will allow urban systems to better cope with and adapt to disturbances and chronic stresses, such as those induced, for example, by climate change, and even to transform the entire system. As Meerow and Newell (2016) point out, the provision and deployment of these resources must not only consider what resources are needed and for whom but also when and where these are needed (e.g., before, during, after a disaster; in vulnerable areas), and not least for which purpose (e.g., to increase economic, social, and/or ecological resilience; at the level of neighbourhoods, city, or city regions; in an engineering, ecological, or evolutionary resilience perspective).

Figure 1.4 depicts the relationship between human recovery and urban resilience. Human recovery can benefit from urban resilience strategies that strengthen physical, social, institutional, and attitudinal resources/assets. These strategies should develop an evolutionary resilience of the urban system to face the ongoing dramatic changes of the earth system. Simultaneously, they should support personal strategies with resources and affordances that strengthen the

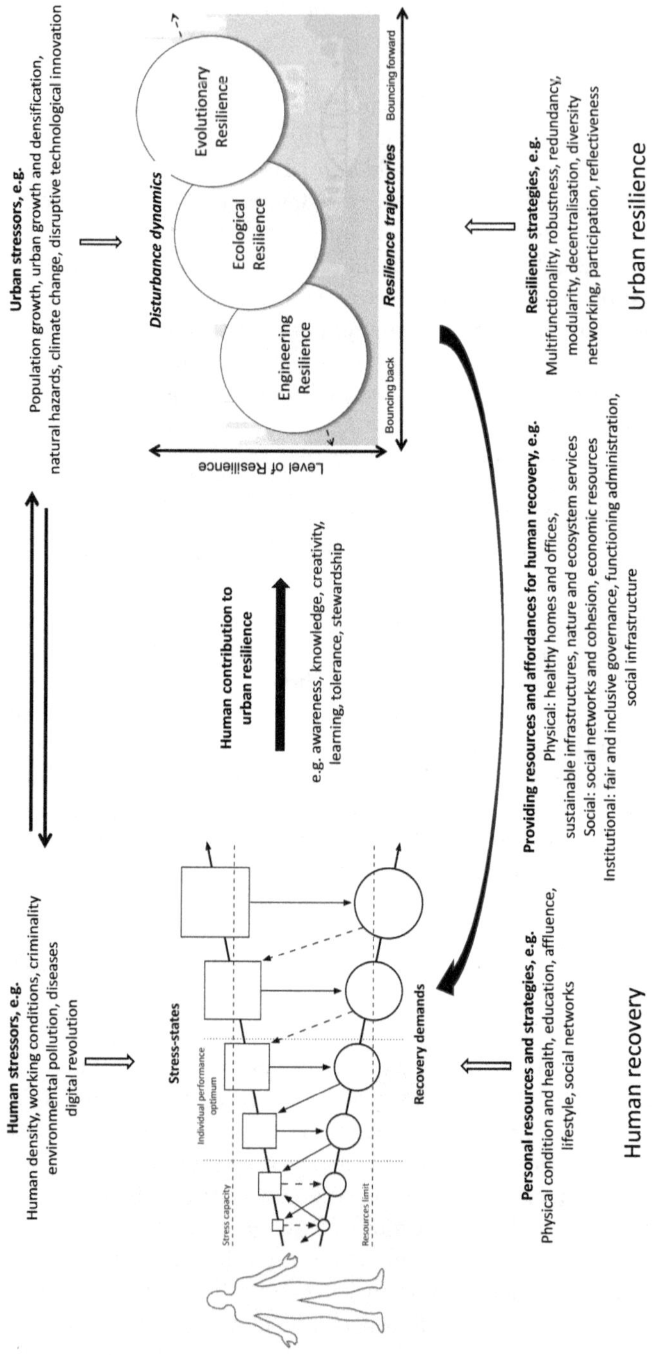

Figure 1.4 Relating human recovery and urban resilience.

individual's capacity to recover from stress by, for example, increasing physical fitness and health, building up economic resources, and providing stimuli for behavioural changes. Humans, then, will be better able to contribute to urban resilience as individuals or in organisations by, for example, enhanced knowledge, creativity, or a higher interest in becoming stewards of the urban environment ('stewardship').

Putting the concepts of human recovery and urban resilience side by side, there appears to be is a large congruence between the resources needed for human recovery and urban resilience, even though the terminology differs to some degree. Therefore, strategies to strengthen urban resilience can potentially support human recovery by providing the necessary resources and affordances. For instance, Dai et al. (2023) found that catering, retail, and sports facilities were contributing to emotional stability during the Covid-19 pandemic in Shenzhen (China), while open spaces were associated with positive emotion, thus contributing to higher levels of restoration. Provision with social infrastructures, and hence their resilience, is often lower in neighbourhoods of lower socioeconomic status, as, for instance, a study in Boston has shown (Fraser et al., 2024). However, understanding the causal linkages between urban resilience and human well-being, and specifically human recovery from stress, is still in deficit. Only recently have these aspects been brought to the fore, for example, in the book *Restorative Cities – Urban Design Manual for Mental Health and Wellbeing* (Roe & McCay, 2021), which describes seven fields of action for promoting mental health in cities and recognises them as an essential contribution to urban resilience.

It should be cautioned, however, that strategies for increasing the resilience of urban systems may ignore the needs of individuals or groups with their specific personal, social, economic, and cultural situations, as well as their different access to power in decision-making. Therefore, there is no automatic 'resilience dividend' for human health and well-being, but the latter needs to be targeted in urban resilience strategies (Martinez et al., 2020). Socially inclusive planning and collaborative governance for urban resilience, which are sensitive to social and environmental injustices, are advocated for this purpose (Mahajan et al., 2022).

Conclusion and recommendations for practice

Human recovery and urban resilience are two complementary concepts with a human-centred and urban systems–centred focus, respectively. The promotion of human recovery and urban resilience is key for healthy living in cities in times of fundamental technological, societal, and climatic changes. Therefore, these two concepts should be systematically related to the design and management of urban areas towards human health and urban resilience. The framework of human recovery and urban resilience relationships offered in this chapter can only be considered as a beginning in this regard but requires further understanding of the causal pathways. This calls for inter- and transdisciplinary efforts in research and practice. Nevertheless, at this stage, the following recommendations can be made for urban design and human health practices:

- Consider the requirements and the need for human recovery in urban planning and governance, and explore systematically how these can be integrated into strategies for urban resilience in order to create synergies and minimise trade-offs.
- The systemic nature of stress and recovery must be well understood to design effective interventions and policies.
- Pay special attention to the resources and affordances for human recovery and how these relate to strengthening resources/assets for urban resilience.
- Promote the just provision of and access to essential social and environmental infrastructures, in particularly urban green infrastructure and its multiple ecosystem services, as a key strategy for human recovery and urban resilience.
- Adopt socially inclusive approaches to participation in urban governance that particularly target society's most vulnerable groups of for enhancing human recovery and urban resilience.
- Recognise the design and management of urban spaces for human recovery as a main goal in sectoral urban health strategies.

References

Ahern, J. (2011). From fail-safe to safe-to-fail: Sustainability and resilience in the new urban world. *Landscape and Urban Planning, 100*(4), 341–343.

Antonovsky, A. (1979). *Health, stress, and coping.* Jossey-Bass.

Antonovsky, A. (1987). *Unraveling the mystery of health.* Jossey-Bass.

ARUP. (2014). *City Resilience Framework: ARUP & the Rockefeller Foundation.* Retrieved November 11, 2023 from https://www.rockefellerfoundation.org/wp-content/uploads/City-Resilience-Framework-2015.pdf

Beckmann, J. (2023). Self-regulation of recovery. In M. Kellmann, S. Jakowski, & J. Beckmann (Eds.), *The importance of recovery for physical and mental health: Negotiating the effects of underrecovery* (pp. 53–69). Routledge.

Beckmann, J., & Heckhausen, H. (2024). Situational determinants of behavior. In J. Heckhausen & H. Heckhausen (Eds.), *Motivation and action* (4th ed., pp. 113–162). Springer.

Beckmann, J., Huber, M., & Andonian-Dierks, C. S. (2024). Chronic illness and well-being: Promoting quality of life with a broadened concept of recovery. In M. Kellmann & J. Beckmann (Eds.), *Fostering recovery and well-being in a healthy lifestyle: Psychological, somatic, and organizational prevention approaches* (pp. 3–23). Routledge.

Beckmann, J., & Kellmann, M. (2024). Fostering recovery and well-being: A concluding summary. In M. Kellmann & J. Beckmann (Eds.), *Fostering recovery and well-being in a healthy lifestyle: Psychological, somatic, and organizational prevention approaches* (pp. 218–222). Routledge.

Beckmann, J., Kellmann, M., & Jakowski, S. (2023). Recovery is more than just healing: Advocating a broader perspective on recovery in physical and mental health. In M. Kellmann, S. Jakowski, & J. Beckmann (Eds.), *The importance of recovery for physical and mental health: Negotiating the effects of underrecovery* (pp. 266–270). Routledge.

Biernacka, M., & Kronenberg, J. (2019). Urban green space availability, accessibility and attractiveness, and the delivery of ecosystem services. *Cities and the Environment (CATE)*, *12*(1), Article 5. Retrieved November 11, 2023 from https://digitalcommons.lmu.edu/cate/vol12/iss1/5

Birtchnell, T., Gill, N., & Sultana, R. (2019). Sleeper cells for urban green infrastructure: Harnessing latent competence in greening Dhaka's slums. *Urban Forestry & Urban Greening*, *40*, 93–104.

Bratman, G. N., Hamilton, J. P., & Daily, G. C. (2012). The impacts of nature experience on human cognitive function and mental health. *Annals of the New York Academy of Sciences*, *1249*, 118–136.

Breslau, J., Marshall, G. N., Pincus, H. A., & Brown, R. A. (2014). Are mental disorders more common in urban than rural areas of the United States? *Journal of Psychiatric Research*, *56*, 50–55. https://doi.org/10.1016/j.jpsychires.2014.05.004

Brown, K., & Westaway, E. (2011). Agency, capacity, and resilience to environmental change: Lessons from human development, well-being, and disasters. *Annual Review of Environment and Resources*, *36*, 321–342.

Burton, I. (1990). Factors in urban stress. *The Journal of Sociology and Social Welfare*, *17*(1), 79–93.

Cao, Y., Wilkinson, E., Pettinotti, L., Colenbrander, S., & Lovell, E. (2021). *A decade of urban resilience: An analytical review*. United Nations Development Program (UNDP). Retrieved November 11, 2023 from www.undp.org

Castells, M. (1996). *The rise of the network society*. Blackwell.

City of Melbourne. (2016). *Resilient Melbourne*. Retrieved November 11, 2023 from https://www.melbourne.vic.gov.au/sitecollectiondocuments/resilient-melbourne-strategy.pdf

Coutts, C. (2016). *Green infrastructure and mental health*. Routledge.

Dai, D., Dong, W., Wang, Y., Liu, S., & Zhang, J. (2023). Exploring the relationship between urban residents' emotional changes and built environment before and during the COVID-19 pandemic from the perspective of resilience. *Cities*, *141*, 104510. https://doi.org/10.1016/j.cities.2023.104510

Davoudi, S. (2012). Resilience: A bridging concept or a dead end? *Planning Theory & Practice*, *13*(2), 299–307.

DeVylder, J. E., Kelleher, I., Lalane, M., Oh, H., Link, B. G., & Koyanagi, A. (2018). Association of urbanicity with psychosis in low- and middle-income countries. *JAMA Psychiatry*, *75*(7), 678–686.

Donnelly, A. A., & MacIntyre, T. E. (Eds.). (2019). *Physical activity in natural settings: Green and blue exercise*. Routledge.

Fraser, T., Feeley, O., Ridge, A., Cervini, A., Rago, V., Gilmore, K., Worthington, G., & Berliavsky, I. (2024). How far I'll go: Social infrastructure accessibility and proximity in urban neighborhoods. *Landscape and Urban Planning*, *241*, 104922. https://doi.org/10.1016/j.landurbplan.2023.104922

Geels, F. W. (2004). From sectoral systems of innovation to socio-technical systems. *Research Policy*, *33*(6–7), 897–920.

Gerges, F., Assaad, R. H., Nassif, H., Bou-Zeid, E., & Boufadel, M. C. (2023). A perspective on quantifying resilience: Combining community and infrastructure capitals. *Science of the Total Environment*, *859*, 160187. https://doi.org/10.1016/j.scitotenv.2022.160187

Gibson, J. J. (1979). *The ecological approach to visual perception*. Houghton Mifflin Harcourt.

Grahn, P., & Stigsdotter, U. A. (2003). Landscape planning and stress. *Urban Forestry & Urban Greening*, *2*(1), 1–18.

Hammoud, R., Tognin, S., Bakolis, I., Ivanova, D., Fitzpatrick, N., Burgess, L., Smythe, M., Gibbons, J., Davidson, N., & Mechelli, A. (2021). Lonely in a crowd: Investigating the association between overcrowding and loneliness using smartphone technologies. *Scientific Reports, 11*, 24134. https://doi.org/10.1038/s41598-021-03398-2

Herslund, L. B., Jean-Baptiste, N., Jalayer, F., Jørgensen, G., Kabisch, S., Lindley, S., Nyed, P. K., Pauleit, S., Printz, A., & Vedeld, T. (2016). Developing multiple-dimensional assessment of urban vulnerability to climate change in Sub-Saharan Africa. *Natural Hazards, 82*, 149–172.

Holling, C. S. (1973). Resilience and stability of ecological systems. *Annual Review of Ecology and Systematics, 4*, 1–23.

Jacobs, M. (1999). Sustainable development as a contested concept. In A. Dobson (Ed.), *Fairness and futurity: Essays on environmental sustainability and social justice* (pp. 21–45). Oxford University Press.

Kallus, K. W. (2016). Stress and recovery: An overview. In K. W. Kallus & M. Kellmann (Eds.), *The Recovery-Stress Questionnaires: User manual* (pp. 27–48). Pearson Assessment.

Kallus, K. W., & Kellmann, M. (2000). Burnout in athletes and coaches. In Y. Hanin (Ed.), *Emotions in sport* (pp. 209–230). Human Kinetics.

Kaźmierczak, A. (2013). The contribution of local parks to neighbourhood social ties. *Landscape and Urban Planning, 109*, 31–44.

Kellmann, M. (2002). Underrecovery and overtraining: Different concepts – similar impact? In M. Kellmann (Ed.), *Enhancing recovery: Preventing underperformance in athletes* (pp. 3–24). Human Kinetics.

Kellmann, M., Bertollo, M., Bosquet, L., Brink, M., Coutts, A. J., Duffield, R., Erlacher, D., Halson, S. L., Hecksteden, A., Heidari, J., Kallus, K. W., Meeusen, R., Mujika, I., Robazza, C., Skorski, S., Venter, R., & Beckmann, J. (2018). Recovery and performance in sport: Consensus statement. *International Journal of Sports Physiology and Performance, 13*, 240–245.

Kellmann, M., Jakowski, S., & Beckmann, J. (Eds.). (2023). *The importance of recovery for physical and mental health: Negotiating the effects of underrecovery*. Routledge.

Kellmann, M., & Kallus, K. W. (2001). *The Recovery-Stress Questionnaire for Athletes: User manual*. Human Kinetics.

Lavie, C. J., Ozemek, C., Carbone, S., Katzmarzyk, P. T., & Blair, S. N. (2019). Sedentary behavior, exercise, and cardiovascular health. *Circulation Research, 124*(5), 799–815.

Lederbogen, F., Kirsch, P., Haddad, L., Streit, F., Tost, H., Schuch, P., Wüst, S., Pruessner, J. C., Rietschel, M., Deuschle, M., & Meyer-Lindenberg, A. (2011). City living and urban upbringing affect neural social stress processing in humans. *Nature, 474*(7352), 498–501.

Lewin, K. (1935). *A dynamic theory of personality*. McGraw-Hill.

Loorbach, D., Frantzeskaki, N., & Avelino, F. (2017). Sustainability transitions research: Transforming science and practice for societal change. *Annual Review of Environment and Resources, 42*(1), 599–626.

Lyndhurst, B. (2003). *London's ecological footprint: A review*. Greater London Authority.

Mahajan, S., Hausladen, C., Sánchez-Vaquerizo, J. A., Korecki, M., & Helbing, D. (2022). Participatory resilience: Surviving, recovering and improving together. *Sustainable Cities and Society, 83*, 103942. https://doi.org/10.1016/j.scs.2022.103942

Markevych, I., Schoierer, J., Hartig, T., Chudnovsky, A., Hystad, P., Dzhambov, A. M., de Vries, S., Triguero-Mas, M., Brauer, M., Nieuwenhuijsen, M. J., Lupp, G., Richardson, E. A., Astell-Burt, T., Dimitrova, D., Feng, X., Sadeh, M., Standl, M.,

Heinrich, J., & Fuertes, E. (2017). Exploring pathways linking greenspace to health: Theoretical and methodological guidance. *Environmental Research, 158*, 301–317.

Marselle, M. R. (2019). Theoretical foundations of biodiversity and mental wellbeing relationships. In M. R. Marselle, J. Stadler, H. Korn, K. N. Irvine, & A. Bonn (Eds.), *Biodiversity and health in the face of climate change* (pp. 133–158). Springer.

Martinez, L., Leon, E., Al Youssef, S., & Karaan, A. K. (2020). Strengthening the health lens in urban resilience frameworks. *Cities & Health, 4*(2), 229–236.

McPhearson, T., Andersson, E., Elmqvist, T., & Frantzeskaki, N. (2015). Resilience of and through urban ecosystem services. *Ecosystem Services, 12*, 152–156.

Meerow, S., & Newell, J. P. (2016). Urban resilience for whom, what, when, where, and why? *Urban Geography, 40*(3), 309–329.

Meerow, S., Newell, J. P., & Stults, M. (2016). Defining urban resilience: A review. *Landscape and Urban Planning, 147*, 38–49.

Mental Health Foundation. (2018). *Stress: Are we coping?* Retrieved November 11, 2023 from https://www.mentalhealth.org.uk/sites/default/files/2022-08/stress-are-we-coping.pdf

Mukim, M., & Roberts, M. (Eds.). (2023). *Thriving: Making cities green, resilient, and inclusive in a changing climate*. World Bank Group.

Norman, D. (1988). *The psychology of everyday things*. Basic Books.

OECD. (2019). *Going digital: Shaping policies, improving lives*. Retrieved November 11, 2023 from https://www.oecd.org/digital/going-digital-synthesis-summary.pdf

Owen, N., Healy, G. N., Matthews, C. E., & Dunstan, D. W. (2010). Too much sitting: The population-health science of sedentary behavior. *Exercise and Sport Sciences Reviews, 38*(3), 105–113.

Pauleit, S., Hansen, R., Rall, E. L., Zölch, T., Andersson, E., Luz, A., Santos, A., Szaraz, L., Tosics, I., & Vierikko, K. (2017). Urban landscapes and green infrastructure. In H. Shugart (Ed.), *Oxford research encyclopedia of environmental science*. Oxford University Press. Retrieved November 11, 2023 from https://doi.org/10.1093/acrefore/9780199389414.013.23

Pauleit, S., Zölch, T., Hansen, R., Randrup, T. B., & Konijnendijk van den Bosch, C. (2017). Nature-based solutions and climate change – four shades of green. In N. Kabisch, H. Korn, J. Stadler, & A. Bonn (Eds.), *Nature-based solutions to climate change adaptation in urban areas: Linkages between science, policy and practice* (pp. 29–50). Springer.

Peen, J., Schoevers, R. A., Beekman, A. T., & Dekker, J. (2010). The current status of urban-rural differences in psychiatric disorders. *Acta Psychiatrica Scandinavica, 121*(2), 84–93.

Rainie, L., & Wellman, B. (2012). *Networked: The new social operating system*. MIT Press.

Revi, A., Satterthwaite, D. E., Aragón-Durand, F., Corfee-Morlot, J., Kiunsi, R. B. R., Pelling, M., Roberts, D. C., & Solecki, W. (2014). Urban areas. In C. B. Field, V. R. Barros, D. J. Dokken, K. J. Mach, M. D. Mastrandrea, T. E. Bilir, M. Chatterjee, K. L. Ebi, Y. O. Estrada, R. C. Genova, B. Girma, E. S. Kissel, A. N. Levy, S. MacCracken, P. R. Mastrandrea, & L. L. White (Eds.), *Climate change 2014: Impacts, adaptation, and vulnerability* (pp. 535–612). Cambridge University Press.

Ribeiro, P. J. G., & Gonçalves, L. (2019). Urban resilience: A conceptual framework. *Sustainable Cities and Society, 50*, 101625. https://doi.org/10.1016/j.scs.2019.101625

Roe, J., & McCay, L. (2021). *Restorative cities – urban design manual for mental health and wellbeing*. Bloomsbury Publishing.

Rollo, S., Gaston, A., & Prapavessis, H. (2016). Cognitive and motivational factors associated with sedentary behavior: A systematic review. *AIMS Public Health, 3*(4), 956–984.

Solmi, F., Dykxhoorn, J., & Kirkbride, J. B. (2017). Urban-rural differences in major mental health conditions. In N. Okkels, C. B. Kristiansen, & P. Munk-Jørgensen (Eds.), *Mental health and illness in the city* (pp. 27–132). Springer Science + Business Media.

Therrien, M.-C., Tanguay, G. A., & Beauregard-Guérin, I. (2015). Fundamental determinants of urban resilience: A search for indicators applied to public health crisis. *Resilience: International Policies, Practices and Discourses, 3*(1), 18–39.

Thivel, D., Tremblay, A., Genin, P. M., Panahi, S., Rivière, D., & Duclos, M. (2018). Physical activity, inactivity, and sedentary behaviors: Definitions and implications in occupational health. *Frontiers in Public Health, 6*, 288. https://doi.org/10.3389/fpubh.2018.00288

United Nations. (2019). *World urbanization prospects: The 2018 revision*. Department of Economic and Social Affairs, Population Division. Retrieved November 11, 2023 from https://www.un.org/development/desa/publications/2018-revision-of-world-urbanization-prospects.html

van den Berg, M., Wendsel-Vos, W., van Poppel, M., Kemper, H., van Mechelen, W., & Maas, J. (2015). Health benefits of green spaces in the living environment: A systematic review of epidemiological studies. *Urban Forestry & Urban Greening, 14*, 806–816.

Ventriglio, A., Torales, J., Castaldelli-Maia, J. M., De Berardis, D., & Bhugra, D. (2020). Urbanization and emerging mental health issues. *CNS Spectrums, 26*(1), 43–50.

VicHealth. (2019). *VicHealth mental wellbeing strategy 2019–2023*. Retrieved November 11, 2023 from https://www.vichealth.vic.gov.au/sites/default/files/Mental-Wellbeing-Strategy-2019.pdf

Walker, B., & Salt, D. (2006). *Resilience thinking: Sustaining ecosystems and people in a changing world*. Island Press.

White, M. P., Elliott, L. R., Grellier, J., Economou, T., Bell, S., Bratman, G. N., Cirach, M., Gascon, M., Lima, M. L., Löhmus, M., Nieuwenhuijsen, M., Ojala, A., Roiko, A., Schultz, P. W., van den Bosch, M., & Fleming, L. E. (2021). Associations between green/blue spaces and mental health across 18 countries. *Scientific Reports, 11*, 8903. https://doi.org/10.1038/s41598-021-87675-0

White, M. P., Hartig, T., Martin, L., Pahl, S., van den Berg, A. E., Wells, N. M., Costongs, C., Dzhambov, A. M., Elliott, L. R., Godfrey, A., Hartl, A., Konijnendijk, C., Litt, J. S., Lovell, R., Lymeus, F., O'Driscoll, C., Pichler, S., Pouso, C., Razani, N., . . . van den Bosch, M. (2023). Nature-based biopsychosocial resilience: An integrative theoretical framework for research on nature and health. *Environment International, 181*, 108234. https://doi.org/10.1016/j.envint.2023.108234

Wilkinson, C. (2012). Social-ecological resilience: Insights and issues for planning theory. *Planning Theory, 11*(2), 148–169.

Xu, J., Liu, N., Polemiti, E., Garcia-Mondragon, L., Tang, J., Liu, X., Lett, T., Yu, L., Nöthen, M. M., Feng, J., Yu, C., Marquand, A., Schumann, G., & The environMENTAL Consortium. (2023). Effects of urban living environments on mental health in adults. *Nature Medicine, 29*, 1456–1467.

2 Commuting to work by car

Is travel time leisure time?

Achim Elfering and Fabrice Huber

Introduction

Commuting to and from work and home is part of most employees' working lives. Before the Covid-19 pandemic, average commuting time increased in many industrialised countries, including Germany (Wöhrmann et al., 2023) and Switzerland. According to the Swiss Federal Statistical Office (Bundesamt für Statistik; BFS, 2024), the duration of the average commute in one direction increased from 23 to 30 minutes between 2000 and 2022, and the percentage of 'longer commutes' (>60 minutes) increased from 2.4% to 8.3% between 2000 and 2022 (BFS, 2024). The trend towards longer commutes in Switzerland is similar to those of other countries, with a Covid-19-related decrease in commutes and a rising commuting rate after the Covid-19 pandemic (BFS, 2024).

Breaks at work and leisure time are the primary opportunities for recovery from work demands (Kallus, this volume, Chapter 3; Semmer et al., 2010). Thereby, recovery can be defined as "an inter- and intraindividual multilevel (e.g., psychological, physiological, social) process in time for the re-establishment of personal resources and their full functional capacity" (according to Kallus, 2016, p. 42; Pauleit et al., this volume, Chapter 1). Among other moderating conditions, recovery depends on situational characteristics, like social interaction (Pauleit et al., this volume, Chapter 1). Hence, commuting can function like a break from work demands, given that commuters detach from work issues and do not engage mentally in work tasks (Elfering et al., 2012). Thus, a characterisation of commuting travel time as leisure time includes the view of commuting as a break that helps detach from private and work demands (Balk, 2024). Such a commuting break would help replenish resources that could serve as a buffer to following stressors at work or at home (Kallus, 2016; Kellmann et al., 2018). Commuting time is an opportunity for recovery experiences, including detachment from work (Balk, 2024), experiences of mastery and control, and relaxation (McAlpine & Piszczek, 2023). Psychological detachment includes a

Elfering, A., & Huber, F. (2025). Commuting to work by car: Is travel time leisure time? In S. Pauleit, M. Kellmann, & J. Beckmann (Eds.), *Creating Urban and Workplace Environments for Recovery and Well-being* (pp. 21–36). Routledge.

DOI: 10.4324/9781003435471-3

mental distancing from work issues that can be achieved by listening to a podcast. Mastery is an experience of progress by meeting challenges and learning. Control refers to the experience of autonomy in acting, and deciding, for example, deciding between alternative routes of driving. Finally, relaxation characterises low mental and physical activation by, for example, listening to music (Sonnentag et al., 2022). Commuting time may also function as a helpful transition break between life domains, as a liminal space between the work domain and private domain that facilitates a smooth transition between the work role and private role (McAlpine & Piszczek, 2023). Thereby, commuting time could help prepare the switch to the other role, allowing commuting employees to unwind psychologically from the previous role. In this sense, commuting time is a schematised exit-and-entry sequence used to disengage from one role and re-engage with another. Such 'rites of separation' may involve, for example, switching attention, adopting a role-appropriate cognitive frame (employee vs other roles, such as husband, partner, friend), and role-appropriate arousal; they may constitute useful and enjoyable preparation for entry to another role (Ashforth et al., 2000). The commute may facilitate transitions in both directions; in a diary study by Sonnentag and Kühnel (2016), morning reattachment (i.e., mentally reconnecting to work before actually starting to work) positively predicted work engagement throughout the day.

In contrast to such positive potential of commuting, the (morning) commute is considered to range among the least enjoyable daily activities (Kahneman & Krueger, 2006). Commuters had lower overall life satisfaction, lower happiness, and more anxiety than non-commuters in research by the Office for National Statistics of the United Kingdom with over 60,000 respondents (UK Office for National Statistics, 2014). Indeed, commute time simply depletes individual resources (Elfering et al., 2020). A salient feature of commuting is that it creates additional demands and often constitutes a stressor (Koslowsky et al., 1996; Stutzer & Frey, 2008). Many authors do not explain why exactly they consider commuting a demand. When they do, they often refer to hassles frequently, but not necessarily associated with commuting, such as traffic jams (Koslowsky et al., 1996; Stutzer & Frey, 2008). From the perspective of the *Job Demands–Control Theory* (Theorell & Karasek, 1996) and its extension, the *Job Demands–Resources Theory* (Bakker & Demerouti, 2016), as well as from the perspective of the *Conservation of Resources* (COR; Hobfoll & Shirom, 2001) model, commuting may be regarded as a demand simply because it requires effort and consumes resources (self-regulation, time, and money). Hence, commuting time limits the time for later exercise, sports, social activities, and other individually preferred recovery experiences (Jung et al., 2024). Hämmig et al. (2009) analysed cross-sectional data from the nationally representative Swiss Household Panel and found that commuting time was one of the variables that affected work–life conflict. Fichter (2015) conducted an online survey including 1,600 Swiss people from the German-language region. People were asked about their life satisfaction; work, life, and living situation; commuting behaviour; and commuting experience. The author reported that the most negatively rated aspects of commuting were unexpected delays, crowding in public transport, and traffic jam. Fichter's (2015) main conclusion is that life satisfaction is influenced only in case of long-distance commuting.

Concerning the morning commute from home to work, two recent diary studies of Gerpott and colleagues (2022) showed that interruptions of automated travel behaviours are resource-depleting and increase self-regulation demands, and such demanding commuting may reduce flow experiences at work and predict less engagement at work, especially when self-control demands at work are high (Gerpott et al., 2022). Thus, work conditions are related to commuting, and vice versa. For instance, work stressors like time pressure seem to predict more risky commuting behaviour, with cognitive failure as a mediating process involved (Elfering et al., 2012, 2013). Whether commuting is experienced as demand or even a stressor seems to depend on commuting experiences that deviate from the usual, automated, and therefore, expected commuting experience, or as Gerpott and colleagues (2022, p. 169) formulated, "your commute may have been slow or unpleasant or may have knocked you out of rhythm, for example, because the traffic flow was interrupted by stop-and-go driving". Such deviating experiences are what Novaco and coworkers (1990) described as an impedance to commutes by car in California, USA. The usual average commute has been experienced many times, and the action regulation is automatic and, therefore, only consumes a few resources, but traffic impedances increase the regulation effort (Elfering et al., 2012).

The potential of commuting to be experienced positively as a recovery time (McAlpine & Piszczek, 2023; Pindek et al., 2023) might depend – among other influences – on an undisturbed commuting rhythm, that is, a highly automated commute that does not deviate from expected traffic and travel speed and traffic experience. During such usual regular commuting, attention could be spent on other activities, for example, in the method of 'off-job crafting', as discussed by de Bloom et al. (2020), which may offer a potential means to utilise commuting time for planning free time, which might aid in role transitions and additionally enhance recovery during leisure hours. In summary, a normal commuting experience could enable individuals to manage their roles better and prepare for improved leisure time utilisation (McAlpine & Piszczek, 2023).

So far, it seems justified to characterise commuting for most commuters as a demanding experience rather than a resource-replenishing leisure time, and a recent meta-analysis proposes that commuting is a demand – a demand, however, that can have both negative and positive effects on outcomes through commuting appraisals (Murphy et al., 2023).

Undisturbed commuting vs commuting impedances

Between persons and within the same individual experience, the same commuting time of 30 minutes may differ depending on the expected (usual) commuting duration, which may be called a relational deviation perspective on commuting time. Delays in commuting times may be appraised often as unnecessary delays.

Commuting time may be unnecessary for many reasons, including unforeseen daily events during commuting, but also because of the lack of possibility to work at different places and times that would allow for reduced commuting times (Elfering et al., 2020). Concerning the individual commutes, the tolerance to delays in commuting times might differ inter- and intraindividually. The commuting time reference is the reasonably expected commuting duration (Morrow, 2010). Other commuting time references might also exist in parallel; for example, Bai and colleagues (2021) measured relative commuting time as the ratio between the specific individual's commute time and the average commute time of all working neighbours (commute ratio), that is, commuting time appraisal is absolute, but also relative (Bai et al., 2021). Hence, there needs to be more than absolute commuting time to capture all the demands associated with commuting; whether the commute is smooth and unproblematic or associated with hassles, such as traffic jams, matters (Pindek et al., 2023). To the extent that delays in commuting time deviate from the expected commuting duration, the delay may increase its probability of acting as a work stressor and prevent commuting from being instrumented as a recovery experience, or what Pindek and colleagues (2023) labelled 'me time'.

The concept of absolute and relative commuting time

How much of a commute time is considered long? Morrow (2010), in her dissertation, uses a measure of relative commuting time defined as the difference between one's current commute time and one's subjective appraisal of a 'reasonable' commute time, and in her works, relative commuting time was a more salient predictor of commuting stress than absolute commute time.

Other than self-report measures of relative commuting effort

Novaco et al. (1990) differentiated between physical and subjective impedance to commutes by car in California, USA. First attempts on behavioural measures of physical impedance, including the amount of braking, were tested by the authors but were found to have no effects. Thus, Novaco and colleagues used self-reports of reduction of speed due to low traffic flow, frequent necessity of braking, and interference from other cars as measurements. Noteworthy, they found physical impedance to predict higher values on various illness measures and job satisfaction beyond the effects of subjectively perceived impedance (e.g., pleasantness or aversive commuting experiences). One may consider commuting time or distance as objective commuting efforts might be easier to estimate than objective impeding commuting events. So far, commuting has often been operationalised in terms of time or distance, or sometimes in terms of a time-based dichotomous categorisation of commuters versus non-commuters. Other authors, however, have used commuters' addresses to define commuting distance; for example, a long commute has been defined as a journey of more than 16 kilometres, or 9.94 miles (Koslowsky et al., 1996), or between 18 and

50 miles (Novaco et al., 1990). However, research has shown that commuting distance is less closely related to outcomes such as health than commuting time (Stutzer & Frey, 2008). Cut-off values, however, should be justified by nonlinear correspondence of commuting time and distance with outcomes, since unjustified cut-off values unnecessarily reduce the information in data and should be avoided if possible (MacCallum et al., 2002). Previous research on commuting time has mainly relied on self-reported data, with all known biases to self-report (Semmer et al., 2004). Some technologies may help researchers derive indicators of relative commuting time that are not based solely on self-reports. When the distance between home and work locations is known, estimates for travel times from software like Google Maps (GM) may be used to calculate objective estimates of undisturbed ('reasonable') commuting times with low impedance. They could be compared with subjective self-reports of travel times. The positive deviation between both travel times (self-reported times longer than GM-estimated time) could be used to estimate a relative commuting time that is not solely based on self-report (Brüßler et al., 2024; Elfering et al., 2020).

Mode of commuting and recovery

Commuting by car is bound to less physical activity compared to other ways of commuting, like public transport, riding on a bicycle, or walking. Compared to those who take public transport, commuters travelling by car were shown to walk 30% fewer steps per day (Wener et al., 2005). Commuting by bicycle has many benefits, which include not only a form of daily exercise but also a cost-effective travelling method (Heinen et al., 2010). Even though obviously beneficial, this travelling method may not be the primary choice for many commuters, for several reasons; a suitable environment, short distances, storage facilities at the workplace, and reasonable weather must be given for an employee to consider this commuting method (Heinen et al., 2010). In Switzerland, around 18% are active commuters who use a bicycle or walk (BFS, 2024). After using motorised private vehicles (half of commuters in 2022), public transport is the second most frequent way of commuting in Switzerland (BFS, 2024). Thus, commuting by car is slightly decreasing. Koslowsky et al. (1996) found that perceived control (on the commuting experience) was higher for people commuting by car than for people using public transportation. Stutzer and Frey (2008) found a larger estimated negative effect of one hour of commuting for users of public transport than for car drivers. Active commuters are generally more satisfied with their commute than those who travel by car, and especially those who use public transport (Chatterjee et al., 2020). Fichter (2015) reported that people commuting by bicycle reported higher levels of life satisfaction than people not commuting by bicycle. He argued that, according to positive psychology (Seligman & Csikszentmihalyi, 2014), physical activity, outdoor activities, and a decelerated lifestyle may have positive impacts on life satisfaction. Moreover, active commuting might affect perceived control on the commuting situation. Finally, one might add that cycling and walking to work and back home can also be characterised as active recovery that involves mainly physical activities "aimed at compensating the metabolic responses of physical fatigue" (Kellmann et al., 2018, p. 240). In summary, evidence is increasing that the positive effects of commuting could depend to a considerable degree on the mode of commuting and mode of recovery. The data analyses reported next are restricted to commuting by car in order to keep commuting mode constant. Moreover, public transport in Switzerland is quite reliable (Schweizerische Bundesbahn, 2024), so that the self-estimated public commuting time and the objective travel times may differ on a daily basis, but across a longer period of time, timeliness in public transport is quite good. Usually, the difference between expected and real travel time in public transport is small and, therefore, limits the eligibility of public transport in the current study of relative commuting time as a unique commuting stressor in Switzerland.

An empirical test of relative commuting time by car as a unique stressor

In a recent survey on working conditions and health in Swiss working population, we asked for information on commuting and tested self-reported commuting (among other predictors) as a predictor of health indicators (Galliker et al., 2024). Huber (2022) added objective commuting time estimates to the dataset, which were generated with GM, a free web-mapping service developed by Google, as well as GM data for commuters who commuted solely by car. GM offers real-time route-planning information for travel by car (time and distance), public transport, and active commuting modes based on maps, real-time traffic information, and public transport information. All data were collected in 2020 and 2021 (for more information on the sample, sampling procedure, and measures, see Galliker et al., 2021, 2024). The research is part of an ongoing collaboration between 'Gesundheitsförderung Schweiz' (Health Promotion Switzerland), a foundation funded by Swiss health insurance, and the Department of Psychology at the University of Bern, as well as the Department of Economy at the University of Applied Sciences in Winterthur (Elfering et al., 2018). The research question on relative commuting is whether relative commuting time is a unique predictor of work-related attitude (job satisfaction, affective commitment, and turnover intention) and health indicators (lack of detachment from work as an indicator of an impeded recovery process, emotional exhaustion, and psychosomatic complaints). The hypothesis is that relative commuting time significantly predicts the outcomes in 2021 beyond self-reported commuting time and work-related predictors, like the Job-Stress Index (JSI; a measure that indicates the balance or imbalance between work-related stressors and job resources, with higher values indicating an imbalance with more stressors than resources; Galliker et al., 2024), and Covid-19-related demands, including an infection with Covid-19 between February 2020 and February 2021, working from home, and the worry of losing the job because of Covid-19. Data from 753 participants (53.8% men, *M* age = 46 years,

SD = 11 years, all with no change in home address and work address and no turnover in the year under study) were analysed in multiple linear regression. All outcome variables were described in previous publications (Elfering et al., 2020, for affective commitment, and turnover intention; see Galliker et al., 2024, for job satisfaction, lack of detachment, emotional exhaustion, and psychosomatic complaints) and psychometrically validated with extensive datasets in German, French, and Italian. Standardised questionnaire instruments were carefully compiled (Igic et al., 2017) and, as a questionnaire tool, independently evaluated and certified (Klumb & Thielsch, 2019).

GM was used to gather objective information about the fastest commuting time in the evening (without traffic peaks). GM offers real-time route-planning information for travel by car (time and distance). When mapping postal codes, GM uses the geographical centre of each postal code area (Google, n.d.). Home and workplace postal codes were among the items of demographic information that participants provided. This information was used to generate estimates of one-way commuting time, which were doubled to estimate total daily commuting time and multiplied by the number of days on which the participants commuted, which was also asked in the questionnaire, to have the weekly commuting time. The authors created a code for the GM commuting time assessment, which automates this process. The self-reported commuting time was assessed with a single item ("How many minutes in total do you usually spend travelling from home to work and back each day?"; Grebner et al., 2010). Relative commuting time was calculated as the difference between self-reported and GM commuting time. The correspondence between self-reported and GM commuting time was $r = .48\left(p < .001\right)$, while self-reported commuting time and relative commuting time were also positively related $\left(r = .58, p < .001\right)$.

Longer (absolute) self-reported duration of daily commuting significantly predicted lower job satisfaction and higher turnover intentions, but not lower affective commitment, which was significantly predicted by longer relative commuting duration (Table 2.1). More lack of detachment was predicted by longer absolute commuting durations, but not by relative commuting time (Table 2.2).

In the prediction of emotional exhaustion, absolute and relative commuting times were not predictive, while more psychosomatic complaints, including headaches, neck or shoulder pain, back or lower back pain, joint or limb pain, loss of appetite, stomach problems, indigestion, skin problems/skin diseases, itching, and eye problems (burning, redness, itching, tearing of the eyes), tended to be predicted by longer relative commuting times (Table 2.2). Generally, effect sizes of absolute and relative commuting time were small. However, considering the JSI and the worry of losing the job as strong predictors, the effect sizes of absolute and relative commuting do point towards commuting time to be a demand rather than a resource, and relative commuting time has a unique stressor potential beyond absolute commuting time, work stressors, and Covid-19-related stressors.

Table 2.1 Multiple linear regression of work attitudes on the Job-Stress Index, Covid-19-related demands, and absolute and relative commuting times.

	Job satisfaction 2021				*Affective commitment 2021*				*Turnover intentions 2021*			
Predictor	B	SE	Beta	*p*	B	SE	Beta	*p*	B	SE	Beta	*p*
Constant	11.071	0.421		.000	9.316	0.517		.000	0.309	0.361		.392
Age (years)	−0.0002	0.003	−.017	.567	0.002	0.004	.019	.572	−0.006	0.003	−.076	.022
Sex (0 = f, 1 = m)	0.062	0.072	.026	.393	−0.223	0.089	−.085	.012	0.010	0.062	.006	.869
Covid-19 infection between 2020 and 2021	−0.091	0.123	−.021	.458	−0.061	0.151	−.013	.685	−0.131	0.106	−.040	.216
Worry of job loss because of pandemic between 2020 and 2021	−0.039	0.021	−.055	.070	−0.007	0.026	−.008	.805	0.065	0.018	.120	.000
Job-Stress Index between 2020 and 2021	−0.105	0.005	−.583	.000	−0.086	0.007	−.435	.000	0.047	0.005	.346	.000
Days of commuting per week between 2020 and 2021	0.012	0.024	.015	.615	0.054	0.029	.062	.064	−0.064	0.020	−.107	.002
Absolute self-reported duration of daily commuting between 2020 and 2021	−0.003	0.001	−.090	.013	−0.001	0.001	−.027	.497	0.003	0.001	.133	.001
Relative commuting time (self-report minus Google Maps) between 2020 and 2021	−0.001	0.001	−.024	.512	−0.003	0.002	−.086	.032	0.001	0.001	.026	.524

Note: $N = 750$; prediction of job satisfaction: $R2 = 0.382$, $F_{(8, 641)} = 57.17$, $p < .001$; prediction of affective commitment: $R2 = 0.226$, $F_{(8, 641)} = 26.98$, $p < .001$; prediction of turnover intentions: $R2 = 0.215$, $F_{(8, 641)} = 25.32$, $p < .001$.

Table 2.2 Multiple linear regression of lack of detachment, emotional exhaustion, and psychosomatic complaints on Job-Stress Index, Covid-19-related demands, and absolute and relative commuting times.

	Lack of detachment 2021				*Emotional exhaustion 2021*				*Psychosomatic complaints 2021*			
Predictor	B	SE	Beta	*p*	B	SE	Beta	*p*	B	SE	Beta	*p*
Constant	0.698	0.765		.362	0.007	0.209		.972	0.721	0.255		.005
Age (years)	−0.011	0.006	−.069	.057	−0.003	0.002	−.050	.116	<0.001	0.002	.002	.963
Sex (0 = f, 1 = m)	−0.040	0.132	−.011	.760	0.080	0.036	.072	.026	0.291	0.044	.230	.000
Covid-19 infection between 2020 and 2021	0.253	0.224	.040	.257	0.048	0.061	.024	.438	−0.035	0.075	−.016	.641
Worry of job loss because of pandemic between 2020 and 2021	0.097	0.039	.093	.013	0.034	0.011	.103	.002	0.031	0.013	.084	.017
Job-Stress Index between 2020 and 2021	0.046	0.010	.172	.000	0.039	0.003	.473	.000	0.028	0.003	.302	.000
Day of commuting per week between 2020 and 2021	−0.012	0.043	−.010	.783	0.007	0.012	.019	.564	−0.016	0.014	−.039	.254
Self-reported duration of daily commuting between 2020 and 2021	0.004	0.002	.086	.050	<0.001	0.001	.030	.444	<0.001	0.001	−.001	.982
Relative commuting time (self-report minus Google Maps) between 2020 and 2021	<0.001	0.002	.001	.975	<0.001	0.001	.030	.431	0.001	0.001	.074	.076

Note: $N = 750$; prediction of lack of detachment: $R2 = 0.058$, $F_{(8,641)} = 6.78$, $p < .001$; prediction of emotional exhaustion: $R2 = 0.288$, $F_{(8, 641)} = 37.40$, $p < .001$; prediction of psychosomatic complaints: $R2 = 0.173$, $F_{(8, 541)} = 20.55$, $p < .001$.

Discussion

In line with the overall impression that absolute and relative commuting times function as a demand rather than a resource, relative commuting was found in the current data to be a unique predictive commuting stressor. Note that, irrespective of commuting mode, a large review reported longer commuting time to relate to lower well-being (Chatterjee et al., 2020). However, the interpretation of relative commuting only as a stressor is also a shortcoming: needing less time to commute than expected predicts more favourable outcomes, while needing more time than expected predicts more negative outcomes. Relativity means deviations from a stored reference value, one source of expected commuting time. This internal reference value was found to be a bit too optimistic in many commuters who use a car (Flade, 2013). An individual bias towards too optimistic travel time expectations would result in longer potentially frustrating relative commuting times. Hence, a fruitful intervention could be a 'correction' of unrealistic travel time expectations in car drivers. At the same time, commuters who use a car do overestimate commuting times by public transport (Flade, 2013). Again, that internal bias might contribute to their commuting experience by car ("It is awful, but it would be even worse with public transport") also refers to such an internal reference standard. The reference standard may change intraindividually with experience (Elfering, 2007; Elfering & Grebner, 2010, 2011). For instance, a transitory increase of commuting times (e.g., due to a construction site) will result in a corresponding increase of the internal reference standard. After the end of construction, the same small delay is experienced less negatively than before the construction period. Such internal reference standards are known in visual perception of stimulus size (Elfering & Sarris, 2006), and job satisfaction ratings (Bowling et al., 2005). Thus, an interesting question is whether internal reference standards systematically change with more flexibility in working times and working places. Increase of work from home days should decrease the internal reference standard of commuting times, and the same delay during commuting now would be worse than in previous times of permanent onsite work. If future studies do confirm such shift in individual reference point, this shift would limit the advantages of work from home. Nevertheless, flexible work times and places have the potential to reduce not only absolute commuting times (Wöhrmann et al., 2023) but also even more relative commuting times when traffic peaks and other computing impedances can be prevented and necessary commutes are often even shorter than expected.

Are the discussed results important for urban planning? Consider a temporary road construction that causes delay across some period; the internal reference standard, as estimated in the absolute commuting time, will increase and persist upon return after the road construction is finished. In the first days of commuting after this finished construction period, shorter commuting time will be a source of joy, because actual commuting time is valued against the old internal reference time that still refers to the construction period. Thus, the absolute and relative quality of commuting time helps explain why improved infrastructures may not improve satisfaction with commuting across more extended periods. Noteworthy, even the relative commuting time may differ in predictability and controllability. Both predictability and controllability are 'psychological' characteristics of an event that are likely to render it into a stressor (Zapf & Semmer, 2004). In addition, lower controllability in commuting time may be experienced to be unfair on the background of social comparison. For instance, individuals who live at the end of a dead end of a narrow street may consider their delay in commuting time to be larger than that of most others living in the same street because they need to wait for others who have to leave first. Other neighbours often block the street, and such delay is experienced as unpredictable and uncontrollable. Moreover, such delay may also be appraised as unnecessary and unreasonable. If so, commuting time might gain specific value as being experienced as disrespectful with respect to the *Stress as Offence to Self* (SOS) model of stress (Ding & Kuvaas, 2023; Semmer et al., 2007, 2015, 2019). Semmer and colleagues (2019) explained that unreasonable tasks are those which one feels one should not have to do, and unnecessary tasks which one feels no one should have to do. Such unreasonable and unnecessary tasks, therefore, are perceived as illegitimate tasks (Semmer et al., 2007). According to the SOS model of work stress, illegitimate tasks do not match the employees' occupational role and pose a threat to occupational self-esteem (Semmer et al., 2015). Illegitimate tasks can be considered as an established stressor (Semmer et al., 2019) and affect recipients with emotions similar to blame, such as feelings of resentment, desire for revenge, and sadness (Semmer et al., 2021). At work, some unnecessary commuting time may be caused by colleagues who always reserve parking places near the workplace while their parking is farther from the workplace, and all efforts to get one of the nearer parking are rejected. During commuting, avoidable conditions like drivers who do not react promptly to changing signals or misleading signalisation that causes slow traffic can be experienced as causing unnecessary commuting time. In such cases, experiencing delays in commuting time because of illegitimate reasons should threaten the self-esteem of commuters (Huber, 2022). Future studies should explore whether unnecessary relative commuting time threatens organisational self-esteem and has a solid impeding influence on recovery from work demands during work breaks and after work (de Jonge & Taris, 2024). Evidence that the appraisal of illegitimate reasons can magnify the stressful effects of stressors at work is increasing. Grotto and Mills (2023) found illegitimate interruptions from work that are inappropriate, avoidable, unnecessary, or unreasonable interruptions to induce unnecessary strain beyond the effects of interruptions per se. A recent study by Kern and colleagues (2023) showed illegitimate time pressure at work to alter the appraisal of time pressure away from being a (less stressful) challenge stressor towards being a (more stressful) hindrance stressor. Hence, considering commuting, future studies should test illegitimate interruption and illegitimate delay that causes illegitimate time pressure to magnify the stressful effect of commuting.

Mental detachment instead of affective rumination about work issues during commuting seems a primary aim, not only to facilitate recovery during commutes, but also to prevent risky commuting safety behaviours (Burch & Barnes-Farrell, 2020).

A change towards active commuting modes seems the silver bullet to improve satisfaction with commuting (Chatterjee et al., 2020), well-being, and health. In Switzerland, the number rose from 15% in 2015 to 18% in 2022 for those who were active commuters and used a bicycle or walked (BFS, 2024). Further increase is eligible, just in light of findings of a large sample of commuters in Korea showing physical inactivity during leisure time and long commuting times to be associated with work-related low back pain (Jung et al., 2024).

Conclusion

To summarise, commuting is a pivotal aspect of modern life, exerting profound influences on individuals, societies, and economies. Its significance extends beyond mere travel time, necessitating a comprehensive examination of its multifaceted impacts. While conventional wisdom often perceives commuting solely through the lens of time spent travelling, adopting a broader perspective encompassing relative dimensions is imperative. The discourse surrounding commuting as a stressor underscores the complexity inherent in its assessment. Studies frequently yield disparate findings, reflecting the nuanced interplay between commuting and well-being. A nuanced delineation of commuting's sub-aspects is imperative to elucidate this intricate relationship. Beyond temporal considerations, factors such as mode of transportation, work arrangement, the voluntariness of the commute, and the potential for utilising travel time for personal pursuits or role transitions emerge as critical determinants of its impact.

Central to this discourse is the notion of unnecessary or unreasonable commuting time, exemplifying the need for a refined understanding of commuting dynamics. Consequently, future research endeavours should prioritise the development of robust measurement tools capable of capturing the intricacies of commuting experiences. Scholars can elucidate how commuting influences them by delineating distinct sub-constructs and exploring their moderating effects on well-being and motivation. Moreover, a paradigm shift is warranted in conceptualising commuting as a demand and a potential resource. By identifying factors that contribute to its transformation from a stressor to a facilitator of well-being and motivation, interventions can be devised to optimise commuting experiences. Such a paradigm shift necessitates a concerted effort to mitigate negative aspects while leveraging commuting as an opportunity for personal growth and fulfilment. In summary, exploring commuting as a phenomenon transcends conventional paradigms, demanding a holistic understanding considering its multiple dimensions. We can illuminate the intricate interplay between commuting and individual well-being through rigorous empirical inquiry and theoretical refinement, paving the way for interventions that harness its transformative potential.

References

Ashforth, B. E., Kreiner, G. E., & Fugate, M. (2000). All in a day's work: Boundaries and micro role transitions. *Academy of Management Review, 25*(3), 472–491.

Bai, B., Gopalan, N., Beutell, N., & Ren, F. (2021). Impact of absolute and relative commute time on work–family conflict: Work schedule control, child care hours, and life satisfaction. *Journal of Family and Economic Issues, 42*, 586–600.

Bakker, A. B., & Demerouti, E. (2016). Job demands–resources theory: Taking stock and looking forward. *Journal of Occupational Health Psychology, 22*(3), 273–285.

Balk, Y. A. (2024). 'Switch off when not in use': The benefits of detachment from work and sport for recovery. In M. Kellmann & J. Beckmann (Eds.), *Fostering recovery and well-being in a healthy lifestyle: Psychological, somatic, and organizational prevention approaches* (pp. 59–72). Routledge.

Bowling, N. A., Beehr, T. A., Wagner, S. H., & Libkuman, T. M. (2005). Adaptation-level theory, opponent process theory, and dispositions: An integrated approach to the stability of job satisfaction. *Journal of Applied Psychology, 90*(6), 1044–1053.

Brüßler, S., von Haaren-Mack, B., Vogelsang, A., & Reichert, M. (2024). Ambulatory assessment for recovery and stress monitoring in the general population. In M. Kellmann & J. Beckmann (Eds.), *Fostering recovery and well-being in a healthy lifestyle: Psychological, somatic, and organizational prevention approaches* (pp. 38–55). Routledge.

Bundesamt für Statistik (BFS). (2024). *Pendlermobilität* [Commuter mobility]. Retrieved February 17, 2024 from https://www.bfs.admin.ch/bfs/de/home/statistiken/mobilitaet-verkehr/personenverkehr/pendlermobilitaet.html

Burch, K. A., & Barnes-Farrell, J. L. (2020). When work is your passenger: Understanding the relationship between work and commuting safety behaviors. *Journal of Occupational Health Psychology, 25*(4), 259–274.

Chatterjee, K., Chng, S., Clark, B., Davis, A., De Vos, J., Ettema, D., Handy, S., Martin, A., & Reardon, L. (2020). Commuting and wellbeing: A critical overview of the literature with implications for policy and future research. *Transport Reviews, 40*(1), 5–34.

de Bloom, J., Vaziri, H., Tay, L., & Kujanpää, M. (2020). An identity-based integrative needs model of crafting: Crafting within and across life domains. *Journal of Applied Psychology, 105*(12), 1423–1446.

de Jonge, J., & Taris, T. W. (2024). Off-job and on-job recovery as predictors of employee health. In M. Kellmann & J. Beckmann (Eds.), *Fostering recovery and well-being in a healthy lifestyle: Psychological, somatic, and organizational prevention approaches* (pp. 24–37). Routledge.

Ding, H., & Kuvaas, B. (2023). Illegitimate tasks: A systematic literature review and agenda for future research. *Work & Stress, 37*(3), 397–420.

Elfering, A. (2007). How fast small things become large: Dynamic change in judgment. *International Journal of Psychology, 42*, 274–284.

Elfering, A., Brunner, B., Igic, I., Keller, A. C., & Weber, L. (2018). Gesellschaftliche Bedeutung und Kosten von Stress [Social significance and costs of stress]. In R. Fuchs & M. Gerber (Eds.), *Handbuch Stressregulation und Sport* (pp. 123–141). Springer.

Elfering, A., & Grebner, S. (2010). A smile is just a smile: But only for men. Sex differences in meaning of faces scales. *Journal of Happiness Studies, 11*, 179–191.

Elfering, A., & Grebner, S. (2011). On intra- and interindividual differences in the meaning of smileys: Does this face show job satisfaction? *Swiss Journal of Psychology, 70*, 13–23.

Elfering, A., Grebner, S., & de Tribolet-Hardy, F. (2013). The long arm of time pressure at work: Cognitive failure and commuting near-accidents. *European Journal of Work and Organizational Psychology, 22*, 737–749.

Elfering, A., Grebner, S., & Haller, M. (2012). Railway-controller-perceived mental work load, cognitive failure and risky commuting. *Ergonomics, 55*(12), 1463–1475.

Elfering, A., Igic, I., Kritzer, R., & Semmer, N. K. (2020). Commuting as a work-related demand: Effects on work-to-family conflict, affective commitment, and intention to quit. *PsyCh Journal, 9*(4), 562–577.

Elfering, A., & Sarris, V. (2006). Memory and assimilation to context in delayed matching-to-sample. *Psychology Science, 48*, 17–38.

Fichter, C. (2015). Mobilität: Macht Pendeln unglücklich? [Mobility: Does commuting cause unhappiness?]. *Wirtschaftspsychologie Aktuell, 2*, 23–26.

Flade, A. (2013). *Der Rastlose Mensch: Konzepte und Erkenntnisse der Mobilitätspsychologie* [The restless human being: Concepts and findings of mobility psychology]. Springer.

Galliker, S., Igic, I., Semmer, N. K., & Elfering, A. (2024). Stress at work and well-being before and during the COVID-19 pandemic: A 1-year longitudinal study in Switzerland. *Journal of Occupational and Environmental Medicine, 66*(1), 56–70.

Galliker, S., Nyffenegger, D., Semmer, N. K., & Elfering, A. (2021). Women and men in leadership positions: Health and work-related attitudes and their associations with work-related stressors, private stressors, and privacy-work conflict. *Zeitschrift für Arbeitswissenschaft, 75*, 29–45.

Gerpott, F. H., Rivkin, W., & Unger, D. (2022). Stop and go, where is my flow? How and when daily aversive morning commutes are negatively related to employees' motivational states and behavior at work. *Journal of Applied Psychology, 107*(2), 169–192.

Google. (n.d.). *Google maps-help*. Retrieved May 23, 2018 from https://support.google.com/maps-topic=3092425

Grebner, S., Berlowitz, I., Alvarado, V., & Cassina, M. (2010). *Stress-Studie 2010. Stress bei Schweizer Erwerbstätigen. Zusammenhänge zwischen Arbeitsbedingungen, Personenmerkmalen, Befinden und Gesundheit* [Stress study 2010: Stress among Swiss employees. Relationships between working conditions, personal characteristics, well-being and health]. Staatssekretariat für Wirtschaft (seco).

Grotto, A. R., & Mills, M. J. (2023). Crossing the line: The violating effects of illegitimate interruptions from work and the differential impact on work-to-family conflict by gender. *Journal of Organizational Behavior, 44*(4), 700–716.

Hämmig, O., Gutzwiller, F., & Bauer, G. (2009). Work-life conflict and associations with work-and nonwork-related factors and with physical and mental health outcomes: A nationally representative cross-sectional study in Switzerland. *BMC Public Health, 9*, 435. https://doi.org/10.1186/1471-2458-9-435

Heinen, E., van Wee, B., & Maat, K. (2010). Commuting by bicycle: An overview of the literature. *Transport Reviews, 30*(1), 59–96.

Hobfoll, S. E., & Shirom, A. (2001). Conservation of resources theory: Applications to stress and management in the workplace. In R. T. Golembiewski (Ed.), *Handbook of organizational behavior* (pp. 57–80). Dekker.

Huber, F. (2022). *Commutes and their effects on work-related stress: A longitudinal analysis in the Swiss working population during Covid-19* [Unpublished master's thesis, University of Bern].

Igic, I., Semmer, N. K., Elfering, A., Zumstein, N., & Lötscher, D. (2017). *Test manual – S-tool (Friendly work space job-stress-analyses).* Gesundheitsförderung Schweiz.

Jung, J., Park, J. B., Lee, K.-J., Seo, Y., & Jeong, I. (2024). Association between commuting time and work-related low back pain with respect to sports and leisure activities in Korean workers. *Industrial Health, 62*(2), 133–142.

Kahneman, D., & Krueger, A. B. (2006). Developments in the measurement of subjective well-being. *Journal of Economic Perspectives, 20*(1), 3–24.

Kallus, K. W. (2016). Stress and recovery: An overview. In K. W. Kallus & M. Kellmann (Eds.), *The Recovery-Stress Questionnaires: User manual* (pp. 27–48). Pearson Assessment.

Kellmann, M., Bertollo, M., Bosquet, L., Brink, M., Coutts, A. J., Duffield, R., Erlacher, D., Halson, S. L., Hecksteden, A., Heidari, J., Kallus, K. W., Meeusen, R., Mujika, I., Robazza, C., Skorski, S., Venter, R., & Beckmann, J. (2018). Recovery and performance in sport: Consensus statement. *International Journal of Sports Physiology and Performance, 13*(2), 240–245.

Kern, M., Semmer, N. K., & Baethge, A. (2023). Energized or distressed by time pressure? The role of time pressure illegitimacy. *European Journal of Work and Organizational Psychology, 32*(4), 575–598.

Klumb, P. L., & Thielsch, M. T. (2019). TBS-DTK-Rezension: "S-Tool – Ein Online-Befragungsinstrument zur Erhebung von Belastungen, Ressourcen und Befinden am Arbeitsplatz" [TBS-DTK review: 'S-Tool – an online survey instrument for assessing stress, resources and well-being in the workplace']. *Psychologische Rundschau, 70*, 232–234.

Koslowsky, M., Aizer, A., & Krausz, M. (1996). Stressor and personal variables in the commuting experience. *International Journal of Manpower, 17*(3), 4–14.

MacCallum, R. C., Zhang, S., Preacher, K. J., & Rucker, D. D. (2002). On the practice of dichotomization of quantitative variables. *Psychological Methods*, 7(1), 19–40.

McAlpine, K. L., & Piszczek, M. M. (2023). Along for the ride through liminal space: A role transition and recovery perspective on the work-to-home commute. *Organizational Psychology Review, 13*(2), 156–176.

Morrow, S. L. (2010). *The psychosocial costs of commuting: Understanding relationships between time, control, stress, and well-being* [Doctoral Dissertation, University of Connecticut]. Retrieved February 17, 2024 from https://opencommons.uconn.edu/dissertations/AAI3415559

Murphy, L. D., Cobb, H. R., Rudolph, C. W., & Zacher, H. (2023). Commuting demands and appraisals: A systematic review and meta-analysis of strain and well-being outcomes. *Organizational Psychology Review, 13*(1), 11–43.

Novaco, R. W., Stokols, D., & Milanesi, L. (1990). Objective and subjective dimensions of travel impedance as determinants of commuting stress. *American Journal of Community Psychology, 18*(2), 231–257.

Pindek, S., Shen, W., & Andel, S. (2023). Finally, some 'me time': A new theoretical perspective on the benefits of commuting. *Organizational Psychology Review, 13*(1), 44–66.

Schweizerische Bundesbahn (SBB). (2024). *Zugpünkltichkeit im Personenverkehr* [Train punctuality in passenger transport]. Retrieved September 12, 2024 from https://reporting.sbb.ch/puenktlichkeit

Seligman, M. E., & Csikszentmihalyi, M. (2014). Positive psychology: An introduction. In M. Csikszentmihalyi (Ed.), *Flow and the foundations of positive psychology: The collected works of Mihaly Csikszentmihalyi* (pp. 279–298). Springer.

Semmer, N. K., Grebner, S., & Elfering, A. (2004). Beyond self-report: Using observational, physiological, and event-based measures in research on occupational stress. In P. L. Perrewé & D. C. Ganster (Eds.), *Emotional and physiological processes and positive intervention strategies: Research in occupational stress and well-being* (pp. 205–263). JAI.

Semmer, N. K., Grebner, S., & Elfering, A. (2010). "Psychische Kosten" von Arbeit: Beanspruchung und Erholung, Leistung und Gesundheit [The 'psychological costs' of work: Workload, recovery, performance, and health]. In U. Kleinbeck & K.-H. Schmidt (Eds.), *Arbeitspsychologie* (pp. 325–370). Hogrefe.

Semmer, N. K., Jacobshagen, N., Keller, A. C., & Meier, L. L. (2021). Adding insult to injury: Illegitimate stressors and their association with situational well-being, social self- esteem, and desire for revenge. *Work & Stress*, *35*(3), 262–282.

Semmer, N. K., Jacobshagen, N., Meier, L., & Elfering, A. (2007). Occupational stress research: The 'stress-as-offence-to-self' perspective. In J. H. S. McIntyre (Ed.), *Occupational health psychology: European perspectives on research* (Vol. 2, pp. 43–60). ISMAI Publishers.

Semmer, N. K., Jacobshagen, N., Meier, L. L., Elfering, A., Beehr, T. A., Kälin, W., & Tschan, F. (2015). Illegitimate tasks as a source of work stress. *Work & Stress*, *29*(1), 32–56.

Semmer, N. K., Tschan, F., Jacobshagen, N., Beehr, T. A., Elfering, A., Kälin, W., & Meier, L. L. (2019). Stress as offense to self: A promising approach comes of age. *Occupational Health Science*, *3*(3), 205–238.

Sonnentag, S., Cheng, B. H., & Parker, S. L. (2022). Recovery from work: Advancing the field toward the future. *Annual Review of Organizational Psychology and Organizational Behavior*, *9*(1), 33–60.

Sonnentag, S., & Kühnel, J. (2016). Coming back to work in the morning: Psychological detachment and reattachment as predictors of work engagement. *Journal of Occupational Health Psychology*, *21*(4), 379–390.

Stutzer, A., & Frey, B. S. (2008). Stress that doesn't pay: The commuting paradox. *The Scandinavian Journal of Economics*, *110*(2), 339–366.

Theorell, T., & Karasek, R. A. (1996). Current issues relating to psychosocial job strain and cardiovascular disease research. *Journal of Occupational Health Psychology*, *1*(1), 9–26.

UK Office for National Statistics. (2014). *Commuting and personal well-being, 2014*. Retrieved May 15, 2024 from https://webarchive.nationalarchives.gov.uk/ukgwa/20160105231823/http://www.ons.gov.uk/ons/rel/wellbeing/measuring-national-well-being/commuting-and-personal-well-being – 2014/art-commuting-and-personal-well-being.html

Wener, R., Evans, G. W., & Boately, P. (2005). Commuting stress: Psychophysiological effects of a trip and spillover into the workplace. *Transportation Research Record*, *1924*(1), 112–117.

Wöhrmann, A. M., Backhaus, N., & Ducki, A. (2023). Mobiles Arbeiten: Chancen und Risiken [Mobile working: Opportunities and risks]. In B. Badura, A. Ducki, J. Baumgardt, M. Meyer, & H. Schröder (Eds.), *Fehlzeiten-Report 2023* (pp. 255–269). Springer.

Zapf, D., & Semmer, N. K. (2004). Stress und Gesundheit in Organisationen [Stress and health in organisations]. In H. Schuler (Ed.), *Organisationspsychologie* (pp. 1007–1112). Hogrefe.

3 Eight days a week

Long working hours, recovery, and breaks

K. Wolfgang Kallus

Introduction

The reduction of weekly/monthly working hours appears to be a primary goal of union–employer conflicts, while other areas of stressful aspects of work and changes in jobs (e.g., digitalisation, automation, remote work, home office, increasing work compression) receive far less attention. The development in recent decades in Europe shows an interesting paradox: reduced average working hours are associated with a decrease of breaks and recovery phases and increased mental health problems (Dragano et al., 2024). This is accompanied by a change in office designs to more open-space offices and shared workplaces, which offer less privacy for breaks and short work interruptions. A work–recovery culture has been abandoned in many crafts and trades in contrast to an elaboration of cool-down and recovery in sports. The responsibility for finding recovery at work is left to the employees, who often do not know much about balancing stress and recovery. But recovery in and from work should be essential in a culture which tries to foster healthy lifestyles, as working more than 55 hours/week contributes to work-related burden of disease and injury. Pega et al. (2021) documented the impact of long working hours referring to WHO/ILO estimates in 194 countries. A trend to reduced weekly working hours is paradoxically associated with an increase in stressful working conditions, potentially generating an increase in psychosomatic symptoms. However, trends are difficult to interpret due to the recent Covid-19 pandemic and long-Covid problems, which superimpose on the data and hamper comparisons across time. Work schedules should consider that recovery needs suitable boundary conditions, such as break/recovery settings, and an inclusion of biological rhythms, cultural rhythms, and individual psychological activity–recovery rhythms.

In sports, recovery has become integrated in training plans and is systematically scheduled by coaches during the competition periods. In work, the

Kallus, K. W. (2025). Eight days a week: Long working hours, recovery, and breaks. In S. Pauleit, M. Kellmann, & J. Beckmann (Eds.), *Creating Urban and Workplace Environments for Recovery and Well-being* (pp. 37–60). Routledge.

DOI: 10.4324/9781003435471-4

interplay between stress and recovery is potentially more complex than in sports, but normally, no coach will aid employees with recovery–stress planning. This is particularly a problem for self-employed or home office work, which is often scheduled by internet meetings.

Recovery

Currently, no generally accepted definition of recovery exists. Kallus (2016, p. 42) defined recovery as

> an inter- and intraindividual multilevel (e.g., psychological, physiological, social) process in time for the re-establishment of personal resources and their full functional capacity. Recovery includes a broad range of physiological processes like sleep, motivated behavior (like eating and drinking) and goal-oriented components (like relaxation or meeting friends). Recovery activities can be passive or active and in many instances recovery is achieved indirectly by activities, which stimulate recovery processes like active sports.

In sports, a consensus statement has been published to define recovery (Kellmann et al., 2018), which is compatible with the aforementioned characteristics. Mechanical models, like unwinding or bouncing back, have been used as metaphors – but they underestimate the importance of recovery and repair processes in biological and biopsychosocial systems. Recovery is always needed when resources are taxed, depleted, or either lost or out of use. On a theoretical level, the stress model published by Hobfoll (1989, see also Hou & Tao, 2023) states that the endangerment of resources is the source, or one of the most prominent sources, of stress. However, Hobfoll's *Conservation of Resources* model does not address the recovery of resources. When Hobfoll (1989) published his concept on the *Conservation of Resources*, he seemed to have neglected the rule: one good way to conserve one's resources is by taking a break – at best, with regenerative or training activities.

Recovery, like stress, is a biopsychosocial phenomenon which can be addressed on different levels. On the biological level of physiological functions, the human body strives to re-establish a homeostatic equilibrium. Rhythmical phenomena like the sleep–wake cycle represent a basic action–recovery cycle. However, sleep is not a passive event but has its own dynamics and function. Sleep deprivation has severe consequences (Kullik & Kiel, 2024). Disturbed vegetative functions and biological rhythms occur immediately; psychological symptoms up to psychiatric symptoms can be provoked by repeated sleep deprivation, which has been used for the torture of prisoners (van Dongen et al., 2003). During sleep, psychological and physiological recovery processes take place. The humoral system is very active, as can be seen in cortisol (the stress-related hormone, which peaks at the end of the night). Circadian rhythms are the most prominent biological rhythms, which are found on different functional levels. Even standard social activities follow a circadian rhythm, with phases of nourishment and grooming interspersed. During wake time, ultradian cycles (cycles shorter than circadian rhythms) are often integrated in social habits. One example is the 'basic rest–activity cycle', as described by Kleitman (1963), which follows approximate 90 minutes and corresponds to break schedules in many Western educational systems. Breaks for recovery should take such biological rhythms into account.

Recovery of resources is not a passive process, like restoring water in a tank, but a process which is often accompanied by active adaptive processes, like increasing the number of vesicles on a synapse, increasing blood flow capacity, learning and automation of skills, optimising communication, and building up social resources. For psychomotor skills, breaks can improve learning through processes of incubation (Ellwood et al., 2009) or mental rehearsals (Schmidt & Lee, 2020). Recovery will take place as soon as the resource is no longer taxed. This can be achieved by a change of action and activity.

Far more effective is taking a break, which requires suitable boundary conditions and appraisals. Recovery in work settings takes place within the working day, between working days, on weekends, and in vacancies. However, breaks, off-duty times, and free-time activities, and even short vacancies, are only effective if the individual switches off effectively from work to regeneration. In sports, Eberspächer et al. (1993) and Kallus et al. (1992) developed the so-called *Sluice Model* for breaks. This model can be adapted to the needs of a busy working day. Research findings from classical laboratory and field studies show that effective breaks ensure the maintenance of a high level of performance as well as reduce fatigue, errors, and stress symptoms (Allmer, 1996; Graf, 1960; Folkard & Lombardi, 2006; Knauth, 2007; Sato et al., 2020; Vieten et al., 2023).

A common paradox of stress appears when employees or businesspeople claim that with increasing stress they find no time to cope with stress and for recovery. But with an increasing consumption of resources, there is a need to also increase the establishment and recovery of resources. This rule is trivial in the technical domain, but obviously not to the same degree with respect to stress and recovery of humans. The frequently stated paradox that increasing stress leaves no time to recover resources needs to be overcome through an understanding that keeping a balance of stress and recovery is essential.

Long working hours, overtime, and the recovery–stress balance

The need for recovery is clearly reflected in the effects of so-called long working hours. The topic of long working hours would benefit from an internationally accepted definition that differentiates long working hours from overtime work as well as night and shift work. Official regulations make a difference between long working hours and overtime (Kallus & Gaisbachgrabner, 2018). The Council of the European Union (1993, 2000, 2003) defined long working hours in the Directives 93/104/EC, 2000/34/EC, and 2003/88/EC as deviation from normal working hours. Normal working hours comprise:

- Maximum average working week (including overtime) of 48 hours over a 17-week reference period
- Minimum daily rest period of eleven consecutive hours in every 24 hours
- Breaks when the working day exceeds six hours
- Minimum weekly rest period of 24 hours plus the eleven-hour daily rest period in every seven-day period
- Minimum of four weeks paid annual leave
- Night work restricted to an average of eight hours in any 24-hour period

However, empirical studies use different cut-offs to define long working hours. Sudden deaths from heart attacks, the so-called *Karoshi syndrome*, were observed in Japanese workers whose working hours exceeded 60 hours/week (Iwasaki et al., 2006; Kubo et al., 2024). Spurgeon et al. (1997) and Knauth (2007) summarise the empirical evidence and conclude that long working hours between 50 and 55 hours a week are associated with serious health problems. Dex et al. (1995) argue that long working hours may be considered differently for men (over 60 hours per week) and women (over 40 hours a week). Caruso et al. (2004) report that even simple overtime of over 40 hours a week shows negative effects, like elevated risk for neck, shoulder, and back pain disorders, more cardiovascular and musculoskeletal complaints, and fatigue, and is also found to negatively affect performance. According to Nachreiner et al. (2005), psycho-vegetative complaints show a steep linear increase from 40 hours on, while musculoskeletal disorders and others show increased risks especially beyond 60 hours/week (Figure 3.1).

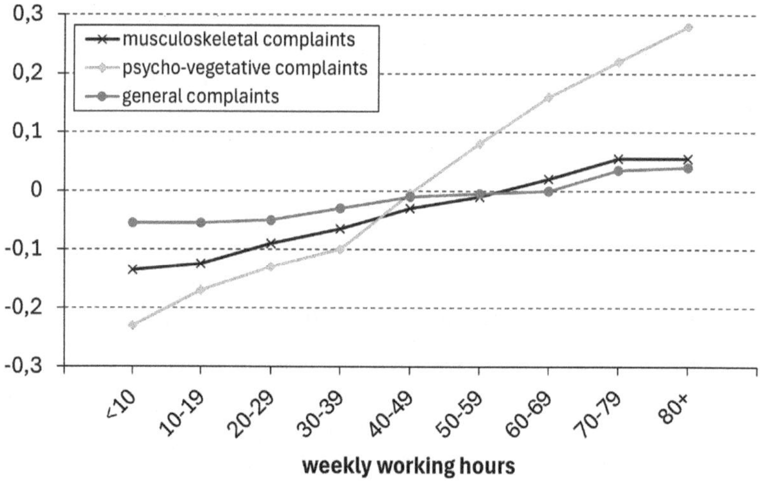

Figure 3.1 Long working hours and complaints.

Source: Adapted from Nachreiner et al. (2005, p. 28).

Long working hours are difficult to define, as working schedules, hours in main job and other jobs, commuting time, business travel time, as well as family or social obligations need to be considered as well. Furthermore, the relation between hours worked and the resulting stress levels can vary considerably for daily, weekly, or annual working hours, with different ways to compensate for peaks in working hours. Overtime can be viewed as the area between regular working schedules and long working hours. This chapter proposes to refer to health-related long working hours beyond 50 hours to 60 hours a week for longer periods or repeated occurrence, which are not compensated directly within a two-month time window. In most instances, however, a restricted view merely on hours spent working is not useful, because a large set of moderators have to be taken into account. One example is long working hours and shift work, which are often confounded, as shift work has unusual working hours, which are often extended beyond eight hours to bridge the nights. Backhaus et al. (2019) conclude that reduced time to recover is one of the most important moderators of the long working hour/health complaint relationship.

Overtime hours are defined as

> work performed by an employee in excess of the normal hours of work which has been officially requested and approved by management. It is work that is not part of an employee's regularly scheduled working week and for which an employee may be compensated.
>
> (Eurofound, 2022, p. 1)

The European Working Time Directive (2003/88/EC; Council of the European Union, 2003) imposes limits on overtime through its provisions on maximum weekly working time (48 hours, including overtime) and a minimum daily rest period (eleven consecutive hours per 24-hour period). Overtime hours cover the area between normal working hours and long working hours. With respect to the recovery–stress profile (Kallus, 2025), overtime showed only marginal effects compared to normal working hours in a study with $(N = 203)$ Austrian blue-collar workers (Gaisbachgrabner, 2014). The Recovery–Stress Questionnaire for Work (RESTQ-Work; Jiménez et al., 2016, 2025) was used to assess the effects of overtime and long working hours in a cross-sectional analysis. The RESTQ-Work assesses twelve general facets of stress (seven scales) and recovery (five scales) and six scales of work-specific stress, like 'burnout', plus nine scales of work-related recovery and resources, like 'efficient breaks'. In the study of Gaisbachgrabner (2014), long working hours resulted in large differences on a couple of scales, such as *General Stress*, *Fatigue*, *Social Recovery*, and *Sleep Quality*, in the basic scales of the RESTQ-Work (Figure 3.2). Also, a couple of differences were found on the work-specific scales. However, no differences occurred on scales that assess classical work resources, like social support, participation, or action latitude.

The effects of long working hours, as indicated in the RESTQ-Work, were also visible in physical stress markers. A very striking effect occurred for thyroid

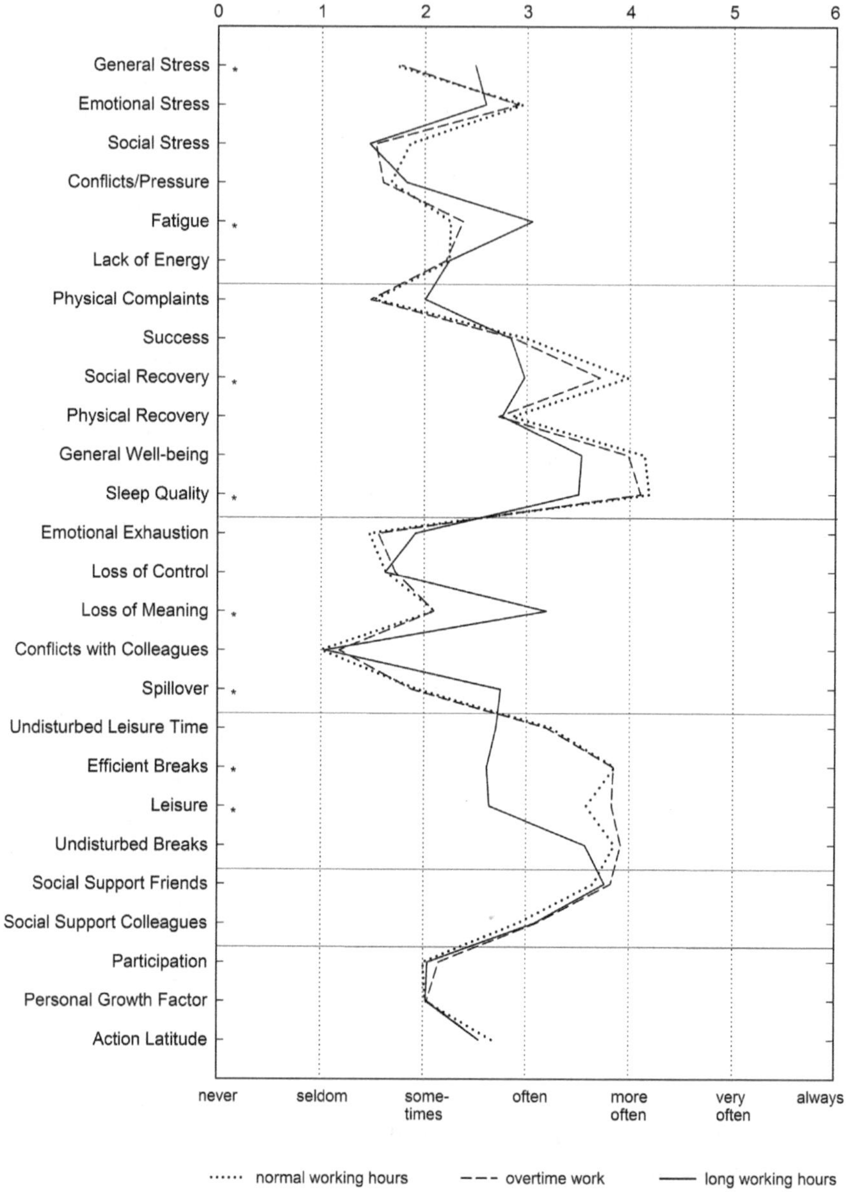

Figure 3.2 RESTQ-Basic scales and different groups of working time: (Manova: $F[2,199] = 4.285$, $p < .0001$, $\eta p^2 = .215$). * = $p < .05$.

Source: Reprinted with permission from Kallus, K. W., & Gaisbachgrabner, K. (2018). Stress and recovery in applied settings: Long working hours, recovery, and breaks. In M. Kellmann & J. Beckmann (Eds.), *Sport, recovery, and performance: Interdisciplinary insights* (pp. 233–246). Routledge.

functions (Kallus & Gaisbachgrabner, 2018). Gaisbachgrabner et al. (2011) detected an odds ratio of 8.5 for thyroid dysfunction in a group of blue-collar workers with long working hours compared to those with normal working hours (overall sample size $N = 203$). This result could be replicated in another study by Gaisbachgrabner (2014) with a lower but still striking odds ratio of 4.5. A quasi-experimental prospective test on long working hours with a small sample $(N = 13)$ supported the results and showed that the change in thyroid function was associated with changes in cortisol awakening values (Dickerson & Kemeny, 2004; Fries et al., 2009; Kirschbaum, 1991). Thus, stress was a crucial factor for the thyroid dysfunction, but changes from recovery towards insufficient recovery (underrecovery) were also visible in the RESTQ-Work profile.

Long working hours beyond 60 hours a week are accompanied by critical situations at work and by critical psychophysiological states of the employees, with health risks in the long run. The most striking effect is sudden cardiac death in Asia, which has been termed *Karoshi* (Kubo et al., 2024). *Karoshi* is associated with intense work, long working hours, and presumably, severe underrecovery. Long working hours can be a strong risk factor for psychosomatic complaints and even sudden cardiac death (Kubo et al., 2024). Simple overtime or exceeding the EU-defined normal workload might not be harmful if the work is well-designed. Working more than 55 hours to 60 hours a week might be stressful or will at least result in recovery problems. Long working hours are often associated with shift work because working hours quickly accumulate in shift work. From a psychological perspective, a decomposition of the combined effects of long working hours and night shifts would be more than worthwhile. It is very difficult to untangle the effects, as many shift systems contain long shifts of twelve or even more hours. At the same time, these shifts encompass relaxation periods and longer breaks. Sometimes the location where shift workers spend these breaks and relaxation periods is the only difference to standby duties. Professional firefighters often stay for 24-hour shifts in the fire station, as this speeds up the time till they reach a fire (Garrett et al., 2024).

Stress and long working hours

The stress concept (McEwen, 1998; Selye, 1936) provides a link between psychological states and physiological changes like blood pressure or changes in immune functioning (Glaser & Kiecolt-Glaser, 1994; Kirschbaum & Hellhammer, 1989). The causal experimental evidence is less convincing for chronic stress and other concepts like chronic fatigue or burnout. Nevertheless, Kubo et al. (2024) discuss long working hours and conclude that the consequences of long working hours and the related unfavourable working conditions can have fatal consequences, as can be seen in *Karoshi*. However, there is still only very sparse experimental evidence, and most data are from cross-sectional, epidemiologic, or health insurance databases. Causal inferences cannot be drawn with high confidence from these data, as not all relevant variables can be included in the statistical models. Thus, there might be a very large portion of the population or age cohort with the same or even more working hours which do not develop cardiovascular or other psychosomatic symptoms. Data are needed to have well-based evidence on protective factors and their boundary conditions. In most instances, long working hours occur in combination with other adverse working conditions, such as shift work, inadequate workspaces as during assembly operations, outdoor work, or psychologically demanding conditions, as in paramedics or firefighters (Le et al., 2022; Sato et al., 2020). A recent study on Chinese courier workers (Hong et al., 2022) shows that working hours, in combination with occupational stress, contribute to the development of depression. The study included a large sample $(N = 1200)$, with more than 66% of the included workers working more than 55 hours a week. However, the study included a broad range of working hours in the correlation-based models, which could have potentially biased the correlations. Interestingly, not only occupational stress but also reduced well-being contributed significantly to the outcome variable. This can be interpreted as an indication of an important contribution of underrecovery and work conditions to the development of depression.

The basic message of this chapter is that the total minutes of a work period or shift are not the most important factor but can be compensated for by good work design, good break plans, and/or a well-functioning team. The problem of long working hours begins with the breakdown of the 24 hours of a normal working day. On a working day, there are paid working periods, periods of commuting to the workplace, and periods with recovery options, like time for grooming, nutrition, and family or social obligations, physical fitness and sports, hobby and personal maintenance, and personal development, as well as periods for sleep and social interactions, communication, and personal recovery. In addition, in modern societies, people spend a considerable time on the internet with social networks, gaming, or media (Fiedler et al., 2023).

Research findings on reduced leisure time (Backhaus et al., 2019) change the view on long working hours, because a pure count of working hours does not provide meaningful results as long as a limit of about 50 hours to 60 hours is not reached. Many athletes, scientists, freelancers, musicians, and most small business enterprises, as well as military personnel and emergency personnel, are affected by long working hours without fatal consequences (Altenmüller et al., in press). However, it might be that they tax their health intensively if they maintain a high stress level over years without balancing recovery and still might have the luck of a stable health. A good balance of stress and recovery in spite of high stress levels due to good coping, clear-cut switches between life domains, good sleep, nutrition, and some regular sports activity might help keep health intact.

Only few researchers focus on repeated stress in their concepts, like McEwen (1998) did with the idea of allostatic load. There is no good reason to explain that recovery–stress concepts have not been extensively studied outside the sports domain. However, missing recovery and inadequate coping might be important to understand the long-term effects of stressful working conditions and individual stress states on health, motivation, and performance.

Underrecovery

Missing or disrupted breaks and disturbed circadian rhythms can result in a state in which recovery from stress is not possible or insufficient. This state can also be the result of non-recreative sleep or disturbed sleep, which is common for young parents or people staying up late (e.g., babies; for bad internet habits, see Heidari & Kellmann, 2024). Underrecovery has not been addressed as a source of aversive effects of long working hours, but periods of regeneration were included in the EU directives for long working hours. Recent publications report a considerable influence of restricted off-duty periods on health and well-being (Backhaus et al., 2019; Kellmann & Beckmann, 2024). The authors state that flexible working time arrangements can result in violations of the 11-hour rule for minimum daily rest periods. Using regression models (sample size $N = 6136$), Backhaus et al. (2019) demonstrate that work–life balance as well as psychosomatic complaints change with restricted off-duty times in a similar way as overtime does. Thus, underrecovery might be an important factor that contributes to the effects of long working hours.

Underrecovery has been described as a precursor of overtraining (Kellmann, 2010), and some basic features have been listed by Davis et al. (2002): negative mood (nervousness, tension, worry, combined with anger, scorn, guilt, self-dissatisfaction, low positive affect, self-dissatisfaction, and sadness), vegetativeness, and hormonal imbalance, with high noradrenalin and elevated cortisol responses, with a subsequent decline to low values. The changes are associated with poor self-regulation. Transferring these symptoms to the working environment shows close parallels to early symptoms of burnout, which might be caused or at least facilitated by underrecovery, following this line of arguments.

Failing to use the off-work time for recovery results in underrecovery, which might become more and more important as off-duty time is increasing. Social obligations in the family, neighbourhood, or for friends, as well as activities in sport or charity associations, as well as internet communication, can be rewarding and help recover from work – but they can be taxing and prevent recovery in some instances (Heidari & Kellmann, 2024). Another source of underrecovery is the tendency to have a second job, which is common for low-wage jobs, students, or retired persons with a small regular income.

Underrecovery might be relevant for fatigue in the subsequent work period or for the development of chronic fatigue. This is a point which is relevant not only for health but also for safety at work and in the occupational system. Health is not the only objective in long working hours. With increasing working hours without an intelligent work–break system, fatigue will appear, which is a major cause of incidents and accidents at work (Austrian Association for Work Medicine, 2019).

Research with the Recovery–Stress Questionnaire (RESTQ; Kallus & Kellmann, 2016; Kellmann & Kallus, 2025) shows that a person could suffer from low recovery without a previous experience of a high-stress state. In sports, underrecovery has received increasing attention; in work settings, other concepts like burnout, chronic fatigue, or stress prevail. However, the perspective of missing or derailed recovery processes and activities might add valuable options to create a healthy life domain system even in high-performance areas. Inadequate recovery or underrecovery is reflected in disturbed sleep and/or disturbed nutrition, a lack of social recovery, options to laugh, physical activity and grooming, and good mood as it occurs in patients with burnout and depression (Agyapong et al., 2022). These symptoms can be but are not necessarily associated with stress. Some symptoms might just be associated with unfavourable working conditions, like shift work, or biorhythmically unfavourable standby times, all of which interfere with proper recovery activity and recovery states.

Underrecovery is not the only causal factor for job-related health or disease. Nevertheless, underrecovery must be considered as an important contributing factor with potential short- and long-term effects on individual well-being and health. However, prolonged, intermittent, or delayed stress symptoms might be one of the most important sources of disturbed recovery processes. Post-traumatic stress symptoms like intrusions are a prominent example of recurring long-term stress effects which interfere with recovery.

Overtime working hours (paid or unpaid) constitute only a part of a stressful week. Non-working hours must **not** be considered as equivalent to recovery time, whereas time for sleep, grooming, and nutrition can be considered as opportunities to recover resources. However, this time needs to be appraised and used properly. An obvious example is a break during a work period. If the break is caused by a technical problem and the duration is unknown, the operator will wait for the system to work again. Thus, a break can be an interruption of activities with an annoying connotation. On the other hand, a break can be a necessary time interval for regaining full attention (similar to switching back from anaerobic to aerobic metabolism in the muscles). Even short breaks filled with positive activities and mood can help to recover at least partly, and especially when they appear in a predictable and uninterrupted manner.

Breaks

Taking measures against underrecovery includes efficient breaks. The aforementioned *Sluice Model* from sports (Eberspächer et al., 1993) is useful in describing efficient breaks, which are an option to cope with extended working hours. Following the *Sluice Model* of breaks, switching from work activity in a work setting to the break activity in a break setting would be optimal. Sometimes recovery in breaks suffers from non-optimal conditions. However, at least mentally switching to the break is mandatory.

A study with rail traffic controllers (Kallus et al., 2009) compared changes from an established and well-designed 12-hour-shift system to an EU-conforming 8-hour-shift roster. Results did not reveal the expected advantages for the 8-hour shifts. The rail traffic controllers in two different locations had very similar activities – but two different shift systems. The shift system is depicted in Figure 3.3. Note that the 12-hour-shift system resulted in 48 working hours

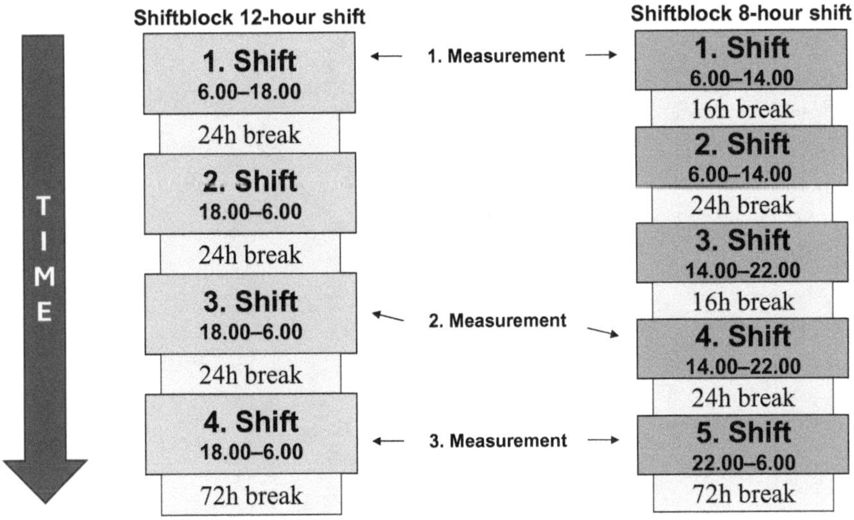

Figure 3.3 Comparison of 12-hour and 8-hour systems of railway workers.

in a shift block, while the 8-hour-shift system resulted in 40 hours worked in a shift block.

Fatigue was assessed with a version of the German Stress-Fatigue Assessment Scales (Beanspruchungs-Mess-Skalen; BMS-Scale; Debitz et al., 2016). After the first shift, both regimes resulted in an increase in fatigue, with higher values at the end of the 12-hour shift, as expected (Figure 3.4). The increase in fatigue continued for the 8-hour-shift system. A complete free 24-hour block allowed the 12-hour shifts a full recovery. Measurements in the final working block showed an increase in fatigue for the 12-hour shift and an accumulation of fatigue for the 8-hour working block, which can be attributed to insufficient recovery in the 8-hour-shift system. The 12-hour-shift system resulted in less-extreme fatigue in the course of the shift block. Figure 3.4 shows that fatigue was larger for the 12-hour work after the first 12-hour work period. For the following work periods (middle and end), the workers experienced higher fatigue in the 8-hour blocks (BMS scores are inverted to indicate stronger fatigue with increasing values). Due to longer times for recovery, the 12-hour shifts show lower fatigue. Results confirm that restricting the analysis to mere working hours results in an incomplete picture of demands. Additionally, recovery options and breaks should be taken into account. Kirchler and Schmidl (2000) published similar results with respect to performance measures. The studies indicate that the 12-hour system with full 24-hour blocks of recovery is superior to the 8-hour system despite 8 hours more working time. In both systems, a 24-hour break preceded the final night shift. However, this is not an experimental result, and it is known from other studies that employees tend to self-select working conditions suiting their life conditions best. Other factors

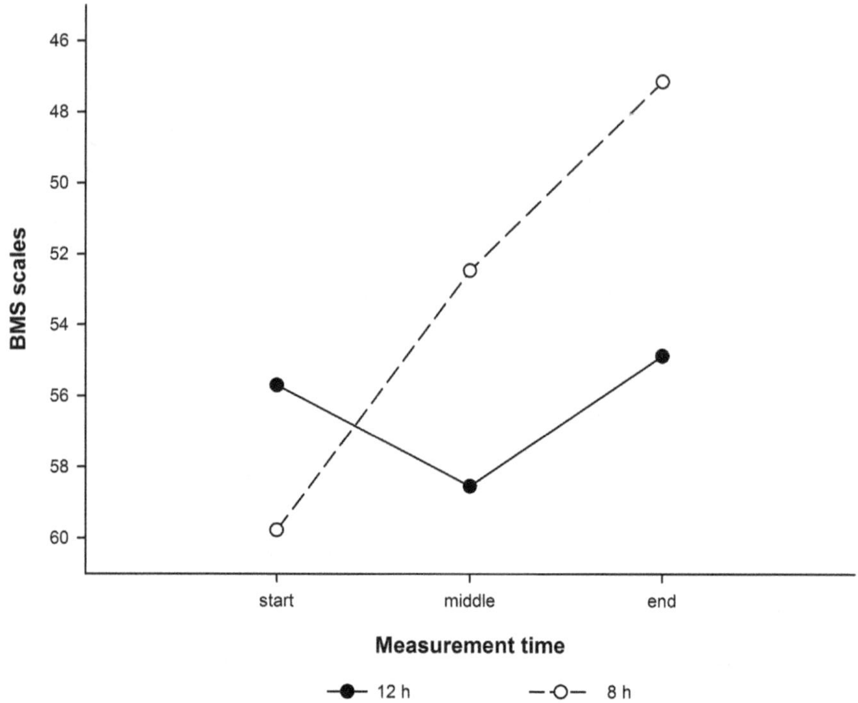

Figure 3.4 Fatigue (end of shift) of 12-hour and 8-hour systems of railway workers.

Note: BMS scale assesses fatigue and stress.

Source: Adapted from Kallus et al. (2009, p. 243).

could have contributed to the results, because no randomisation had been possible. It should also be pointed out that the 8-hour system was new, while the 12-hour system had a longer tradition in the company.

A wide range of jobs with extensive working hours comprises opportunities to actively organise job and working patterns to create recovery options. A switch in tasks or role can result in partial recovery of resources. Data from laboratory and field studies show that intelligent breaks are very effective in providing a high performance level throughout the working day, in addition to reducing negative mood changes and the appearance of physical stress symptoms (Buchegger, 2017).

Classical studies on the effects of breaks on performance have already demonstrated that short, early breaks can be very effective (Graf, 1922, 1960). Resources can be conserved by a proper break schedule (plus other factors). A good break regime is comparable with an intelligent use of resources.

Effective breaks are supported by a change in attention, posture, activity, and also social context. Task analysis conducted in public administrations revealed a tendency to stay at the workplace, consuming legally defined breaks there, observing the computer monitors, and keeping phone and internet active. This can result in breaks without mentally switching off or without 'detachment' (Korunka et al., 2012). An individual-oriented work organisation in many administrative areas prohibits teamwork and sharing resources, especially regarding mutual time for breaks. Furthermore, innovations in technical support can provide increased possibilities for short breaks. Note that breaks always have the feature of interruption as soon as they do not conform with the task structure. However, in the work-specific culture of skilled crafts and trades, systematic breaks for (second) breakfasts and afternoon rests have become a social tradition, like the siesta in Spain. Thus, in some regions of the work environment, recovery–stress cycles within working days are well established. Even stronger social rules govern the weekend culture in our society. In addition, systematic breaks are linked to holidays in schools and universities and create blocks of non-working days, such as Easter and Christmas, in most societies (Kellmann & Heidari, 2020).

Break settings as behaviour settings

The concept of behaviour settings from environmental psychology might be used to design appropriate break settings. A behaviour setting (Barker, 1968; Schoggen, 1989) comprises a set of an external setting with time-space boundaries, typical behaviours, and the suiting environmental features. The behaviour in a behaviour setting follows a common script, which is not individual, such as drinking in a bar or eating in a restaurant or having your hair cut at a barber's shop. These typical behaviours can be observed as 'standing patterns of behaviour'. Different behaviour settings can occur in the same environmental space, as behaviour settings are time-space-bound, like the Friday market or a parish fair in the parking area. Thus, a behaviour setting is defined as a standing pattern of behaviour in a space-time unit of the environment which shows a high degree of synomorphy. A synomorph is a standing pattern of behaviour in a well-fitting setting. A set of synomorphs characterises a behaviour setting. Behaviour settings take place in a defined time-space unit and have boundaries. A behaviour setting follows something like a program, and some of the actors in a behaviour setting take the role to run/and or maintain the setting.

The behaviour setting idea can well be adopted for breaks; suitable break settings will help create regenerative breaks. For effective breaks, a suitable environment must be found, attended to, or improvised in many instances. The setting helps switch or switch off effectively. It is like switching off after work (detachment; Balk, 2024; de Jonge & Taris, 2024; Sonnentag & Fritz, 2015), but the time frame for breaks is different.

The proposed sluice or water gate metaphor, proposed by Eberspächer et al. (1993) for the sports domain, represents a break in the flow of work actions. The *Sluice Model* describes a break as the first step of switching off or relaxing before regeneration can start. At the end of the break, one needs to re-enter the stream of action again by increasing the activation to a level that was predetermined at the beginning of the break. In contrast to sports, efficient breaks must be prepared in the workflow. Particularly, restarting work after a break must often be structured in advance, because breaks interrupt the workflow and require some effort to take up the thread of action again after the break. This might be a reason that breaks are not being taken regularly or may be even overrun by employees. However, an action flow cannot be stopped at any point as, for example, a high jump or golf swing in sports. As a first step, suitable options for stops in the action flow must be identified, sometimes in advance. The example of white-water canoeists can serve as a metaphor, as they determine stop points during inspection of the passage before they enter a long and demanding passage or cascade. In the *Action Regulation Theory* (Hacker, 2003), work is organised in loops, which should be completed sequentially and in a hierarchical direction, which means actions should be planned, anticipated, executed, finished, and evaluated by a person or a group and all psychic functions should be used: perceptive, cognitive, executive, psychomotor, and evaluative. When a sequence or subsequence of an action is finished, options for a break are given. If they do not naturally occur in the activity, the action should be organised with an action plan, defining opportunities to interrupt the activity. Sometimes memory cues will be needed to help a smooth restart of the action after a break.

Starting a break can be achieved by shifting to a break setting, a change in activity, or a change of the attentional focus. Cues and habits can help integrate them into daily routines. Note that recovery is a process which is very susceptible to disturbances (Kallus & Krauth, 1995). Thus, a break can become ineffective for recovery when disturbances occur (Vieten et al., 2023). Coworkers often join for a break. Thus, the positive social situation might play an important role for break settings and, of course, for the duration of working periods and shifts.

Interruption of work will not help recover automatically in all instances. Some interruptions are just annoying, like a breakdown of the computer, and can be mentally switched to a break only when some control over the time is possible and restart options are available.

Breaks as a planned action

Breaks, as well as working periods, profit from a good structure with clear cues for the start of a break, setting and activities during the break, clear cues for the end of the break, and the start of the next working period. Sometimes break habits have been established. If not, they should be provided by the work organisation or leaders. Breaks as well as action periods should have a schedule which can be anticipated well. Action concepts allow to structure work and activities and help establish work–recovery cycles (Wieland-Eckelmann & Baggen, 1994). Planned work–recovery cycles are even an option to prevent burnout. This is of special relevance for New Work (Bergmann, 1977, 2004), that is, the organisation in home office settings. To structure an effective break, the kind of activity during the break needs to be determined in advance, which can be relaxing or demanding physically and mentally. Straussberger (2002) demonstrated in a study with air traffic controllers that break activities which involved screens (computer, mobile devices) were less efficient compared to social activities or physical action.

Breaks and attentional skills

Even short breaks (interspersed early enough) can help extend resources like attention over longer times. Recent studies propose short breaks with naps to reduce the impact of stressful work (Anand et al., in press). This is in line with some of our own research findings showing that even short, early breaks help conserve resources; particularly when long working hours must be expected, early breaks will have long-lasting effects in terms of resource conservation (Kallus & Gaisbachgrabner, 2018). Modern flexible work arrangements and New Work (Bergmann, 1977, 2004) often interfere with effective breaks in proper break settings with social contact and/or physical activity options (Koppen et al., this volume, Chapter 5). Effective break settings require a collective or team-oriented organisation in which the individualised work organisation is 'resocialised'. For the flexible work arrangements and New Work, a new 'break culture' must be developed to make sure that the switching from 'work to break' and from 'break back to work' is smooth and effective. Break habits are a first start to establish a personal 'break culture'.

As known from high-performance athletes, attentional skills play a very important role in break management (Revlin, 2013). Attentional skills are well known in mental training for athletes (Mayer & Hermann, 2011) and in mindfulness training in organisations (Kabat-Zinn, 2003). Attention is controlled automatically by deep brain areas and by self-regulation from the prefrontal cortex. Sometimes the switching of attention requires conscious control when automatic processes take over control. Everyone knows the effect of a catchy tune (earworm music), which is very difficult to switch off. Switching off from work or emotionally impacting events is necessary to have effective breaks (Balk, 2024).

Attentional shifting is a basic mental skill which can be developed with practice in and off the job. A modern variant is mindfulness training (Kabat-Zinn, 2003). A specific set of methods from mindfulness training focuses on the body and is termed centring, which allows to switch attention instantly and allows a good start into the break and to switch back from the break to the next task (Barbarino, 2020; Walsh, 2017). Table 3.1 provides a list of examples of exercises for attentional control.

The problem of breaks in home office settings

Structured breaks are hampered by the modern systems of 24/7 availabilities of services, increasing automation, inter-regional production chains, or worldwide transport systems like aviation. Changes in work organisation and work patterns due to the Covid-19 pandemic, like home office, also cause changes in work–rest schedules. Therefore, it is worthwhile to more closely inspect work–rest cycles in modern work systems. One very important new area is the home

Table 3.1 Examples of exercises for attentional control.

- Directing attention to relaxation-oriented bodily functions, like breathing with deep breathing out.
- Using a relaxation-conditioned mantra.
- Using any skill from mental trainings.
- Directing attention to emotionally positive memories or scenes.
- Converting waiting periods into short breaks for regeneration as often as possible. Waiting times can be lost times – regeneration is valuable.
- Using attentional skills to regenerate even in short breaks.
- Switching to positive mental images which make you smile or laugh.
- Including all senses in a mental scene.
- Centring (Walsh, 2017).
- Breathing exercises also use attentional switches. Broadening and narrowing attention is another exercise.
- Establishing break habits for your personal break culture.
- Writing an intruding thought or image on a sheet of paper and putting it in a drawer for a short but well-defined period of time.

office. Long-term work in the home office should be complemented by office work with colleagues. Online meetings should be complemented by regular face-to-face meetings, as social interaction is one of the highly important aspects of work. For home office work, new skills are required, which comprise self-designed break settings, attentional shifting, and break rituals. One of the central skills is attention control. Especially in home office, a lot of stimuli and signals catch attention and tend to disrupt ongoing work and/or to disturb breaks.

In a proper home office work setting, private stimuli are reduced, and attention is shielded from distractions. However, shifting from work to recovery can be a difficult task in this context. The opposite is true as well, as Sonnentag (2018) stated when discussing the problem of switching off after a work period (problem of detachment). Internet chats and social media can be very time-consuming, which makes them relevant for the discussion of recovery–stress balancing. Liu et al. (2021) show that even sleeping time can be reduced in heavy internet users. The regeneration effect of internet games or social media is often very limited, as a switch from work to leisure is only partly executed when screen work and private PC screens tax the same resources. Eyes and attention are stressed in similar ways. However, some video games seem to help shift from work to non-work and support switching off from work (Sonnentag, 2018). However, from a recovery perspective, spending time at the PC cannot replace physical activity or social contacts, particularly with regards to health.

Breaks as interruption of work

Taking a break is not as easy as it might seem at first glance. Control is an important aspect of work design and seems to be even more important, with reference to breaks, recovery, and recreation. However, prescribing breaks from the organisation did not have the desired positive effect in all instances: prescribed breaks might be interruptions in ongoing work (Wagner-Hartl et al., 2017). Forced breaks in ongoing activities might be a more or less annoying interruption of action. Interruptions of action are a primary source of emotional anger reactions. Furthermore, breaks in action can evoke the state of waiting for continuation (red traffic light). Depending on the perception, the same situation can be an annoying waiting time or a positive break to recover. One crucial difference is the knowledge of the duration of an interruption of the activity. The evaluation of the situation, or better, the appraisal, in the sense of Lazarus (1991), is essential to predict the effect of a break. The appraisal is important to qualify an interruption of action as a break with recovery potential or an annoying waiting time. In addition, breaks during work can serve as opportunities for feedback and debriefing.

Reducing the impact of demands by appropriate breaks in a work period is one way to cope with unusual or long working hours. Shift systems have different ways to prevent underrecovery or long-term stress by off-duty times – within and between working weeks or shift blocks. Nonfunctional off duty activities can occur, like second job hours, conflicts in social relations, difficulties to manage everyday life, health problems, financial problems, and so on. Thus, off-duty at work should not be equated with recovery.

Breaks between work periods can be used to promote skills in a hobby; join some physical activity; meet friends; engage in positive social contacts; enjoy games, love of family, and related others; go for a walk; or do some shopping, enjoy a restaurant, or some leisure facilities, enjoying a good book or internet amusement. The list of moderators for the duration of shifts, shift blocks, and working periods could be extended. Recovery activities are always highly individuum-specific. Time between duty periods or weekends can balance work, obligations, and other life domains (Korunka et al., 2012; Park et al., 2019; Sato et al., 2020; Vieten et al., 2023).

Life domain balance

Life domain balance is often termed 'work–life balance', which ignores the fact that work is an important part of our life (Beckmann & Kellmann, 2024). However, work is a life domain which often conflicts with other domains due to the fact that work can have strict time obligations and long-term contracts, is supported by laws and social norms, and limits the individual options of behaviour more than other domains do. Sometimes, work interferes with other recovery through activities in other domains, to the point where people working in standby mode are signalled with alarms while they are sleeping in order to wake them up. Standby times are an area which shows that working hours are a tricky area. Case reports for the working times of physicians indicate severe problems with standby times. The end of the school holidays is accompanied by increased accident rates on highways. For these times, paramedics must work nearly all their standby time and often are on duty after this, which adds up to extreme working hours – in these instances, adequate and effective recovery opportunities need to be planned and provided.

Sometimes, work and other life domains tax the same resources, and off-work time is not necessarily time for recovery. This might result in a need for recovery or sometimes even lead to underrecovery comparable to debt in oxygen after intense physical exhaustion. Sometimes a separation of life domains is difficult to achieve. Tools like debriefings might be helpful, as debriefings allow a better emotional recovery and detachment (Hogg, 2024).

Conclusion

Long working hours beyond the limit of about 50–60 hours per week for more than 6–8 weeks in a row or similar do not only impair safety at work but also lead to risks of severe health impairment, as demonstrated by health insurance data. Simple overtime for a short period is below the threshold of health risks if the problem of fatigue and other strain symptoms are compensated by a good work design and efficient recovery time. One problem is that subjective fatigue and monotony are perceived only with delay. Thus, a deterioration of performance, health, and well-being might already have occurred when the subjective state becomes eventually aware. Thus, break and recovery regimes need to be planned anticipatorily by a proper work and task design. A good mood and a positive atmosphere are helpful; smiling and laughing might be of great value – a good reason to leave a wholehearted, serious, earnest workplace atmosphere for a break. It can be helpful to have a look at the *Sluice Model* for breaks in sports when breaks are planned for work settings.

Table 3.2 lists the moderators for effective breaks, starting with external factors, continuing with action-related factors, and finally mentioning individual psychological processes.

The idea of the millennium 'faster, better, cheaper' (which has been caricatured by the rule 'select two') seems to become out of fashion, anyway. Cars with more than 200 kilowatts are forced to slow down in many rural areas to less than 20 miles per hour. Highways have speed limits in many sections, and traffic jams are nearly unavoidable in populated areas. Thus, there is a tendency to slow down, which might be useful in many occupational settings.

Taking more breaks and even longer breaks will help keep human resources, mind, and body in better shape and thus help conserve resources. A redesign of tasks and work will be necessary, as increasing automation and economic pressure has to be counteracted by a human-oriented work design, especially in new areas like home office. Effective break settings and new break habits might be an important component. For all 24/7 kinds of business and service, it is important to recognise that night work and shift work often occur together with longer or irregular working hours. Long working hours might be an important stress factor when they occur together with night shifts and disrupted regeneration.

Table 3.2 Moderators for effective breaks.

• Formal aspects: duration of the break, social situation in the break. • Environmental break settings. • Kind of work activity before the break (especially cognitive and physical demands, attentional demands within a working block, physical demands within a working block, social demands within a working block, number and kind of action units in a working block, duration of break-to-break working blocks). • Regeneration, nutrition, and activity options in the break (options for distractions and break activities, which might be compensatory to the demands of work or unrelated but with other demands than the work period). • Options to recover physical and psychological needs. • Options for full recovery between shifts. • Action latitude with respect to timing. • Tools to use in the break. • Mood state. • Psychophysical fitness. • Recovery skills/mental shifting skills. • Preparation and briefing of the following work period.

In these circumstances, states of underrecovery might occur. Their impact is still not fully resolved.

Finally, it should be noted that long working hours and even short overtime can be harmful to the employees in adverse work environments or when conducting health-impairing work. Work medical thresholds and limits always need to be considered in adverse environmental or workplace conditions. Time for recovery should be extended for less-fit or older employees.

Instead of reducing the weekly working hours, employees might try to obtain 45-minute or 50-minute working hours (like in many educational and sports settings), with regular breaks in appropriate break settings, or 90-minute working blocks with 15- to 20-minute breaks interspersed to obtain good work–recovery balances in the workplace.

References

Agyapong, B., Obuobi-Donkor, G., Burback, L., & Wei, Y. (2022). Stress, burnout, anxiety and depression among teachers: A scoping review. *International Journal of Environmental Research and Public Health, 19*(17), 10706. https://doi.org/10.3390/ijerph191710706

Allmer, H. (1996). *Erholung und Gesundheit: Grundlagen, Ergebnisse und Maßnahmen* [Recreation and health: Basics, results and measures]. Hogrefe.

Altenmüller, E., Kellmann, M., Beckmann, J., & Moyle, G. (Eds.). (in press). *Recovery and well-being in the performing arts.* Routledge.

Anand, A., Tóth, R., Doll, J. L., & Singh, S. K. (in press). Wake up and get some sleep: Reviewing workplace napping and charting future directions. *European Management Journal.* https://doi.org/10.1016/j.emj.2024.04.003

Austrian Association for Work Medicine. (2019). *Guidelines for the work-medical evaluation of long working hours* [Leitfaden zur arbeitsmedizinischen Beurteilung langer Arbeitszeiten]. ÖGA.

Backhaus, N., Brauner, C., & Tisch, A. (2019). Auswirkungen verkürzter Ruhezeiten auf Gesundheit und Work-Life-Balance bei Vollzeitbeschäftigten: Ergebnisse der BAuA-Arbeitszeitbefragung 2017 [Quick returns, health, and work-life-balance in full-time employees: Results from the BAuA working time survey 2017]. *Zeitschrift für Arbeitswissenschaft, 73*, 394–417.

Balk, Y. A. (2024). 'Switch off when not in use': The benefits of detachment from work and sport for recovery. In M. Kellmann & J. Beckmann (Eds.), *Fostering recovery and well-being in a healthy lifestyle: Psychological, somatic, and organizational prevention approaches* (pp. 59–72). Routledge.

Barbarino, M. (2020). *Zentrierung* [Centering]. Springer.

Barker, R. G. (1968). *Ecological psychology: Concepts and methods for studying the environment of human behavior.* Stanford University Press.

Beckmann, J., & Kellmann, M. (2024). Fostering recovery and well-being in a healthy lifestyle: A concluding summary. In M. Kellmann & J. Beckmann (Eds.), *Fostering recovery and well-being in a healthy lifestyle: Psychological, somatic, and organizational prevention approaches* (pp. 218–222). Routledge.

Bergmann, F. (1977). *On being free.* University of Notre Dame.

Bergmann, F. (2004). *Neue Arbeit, Neue Kultur* [New work, new culture]. Arbor.

Buchegger, C. (2017). *Eine empirische Untersuchung zum Einfluss des aktuellen Erholungs-Beanspruchungs-Zustands auf den Kurerfolg* [An empirical study on the influence of the current recovery-stress state on the treatment outcome; Unpublished doctoral dissertation]. University of Graz, Austria.

Caruso, C., Hitchcock, E., Dick, R., Russo, J., & Schmit, J. (2004). *Overtime and extended work shifts: Recent findings on illnesses, injuries, and health behaviors.* NIOSH Publications Dissemination.

Council of the European Union. (1993). *Council Directive 93/104/EC of 23 November 1993 concerning certain aspects of the organization of working time.* Retrieved May 17, 2024 from https://eur-lex.europa.eu/legal-content/EN/TXT/?uri=celex%3A31993L0104

Council of the European Union. (2000). *Directive 2000/34/EC of the European Parliament and of the Council of 22 June 2000 amending Council Directive 93/104/EC concerning certain aspects of the organisation of working time to cover sectors and activities excluded from that Directive.* Retrieved May 17, 2024 from https://eur-lex.europa.eu/legal-content/EN/ALL/?uri=celex:32000L0034

Council of the European Union. (2003). *Directive 2003/88/EC of the European Parliament and of the Council of 4 November 2003 concerning certain aspects of the organisation of working time.* Retrieved May 17, 2024 from https://eur-lex.europa.eu/legal-content/EN/TXT/?uri=CELEX:32003L0088

Davis, H., Botterill, C., & MacNeill, K. (2002). Mood and self-regulation changes in underrecovery: An intervention model. In M. Kellmann (Ed.), *Enhancing recovery: Preventing underperformance in athletes* (pp. 161–179). Human Kinetics.

de Jonge, J., & Taris, T. W. (2024). Off-job and on-job recovery as predictors of employee health. In M. Kellmann & J. Beckmann (Eds.), *Fostering recovery and well-being in a healthy lifestyle: Psychological, somatic, and organizational prevention approaches* (pp. 24–37). Routledge.

Debitz, U., Plath, H. E., & Richter, P. (2016). *Beanspruchungs-Mess-Skalen: Verfahren zur Erfassung erlebter Beanspruchungsfolgen: Psychische Ermüdung – Monotonie – Psychische*

Sättigung – Stress. Manual [Methods for assessing experienced consequences of stress: Psychological fatigue – monotony – psychic saturation – stress. Manual]. Hogrefe.

Dex, S., Clark, A., & Taylor, M. (1995). *Household labour supply. Department of Employment Research Series: Vol. 43*. University of Essex.

Dickerson, S. S., & Kemeny, M. E. (2004). Acute stressors and cortisol responses: A theoretical integration and synthesis of laboratory research. *Psychological Bulletin, 130*(3), 355–391.

Dragano, N., Gerö, K., & Wahrendorf, M. S. (2024). Mental health at work after the COVID-19 pandemic – what European figures reveal. Retrieved May 17, 2024 from https://osha.europa.eu/sites/default/files/documents/Mental%20health%20at%20work%20after%20the%20COVID%20pandemic_en_0.pdf

Eberspächer, H., Hermann, H.-D., & Kallus, K. W. (1993). Psychische Erholung und Regeneration zwischen Beanspruchungen [Mental recovery and regeneration between stresses]. In J. R. Nitsch & R. Seiler (Eds.), *Bewegung und Sport: Psychologische Grundlagen und Wirkungen 1* (pp. 237–241). Academia.

Ellwood, S., Pallier, G., Snyder A., & Gallate, J. (2009). The incubation effect: Hatching a solution? *Creativity Research Journal, 21*, 6–14.

Eurofound. (2022). *Overtime in Europe: Regulation and practice*. Publications Office of the European Union, Luxembourg. Retrieved May 17, 2024 from https://www.eurofound.europa.eu/en/publications/2022/overtime-europe-regulation-and-practice

Fiedler, R., Heidari, J., Birnkraut, T., & Kellmann, M. (2023). Digital media and mental health in adolescent athletes. *Psychology of Sport and Exercise, 67*, 102421. https://doi.org/10.1016/j.psychsport.2023.102421

Folkard, S., & Lombardi, D. A. (2006). Modeling the impact of the components of long work hours on injuries and "accidents". *American Journal of Industrial Medicine, 49*(11), 953–963.

Fries, E., Dettenborn, L., & Kirschbaum, C. (2009). The cortisol awakening response (CAR): Facts and future directions. *International Journal of Psychophysiology, 72*(1), 67–73.

Gaisbachgrabner, K. (2014). *Empirische Untersuchungen zu langen Arbeitszeiten und dem Hypothalamus-Hypophysen-Schilddrüsen-System im Mehrebenenansatz* [Empirical studies on the effects of long working hours on the hypothalamus-pituitary-thyroid-system; Unpublished doctoral dissertation]. University of Graz, Austria.

Gaisbachgrabner, K., Kallus, K. W., & Uhlig, T. (2011). *Lange Arbeitszeiten* [Long working hours; Unpublished manuscript]. University of Graz, Austria.

Garrett, L. R., Harveson, A. T., & Ayars, C. (2024). Shift schedule effects on firefighter health and fitness. *Work, 78*(4), 1115-1122.

Glaser, R., & Kiecolt-Glaser, J. (1994). *Handbook of human stress and immunity*. Academic Press.

Graf, O. (1922). Über lohnendste Arbeitspausen bei geistiger Arbeit [Worthwhile rest breaks for mental work]. *Psychologische Arbeiten*, 7, 548–611.

Graf, O. (1960). *Arbeitsphysiologie* [Physiology of work]. Gabler.

Hacker, W. (2003). Action regulation theory: A practical tool for the design of modern work processes? *European Journal of Work and Organizational Psychology, 12*, 105–130.

Heidari, J., & Kellmann, M. (2024). "Use it right": The relationship between digital media and recovery. In M. Kellmann & J. Beckmann (Eds.), *Fostering recovery and well-being in a healthy lifestyle: Psychological, somatic, and organizational prevention approaches* (pp. 103–114). Routledge.

Hobfoll, S. E. (1989). Conservation of resources: A new attempt at conceptualizing stress. *American Psychologist, 44*(3), 513–524.

Hogg, J. M. (2024). Debriefing sport performance: A strategy to enhance mental and emotional recovery and plan for future competition. In M. Kellmann & J. Beckmann (Eds.), *Fostering recovery and well-being in a healthy lifestyle: Psychological, somatic, and organizational prevention approaches* (pp. 73–91). Routledge.

Hong, Y., Zhang, Y., Xue, P., Fang, X., Zhou, L., Wei, F., Lou, X., & Zou, H. (2022). The influence of long working hours, occupational stress, and well-being on depression among couriers in Zhejiang, China. *Frontiers in Psychology, 13*, 928928. https://doi.org/10.3389/fpsyg.2022.928928

Hou, W. K., & Tao, J. T. (2023). Stress. In H. S. Friedman & C. H. Markey (Eds.), *Encyclopedia of mental health* (3rd ed., pp. 382–388). Academic Press.

Iwasaki, K., Takahashi, M., & Nakata, A. (2006). Health problems due to long working hours in Japan: Working hours, workers' compensation (Karoshi), and preventive measures. *Industrial Health, 44*(4), 537–540.

Jiménez, P., Bregenzer, A., & Kallus, K. W. (2025). Recovery-Stress Questionnaire for Work. In M. Kellmann & K. W. Kallus (Eds.), *The Recovery-Stress Questionnaires: A user manual* (pp. 171–205). Routledge.

Jiménez, P., Dunkl, A., & K. W. Kallus (2016). Recovery-Stress Questionnaire for Work. In K. W. Kallus & M. Kellmann (Eds.), *The Recovery-Stress Questionnaires: User manual* (pp. 158–187). Pearson Assessment.

Kabat-Zinn, J. (2003). Mindfulness-based interventions in context: Past, present, and future. *Clinical Psychology: Science and Practice, 10*, 144–156.

Kallus, K. W. (2016). Stress and recovery: An overview. In K. W. Kallus & M. Kellmann (Eds.), *The Recovery-Stress Questionnaires: User manual* (pp. 27–48). Pearson Assessment.

Kallus, K. W. (2025). RESTQ-basic: The general version of the Recovery-Stress Questionnaire. In M. Kellmann & K. W. Kallus (Eds.), *The Recovery-Stress Questionnaires: A user manual* (pp. 28–75). Routledge.

Kallus, K. W., Boucsein, W., & Spanner, N. (2009). Eight- and twelve-hour shifts in Austrian rail traffic controllers: A psychophysiological comparison. *Psychology Science Quarterly, 51*(3), 283–297.

Kallus, K. W., Eberspächer, H., & Hermann, H.-D. (1992). Systematische, naive und gestörte Regeneration im Sport [Systematic, naive and disturbed regeneration in sports]. In L. Montada (Ed.), *Bericht über den 38. Kongress der Deutschen Gesellschaft für Psychologie in Trier* (pp. 436–437). Hogrefe.

Kallus, K. W., & Gaisbachgrabner, K. (2018). Stress and recovery in applied settings: Long working hours, recovery, and breaks. In M. Kellmann & J. Beckmann (Eds.), *Sport, recovery, and performance: Interdisciplinary insights* (pp. 233–246). Routledge.

Kallus, K. W., & Kellmann, M. (Eds.). (2016). *The Recovery-Stress Questionnaires: User manual.* Pearson Assessment.

Kallus, K. W., & Krauth, J. (1995). Nichtparametrische Verfahren zum Nachweis emotionaler Reaktionen [Non-parametric methods for the provement of emotional reactions]. In G. Debus, G. Erdmann, & K. W. Kallus (Eds.), *Biopsychologie von Stress und emotionalen Reaktionen* (pp. 23–43). Hogrefe.

Kellmann, M. (2010). Preventing overtraining in athletes in high-intensity sports and stress/recovery monitoring. *Scandinavian Journal of Medicine & Science in Sports, 20*(Suppl. 2), 95–102.

Kellmann, M., & Beckmann, J. (Eds.). (2024). *Fostering recovery and well-being in a healthy lifestyle: Psychological, somatic, and organizational prevention approaches.* Routledge.

Kellmann, M., Bertollo, M., Bosquet, L., Brink, M., Coutts, A. J., Duffield, R., Erlacher, D., Halson, S. L., Hecksteden, A., Heidari, J., Kallus, K. W., Meeusen, R., Mujika,

I., Robazza, C., Skorski, S., Venter, R., & Beckmann, J. (2018). Recovery and performance in sport: Consensus statement. *International Journal of Sports Physiology and Performance, 13*, 240–245.

Kellmann, M., & Heidari, J. (2020). Changes in the perception of stress and recovery in German secondary school teachers. *Teacher Development, 24*, 242–257.

Kellmann, M., & Kallus, K. W. (Eds.). (2025). *The Recovery-Stress Questionnaires: A user manual*. Routledge.

Kirchler, E., & Schmidl, D. (2000). Schichtarbeit im Vergleich: Befindensunterschiede und Aufmerksamkeitsvariation während der 8-Stunden- versus 12-Stunden-Schichtarbeit [Comparison of shifts: Differences in health and attention during the 8-hour versus 12-hour shifts]. *Zeitschrift für Arbeits- und Organisationspsychologie, 44*(1), 2–18.

Kirschbaum, C. (1991). *Cortisolmessung im Speichel – eine Methode der biologischen Psychologie* [Cortisol measurement in saliva – a method of biological psychology]. Huber.

Kirschbaum, C., & Hellhammer, D. H. (1989). Salivary cortisol in psychobiological research – an overview. *Neuropsychobiology, 22*, 150–169.

Kleitman, N. (1963). *Sleep and wakefulness*. University of Chicago Press.

Knauth, P. (2007). Extended work periods. *Industrial Health, 45*, 125–136.

Korunka, C., Kubicek, B., Prem, R., & Cvitan, A. (2012). Recovery and detachment between shifts, and fatigue during a twelve-hour shift. *Work, 41*(Suppl. 1), 3227–3233.

Kubo, T., Liu, X., & Matsuo, T. (2024). Death due to overwork: Problems and solutions. In M. Kellmann & J. Beckmann (Eds.), *Fostering recovery and well-being in a healthy lifestyle: Psychological, somatic, and organizational prevention approaches* (pp. 199–217). Routledge.

Kullik, L., & Kiel, A. (2024). Sleep well! A key strategy beyond sports. In M. Kellmann & J. Beckmann (Eds.), *Fostering recovery and well-being in a healthy lifestyle: Psychological, somatic, and organizational prevention approaches* (pp. 143–162). Routledge.

Lazarus, R. S. (1991). *Emotion and adaptation*. Oxford University Press.

Le, A. B., Balogun, A. O., & Smith, T. D. (2022). Long work hours, overtime, and worker health impairment: A cross-sectional study among stone, sand, and gravel mine workers. *International Journal of Environmental Research and Public Health, 19*(13), 7740. https://doi.org/10.3390/ijerph19137740

Liu, H., Ji, Y., & Dust, S. B. (2021). "Fully recharged" evenings? The effect of evening cyber leisure on next-day vitality and performance through sleep quantity and quality, bedtime procrastination, and psychological detachment, and the moderating role of mindfulness. *Journal of Applied Psychology, 106*(7), 990–1006.

Mayer, J., & Hermann H.-D. (2011). *Mentales Training* [Mental training]. Springer.

McEwen, B. S. (1998). Stress, adaptation and disease: Allostasis and allostatic load. *Annals of the New York Academy of Sciences, 840*, 33–44.

Nachreiner, F., Rädiker, B., Janßen, D., & Schomann, C. (2005). *Untersuchungen zum Zusammenhang zwischen der Dauer der Arbeitszeit und gesundheitlichen Beeinträchtigungen – Ergebnisse einer Machbarkeitsstudie* [Studies on the link between the duration of working hours and health impairments – results of a feasibility study]. GAWO.

Park, S., Lee, J. H., & Lee, W. (2019). The effects of workplace rest breaks on health problems related to long working hours and shift work among male apartment janitors in Korea. *Safety and Health at Work, 10*(4), 512–517.

Pega, F., Náfrádi, B., Momen, N. C., Ujita, Y., Streicher, K. N., Prüss-Üstün, A. M., Technical Advisory Group, Descatha, A., Driscoll, T., Fischer, F. M., Godderis, L., Kiiver, H. M., Li, J., Magnusson Hanson, L. L., Rugulies, R., Sørensen, K., & Woodruff, T. J. (2021). Global, regional, and national burdens of ischemic heart disease and stroke attributable to exposure to long working hours for 194 countries, 2000–2016: A systematic analysis from the WHO/ILO joint estimates of the work-related burden of disease and injury. *Environment International, 154*, 106595. https://doi.org/10.1016/j.envint.2021.106595

Revlin, R. (2013). *Cognition: Theory and practice*. Worth Publishers.

Sato, K., Kuroda, S., & Owan, H. (2020). Mental health effects of long work hours, night and weekend work, and short rest periods. *Social Science & Medicine, 246*, 112774. https://doi.org/10.1016/j.socscimed.2019.112774

Schmidt, R. A., & Lee, T. D. (2020). *Motor learning and performance: From principles to application*. Human Kinetics.

Schoggen, P. (1989). *Behavior settings: A revision and extension of Roger G. Barker's "Ecological Psychology"*. Stanford University Press.

Selye, H. (1936). A syndrome produced by diverse nocuous agents. *Nature, 138*, 32.

Sonnentag, S. (2018). The recovery paradox: Portraying the complex interplay between job stressors, lack of recovery, and poor well-being. *Research in Organizational Behavior, 38*, 169–185.

Sonnentag, S., & Fritz, C. (2015). Recovery from job stress: The stressor-detachment model as an integrative framework. *Journal of Organizational Behavior, 36*(Suppl. 1), 72–103.

Spurgeon, A., Harrington, J. M., & Cooper, C. L. (1997). Health and safety problems associated with long working hours: A review of the current position. *Occupational and Environmental Medicine, 54*, 167–375.

Straussberger, S. (2002). *Auswirkungen von aktiven Kurzpausen auf physiologische, psychologische und Leistungsvariablen in simulierter Flugüberwachung* [Effects of active breaks on physiological, psychological, and performance parameters in simulated air traffic control] [Unpublished master's thesis, University of Graz].

van Dongen, H. P., Maislin, G., Mullington, J. M., & Dinges, D. F. (2003). The cumulative cost of additional wakefulness: Dose-response effects on neurobehavioral functions and sleep physiology from chronic sleep restriction and total sleep deprivation. *Sleep, 26*(2), 117–126.

Vieten, L., Wöhrmann, A. M., Wendsche, J., & Michel, A. (2023). Employees' work breaks and their physical and mental health: Results from a representative German survey. *Applied Ergonomics, 110*, 103998. https://doi.org/10.1016/j.apergo.2023.103998

Wagner-Hartl, V., Pfaffstaller, E., & Kallus, K. W. (2017). How to implement an effective intervention for breaks during working day – a field study. *Psychology, 8*(5), 728–745.

Walsh, M. (2017). *Centering: Why mindfulness isn't enough*. Brighton.

Wieland-Eckelmann, R., & Baggen, R. (1994). Beanspruchung und Erholung im Beanspruchungs-Erholungs-Zyklus [Stress and recovery in the stress-recovery cycle]. In R. Wieland-Eckelmann, H. Allmer, K. W. Kallus, & J. H. Otto (Eds.), *Erholungsforschung* (pp. 102–154). PVU.

4 Designing urban green spaces supporting health and recovery

Anna Bengtsson, Anna Åshage, and Patrik Grahn

Introduction

All over the world, people migrate from the countryside to the cities. The demand for land, especially in the central parts of cities, often leads to densification, where green spaces disappear in favour of workplaces, streets, shopping centres, and housing. Densification is expected to provide many advantages in contrast to urban sprawl, such as shorter distances between homes and workplaces, which, among other things, can lead to a reduction in traffic (Elfering & Huber, this volume, Chapter 2). From a technological-economic perspective, densification at the expense of parkland may seem rational (Artmann et al., 2019; Pelczynski & Tomkowicz, 2019; Pont et al., 2021; Teller, 2021). At the same time, more and more people worldwide are suffering from stress-related illnesses. In fact, the World Health Organization has designated stress-related ill health as "the health epidemic of the 21st century" (Fink, 2017, p. 1). For many decision-makers, the connection between green spaces in urban areas and people's health and well-being may be abstract and difficult to understand, although it has long been known that densely built-up cities with noisy, crowded streets and squares cause stress (Ostfeld & D'Atri, 1975). However, humans are biological beings, where exposure to natural areas affects our health. In this chapter, an urban structure is proposed that is based on people's immediate need for green areas in the places where they live, work, study, or are cared for. The chapter begins by explaining how green areas can lead to recovery, for example, from high stress levels, where the need for green areas starts inside the houses and extends over the entire city.

Humans are physically and psychologically prepared to understand and act on signals in a multisensory natural environment because people have a large number of senses that help them perceive and interpret their surroundings, including sight, hearing, smell, taste, soft touch, pressure, balance, proprioception, temperature sensing, and gravity (Hellier, 2017). During the millions of years of

Bengtsson, A., Åshage, A., & Grahn, P. (2025). Designing urban green spaces supporting health and recovery. In S. Pauleit, M. Kellmann, & J. Beckmann (Eds.), *Creating Urban and Workplace Environments for Recovery and Well-being* (pp. 61–82). Routledge.

DOI: 10.4324/9781003435471-5

human evolution, when people lived in an environment where they depended on finding safe places where they could get food and water, and where they could settle with their families and, at the same time, needed to avoid dangers, e.g., from larger predators, it was necessary to make comprehensive decisions in order to survive (Nicolaides et al., 2014; Russell & Lightman, 2019). Our sensory receptors collect a wealth of information (about eleven million bits of information per second) and communicate this information to the central and peripheral nervous system in a variety of ways. The conscious brain can process about 40 bits of information per second (Wilson, 2004). That is, the majority of the processing of what happens in our environment, and the decisions that are made, happens unconsciously (Dijksterhuis, 2004; Liebowitz, 2020; Wilson, 2004).

If the signals imply demands or even danger, our stress system will be activated (Cannon, 1929; Selye, 1936; Uvnäs-Moberg & Petersson, 2022). It increases our alertness, decreases our need for sleep and feelings of hunger, raises our blood pressure and heart rate, and activates our fight-flight-or-freeze response. This response is needed so humans can adapt to and resolve the situation. Short-term states of stress, such as solving a task at work, winning a competition, or having access to stimulating social environments, are satisfying, not least in terms of our needs for sociality, and also activate our reward system. If the stress system needs to be active for a longer period, it will be dangerous for our health and well-being (Nicolaides et al., 2014; Russell & Lightman, 2019). While the stress system helps people mobilise strength and energy to solve urgent tasks that, in the worst case, can pose a danger to life, there is a counteracting system that instead helps people recover strength, energy, and joy in life. The system is involved in many protective, healing, and health-promoting mechanisms. This *Calm and Connection System* (CCS; Grahn et al., 2021) also contributes to the formation of family and home, bonding with spouse and children, and place attachment. In addition to being used in family and home formation, the system is also activated to protect and monitor areas close to where people stay, especially at home (Grahn et al., 2023; Rigney et al., 2022). Activation of the CCS leads to several reactions in the body, such as reduced stress, increased appetite, better sleep, increased healing ability, increased cognitive ability, and increased happiness and interest in social activities. It is related to how the *Default Mode Network* (DMN) in the brain develops and is maintained. The DMN is a key component of human consciousness and critical to mental health. Among other things, the DMN is the centre of a person's self-concept – including memories of the past and ideas about the future – which e.g., supports communication with others as well as one's own reflections (Kühn et al., 2021; Zheng et al., 2022). The CCS is activated by calm sensory stimuli, such as the sight of a mirror-like surface of water, the scent of flowers, or the soothing sound of the wind in the treetops. People feel calm, trust, and hope and develop a sense of belonging (Buemann & Uvnäs-Moberg, 2020; Uvnäs-Moberg et al., 2015, 2022). When activated, people can create their own secure relationships with different physical environments as well as with other people (Grahn et al., 2021;

Love, 2014). Characteristics that are experienced as calm and safe and/or attract curiosity increase the possibility of connection and the ability to feel empathy (also for oneself) and open new ways of thinking, thereby developing new coping strategies (Grahn et al., 2021, 2022; Liebowitz, 2020).

Long-term stress can lead to many health problems, such as cardiovascular disease and mental illness. However, stress can be caused by many circumstances and is personal. Everyday stress is usually caused when people feel that they are not in control of a situation. The body perceives this as a threat, and our stress system is activated. However, what leads to stress for one person does not necessarily lead to stress for another. It may even be the case that what leads to stress for one is what reduces stress for another. For example, many may become stressed by living in busy urban environments with many stimuli from people and buildings, while others suffer from too little stimuli and long for such environments (Hentschel et al., 2004; Högberg & Strandh, in press; Staats et al., 2024). So it is common that people's needs vary from day to day and may even vary during the day. Sometimes people have a great need to find quiet, safe areas where they can stay, while at other times they need to seek out stimulating environments. Through self-regulation and by seeking out supportive settings in the environment, stress can be alleviated.

The role of private gardens in terms of people's recreation, health, and well-being has unfortunately been overlooked for a long time (de Bell et al., 2020; de Vries & Chalmin-Pui, this volume, Chapter 7). This is despite research showing that unclear boundaries in the immediate environment for what is private, semi-private, or public green space can reduce the feeling of control and thus increase stress levels (Grahn et al., 2023; Nowzari et al., 2023; Rigney et al., 2022). The immediate environment at homes, workplaces, hospitals, etc. often lacks qualities that are in demand and needed in terms of rest or stimulation. The obvious strategy should be to start from how our body works and reacts to stress by designing supportive green areas for stimulation and rest where people stay. Therefore, the model presented here is based on places where people stay: the four zones of contact with the outdoor environment. People have needs that have to be supported frequently and in a nearby environment, while other needs can wait and can be met in environments further away. What these needs are and how they can be supported by qualities in the outdoor environment are presented next. This is followed by a presentation of the tool, as well as some examples of how it can be used in the design and planning of health-promoting green spaces.

It is, of course, impossible to create an environment that suits everyone, but a long series of studies form the basis of the proposal presented here, where the content, distance to, and size of green areas are based on research on people's needs at group level (Bengtsson et al., 2024; Grahn et al., 2023). A review of a number of meta-analyses and systematic research reviews has, in recent years, documented the importance of accessible, nearby, appealing, and well-maintained green areas to attract visitors and thereby stimulate them to stay healthy or recover from, for example, high stress levels or low attention span

(Pauleit et al., this volume, Chapter 1). The qualities of the areas in terms of proximity, size, content, and design are included in the models presented here, to be used by practitioners for the planning, design, and management of health-promoting outdoor environments (Grahn et al., 2023; Jimenez et al., 2021).

Four zones of contact with the outdoor environment

The model *Four Zones of Contact with the Outdoor Environment* (Bengtsson, 2015) is based on research findings on how people perceive and interpret qualities in natural environments and green areas, partly related to recovery from mental fatigue and high stress levels, and partly related to distance, accessibility, content, and size of stimulating or calm and restful outdoor environments from the place where people stay, for example, home, workplace, hospital, or school. To begin with, the four zones are described based on territory and distance from home, school, workplace, etc., and then the qualities are presented.

Zone 0: This zone refers to the interior of buildings without contact with the outside environment and can, for example, be found in workplaces, schools, and hospitals.

Zone 1: Contact with the external environment from inside a building, through a window. When people are stressed and tired, exposure to certain calm and attractive natural environments can quickly and unconsciously lower stress levels and restore attention capacity. This contact has proved to be significant in many contexts – in homes (including homes for the elderly), in workplaces, in schools, and in hospitals (Honold et al., 2016; Koppen et al., this volume, Chapter 5; Korpela et al., 2015; Li & Sullivan, 2016; Lottrup et al., 2013; Ulrich, 1984). Research has shown that the visual contact with green areas through windows is partly health-promoting in itself and partly attracts people to visit public green areas (Ekkel & de Vries, 2017).

Zone 2: This is about the transition between indoors and outdoors – such as balconies, terraces, porches, glazed verandas, and winter gardens. It increases the opportunities for contact with the outdoor environment and for spending time outdoors (de Bell et al., 2020; Honold et al., 2016). In preschools, the availability of simple detached roofs has involved the children being outside more often. In the event of short rain showers, children and staff can seek shelter under the roofs for a short time instead of going indoors, taking off their clothes and shoes, and staying indoors. Zone 2 has also been shown to increase the opportunities for outdoor living in nursing homes and workplaces (Bengtsson, 2015; Bengtsson & Grahn, 2014; Grahn, 2007; Stigsdotter & Grahn, 2004a, 2004b). This is important because it increases exposure to daylight and sunlight on the skin. Daylight releases endorphins, which relieve pain, are generally mood-elevating, and affect our desire to eat, drink, and sleep. Daylight also regulates our biological clock, which means that humans sleep well and wake up alert in the morning (Holick, 2016). When the biological clock works as it should, people become more alert, the body's immune system works better, and the risk of mental illness and cardiovascular diseases decreases. When the sun shines on the skin, vitamin D is formed, which the body needs to build, maintain, and repair various tissues and systems in the body (Holick, 2016; Neville et al., 2021).

Zone 3: The distance from people's residences to nature or public green spaces has often been seen as a main indicator of accessibility. Several research studies also show that people who live near green areas statistically stay significantly healthier and live longer than those who live further from green areas (Rojas-Rueda et al., 2019). However, as mentioned earlier, the role of private gardens has long been overlooked (de Bell et al., 2020). Access to private gardens leads to better mental health as stress levels are lower and mental fatigue is reduced (Collins et al., 2023; de Bell et al., 2020; Grahn & Stigsdotter, 2003; Poortinga et al., 2021; Stigsdotter & Grahn, 2004b). Zone 3 is the green space on the site directly adjacent to the building – the private house, the workplace, the home for the elderly, the school, the preschool, or the hospital. Several studies have found that good access to stays in Zone 3, that is, private gardens (gardens of private houses and terraced houses, as well as gardens at multi-family houses; de Vries & Chalmin-Pui, this volume, Chapter 7), has a significant relationship with increased outdoor activities. The increase is partly due to a high proportion of outdoor activities being performed on a person's own property, and partly to the fact that Zone 3 acts as a stepping stone, so that the frequency of outdoor activities also increases in public parks (de Bell et al., 2020; Grahn & Stigsdotter, 2003; Lenaerts et al., 2021). The same phenomenon is also seen at schools, workplaces, preschools, nursing homes, and hospitals. Those who have access to well-defined Zone 3 gardens stay outdoors with their children, students, residents, patients, and staff much more often than those who do not have their own gardens. In addition, they visit public parks significantly more often than those who do not have their own gardens (de Bell et al., 2020; Grahn, 1991; Ottosson, 2007). In order for Zone 3 to function well based on the needs of the users, however, the site needs to be large enough, contain the necessary qualities, and be undisturbed. Outside users must not interfere with their activities. This applies to individual users as well as, for example, preschools, schools, hospitals, workplaces, and homes for the elderly (Bengtsson, 2015; de Bell et al., 2020; Grahn, 1991; Grahn & Stoltz, 2022; Lottrup et al., 2013; Mårtensson et al., 2009; Stigsdotter & Grahn, 2004a).

Zone 4: This provides access to public parks and natural environments. Many studies support a threshold value regarding the distance to public green areas of 300 metres because the use of the green areas decreases sharply when the distance increases (Grahn & Stigsdotter, 2003; Rojas-Rueda et al., 2019; Triguero-Mas et al., 2015; World Health Organization, 2016). However, a shorter distance than 300 metres is relevant, not least for children, the disabled, and the elderly (Akpinar, 2017; Ayala-Azcárraga et al., 2019; Grahn & Stigsdotter, 2003). Astell-Burt et al. (2022) and Jamalishahni et al. (2023) have found that proximity to smaller green areas right next to the home is significantly related to people meeting more often, which reduces the risk of experiencing loneliness. Activities that enhance social contacts can involve finding a place where people can rest in the sun, breathe fresh air, eat packed lunches, and/or visit a playground with the children, which also works in smaller green areas (Gozalo et al., 2019; Krekel et al., 2016; Nutsford et al., 2013; Pretty et al., 2005). Several factors, in addition to the users' age and health, influence the relationship between distance and use regarding Zone 4. If there are attractive qualities further away, the distance is perceived as shorter, and likewise, if people can see the green space and/or if there is a relatively straight and easy path to a green space, the distance is also perceived as shorter. The attractive qualities can be about size, that the area is perceived as a natural area, or that there are good opportunities for sports (Nilsson et al., 2019; Paquet et al., 2013). The most important factor influencing the relationship between distance and use, however, is safety. If a certain green area is perceived as unsafe, people do not visit it, even if it is close by. Maintenance has a strong impact on perceived security: if there is rubbish, weeds, broken glass, graffiti, or if park benches or playground equipment are broken, the area is perceived as unsafe (Ceccato, this volume, Chapter 10; Evensen et al., 2021; Williams et al., 2020). Likewise, disruptive park visitors affect perceived safety, as does poor lighting. Through an upgrade of the green areas and proper management, the accessibility of the green areas could increase significantly (Evensen et al., 2021; Williams et al., 2020).

Zone 4 is about public parks in cities. Several studies (see later references) indicate that it is relevant to classify these green areas according to people's need for qualities, that is, amenities and what will later in this chapter be described as perceived sensory dimensions in green areas, the proximity to these green areas, and their size. *Urban greenery and small pocket parks* can work well for certain types of experiences, such as social gatherings, to inspire people to move or to get some fresh air and sun. Such greenery should ideally be as close to people as possible, preferably visible from windows and/or entrances to homes. *Neighbourhood parks* should contain more qualities (see earlier text), be within 300 metres, and contain opportunities for play and ball games and should allow people to feel they are in a larger green area, where they can escape the busy life and the sounds of traffic. In addition, there should be *larger district parks and city parks* (Ayala-Azcárraga et al., 2019; Fan et al., 2017; Hooper et al., 2018; Labib et al., 2020; Wood et al., 2017). The smallest, small, medium, and large green areas are thus suggested to have different functions and qualities to meet different needs (Table 4.1).

Table 4.1 Types of green spaces (according to size) and critical distances for potential health-promoting effects.

Green space	*Minimum size (≈ha)*	*Maximum distance from housing (≈m)*
Zone 4.5: Recreation area	>100	>5,000
Zone 4.4: City park	>20	5,000
Zone 4.3: District park	5–7	1,000
Zone 4.2: Neighbourhood park	1–2	300
Zone 4.1: Pocket park/urban greenery	<1	<300

Source: Table adapted from Grahn and Stoltz (2021).

Pyramid of supportive environments

A spectrum of *supportive enriched environments* is needed in a city to be able to satisfy the different needs of a population. Just by looking at the surrounding green areas from the window, people can perceive and judge environments as calming or stimulating (Zone 1: Honold et al., 2016; Li & Sullivan, 2016). Some smaller green areas near the home can serve social purposes and combat loneliness (Astell-Burt et al., 2022; Jamalishahni et al., 2023) and/or can be experienced as quiet, safe, and calm, thereby reducing stress and leading to recovery of attention (Collins et al., 2023; de Bell et al., 2020). Often, however, people need to seek out larger green areas in order to find environments that can properly support the need for stress recovery and recovery of a depleted attention capacity. Many people of all ages worldwide today suffer from stress-related mental illness as well as poor ability to focus attention. Research shows that these people have a great and immediate need to find support from the environment through self-regulation in order to organise their thoughts through inward involvement. They often cannot cope with social contexts; instead, they escape to quiet, secluded areas. There is a range of needs for different types of environments, from those that support inward involvement, emotional participation, and active participation to those that support outgoing involvement. People suffering from stress often cannot cope with social situations and seek to find quiet, secluded areas. Supportive environments can lead to the activation of the CCS, which leads to a reduction of stress, better attention capacity, and that interest in more social environments is awakened (Grahn et al., 2022; Kumar et al., 2020; Zeev-Wolf et al., 2020).

Resting in large, quiet, and safe green spaces has been shown to provide recovery from both high stress levels and depleted capacity for directed attention (Grahn et al., 2023). However, in addition, by walking or running, people can often speed up recovery from stress and poor attention (Ekelund et al., 2016; Kellmann & Beckmann, 2024). Research results show that small green areas next to houses do not support the need for physical activity; larger areas are needed (Wang et al., 2019). These should preferably be varied and hilly. Physical activity positively affects the whole body, when all the senses and neuromotor functions can be used. Through this, growth in the brain can be stimulated, so-called neurogenesis (Kempermann, 2019, 2022). But for it to function optimally, the environment must be enriched in a multisensory manner. Natural environments enable complex interactions with the inherited functions of our bodies, which influence and change the structure and function of the body and brain during a person's lifetime (Gomes-Leal, 2021; Grońska-Pęski et al., 2021; Kemperman, 2019). Kühn et al. (2017) maintain that natural forest environments serve as the best environments for humans. For example, if a person is running on a forest path, there must be hyper-fast communication between the person's eye, brain, and muscles so that the person has time to lift their feet high enough, for example, to both detect and avoid a stone on the road. The eye perceives the stone and primes (that is, prepares and instructs) muscles in the legs and feet for how the runner should meet the obstacle. This occurs in rapid neuromotoric processes of which the person is unaware; they are subconscious, or 'subliminal'. Such subliminal priming processes in nature can stimulate and facilitate healing processes in the body and accelerate neurogenesis in the brain. Even a very old human brain can develop via neurogenesis through stays in diversely enriched environments (Blakemore et al., 2017; Chen et al., 2018; Kempermann, 2019; Lambert et al., 2019; Mohd Sahini et al., 2024). Over the years, many studies have been conducted on mice and rats. In recent years, research in the field has increased significantly, and many results show that the effects on humans and animals are similar, which means great opportunities in both therapy and health promotion and encourages more research (Clemenson et al., 2015; Farioli-Vecchioli et al., 2022; Kempermann, 2022).

Eight multisensory dimensions for an enriched city: The Perceived Sensory Dimensions

In order to be able to plan and design health-promoting and environmentally enriched green areas, it is important to be able to understand the impact of their essential qualities on health in different contexts. These essential qualities must be described holistically, based on sensory information via, for example, vision and hearing, and should be related to the content and the size of the area as well as to people's associations or connotations related to, for example, activities, safety, and symbolism. In order to be manageable, for example, for landscape architects, the qualities must not be too numerous and must be understood intuitively, one by one, and in relation to other qualities. Over several decades, research has developed the *Perceived Sensory Dimensions*, the PSD model (Stoltz & Grahn, 2021a; Table 4.2), which has proved to be valid and reliable in terms of describing the overall characteristics of green areas (An et al., 2022; Chen et al., 2019; Qiu & Nielsen, 2015; Wang & Li, 2024).

Several research studies show that all eight PSDs have supportive functions, but while some PSDs are clearly restorative, such as *Serene* and *Sheltered*, others are more stimulating, such as *Social* and *Cultural*. There is a gradient, from the

Table 4.2 Perceived Sensory Dimensions (PSDs).

PSD	*The environment affords . . .*
Social	A sense of bustling activity, people, and movement. A dense and lively place, with social activities and interactions. Often especially strong in dense urban settings, for example, around cafés, shopping streets, and squares.
Cultural	A sense of fascination with human culture, creativity, labour, and history. The cultivated, crafted, and man-made, as opposed to the 'self-made' or natural.
Open	A sense of openness and freedom. Overviews, prospects, vistas, and stays. Open space for physical activities, room to roam freely, to see far into the distance.
Diverse	A sense of diversity and variation in the environment. A large variety of different species of plants and animals. A multi-layered and diverse vegetation, often in combination with water features.
Cohesive	A sense of spatial cohesion and spaciousness. An experience of a 'world in itself'. An extended, uninterrupted whole, possible to explore.
Natural	Fascination with the natural world, its distinctive shapes and colours, its inherent force and power. A sense of the wild and untouched, of the passage of time.
Sheltered	A sense of shelter, safety, and protection. An enclosed space, a refuge, a hideaway. The possibility to 'be seen without being seen'.
Serene	A sense of serenity, peace, quiet, and stillness. Freedom from noise and disturbances. Peaceful sounds of nature. Absence of other people, signs, signals, and/or threatening or intrusive stimuli.

most stimulating to the most restorative (Bengtsson, 2015; Grahn & Stigsdotter, 2010; Memari et al., 2021; Ottosson & Grahn, 2008; Pálsdóttir et al., 2014; Figure 4.1).

Qualitative and quantitative studies regarding PSDs show that several factors have opposite effects, while other factors are relatively close to each other (Stoltz & Grahn, 2021b). In summary, the eight PSDs can be ordered according to Figure 4.2: the eight PSDs lie along four axes. Each axis has opposite properties and attributes (Stoltz & Grahn, 2021a). There is a gradient along these four axes, from the extremes to more moderate expressions. Adjacent PSDs in the model are synergistic and mutually supportive (Figure 4.2). It is suggested that designing environments where three such adjacent PSDs support each other can contribute to creating places with many supportive functions and low conflict between different experiential values (Stoltz & Grahn, 2021a).

There are two clear gradients in Figure 4.2. *Shelter*, *Natural*, *Serene*, and *Cohesive* provide restorative support, while *Diverse*, *Social*, *Cultural*, and *Open* provide stimulating support. On another gradient, *Natural*, *Serene*, *Cohesive*, and *Open* often appear most clearly in large green areas, while *Shelter*, *Diverse*, *Social*, and *Cultural* can also appear in smaller green areas. These gradients regarding the

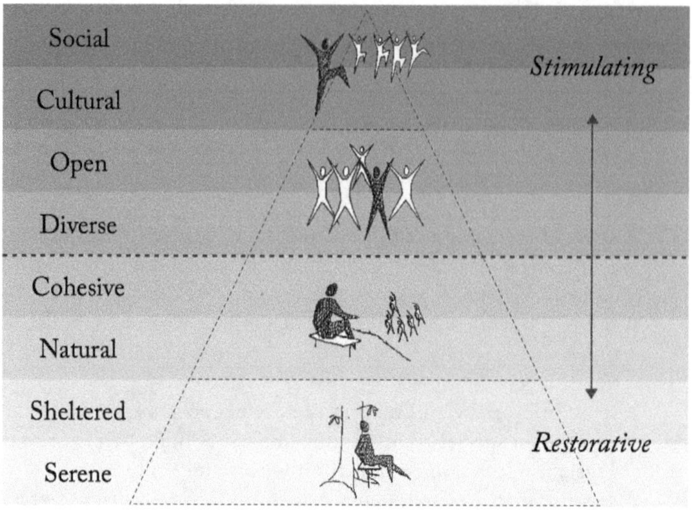

Figure 4.1 The model of supportive environments integrated with the *Perceived Sensory Dimensions* (PSDs). The eight PSDs are placed on a scale from the most stimulating to the most restorative.

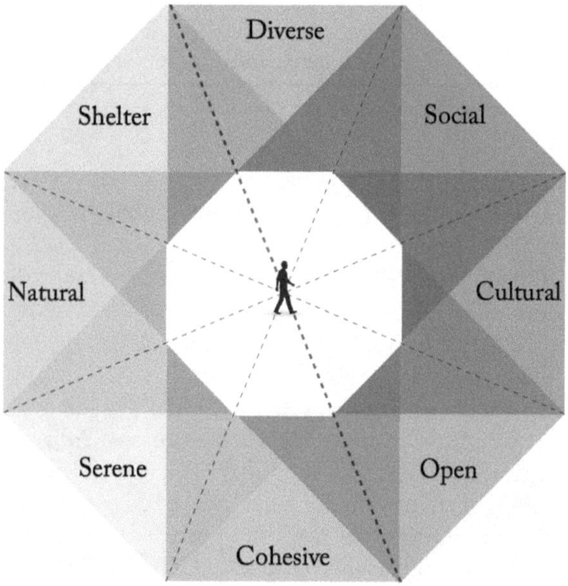

Figure 4.2 Relationships between the eight *Perceived Sensory Dimensions* (PSDs), explained through four axes of opposing characteristics and complementary characteristics to the adjacent PSDs. The closer the PSDs are in the model, the closer the associations between them.

eight PSDs can be used in the planning and design of health-promoting environments (Stoltz & Grahn, 2021b).

The Quality Evaluation Tool

The Quality Evaluation Tool (QET; Bengtsson & Grahn, 2014) is an evidence-based design model designed to help practitioners analyse qualities related to the target group, the activity, and the physical environment, for instance, in the design of workplaces, schools, hospitals, or homes for the elderly. The tool is often used in dialogues, and the output supports design that leads to 1) environments that benefit user health and well-being, 2) environments that meet a variety of user needs and desires, and 3) environments that are accessible and usable. QET is based on and synthesises research findings, such as the *Pyramid of Supportive Environments*, the *Perceived Sensory Dimensions*, *Four Zones of Contact with the Outdoor Environment*, as well as research results regarding accessibility and safety.

QET has been developed to cover a wide range of needs and preferences regarding people in general, as well as people with special needs (Bengtsson & Grahn, 2014). There are 19 evidence-based environmental qualities included in the tool, which are divided into two main groups:

1. Environmental qualities related to people feeling comfortable using outdoor environments
2. Environmental qualities related to people experiencing positive contact with outdoor environments in the form of stimulation or rest and recovery

The first group contains six environmental qualities that designers should strive for in order to increase the comfort of people in outdoor environments, that is, comfortable design. These features support people's ability to use the outdoor environments and are important to consider throughout the green space. The second group contains 13 environmental qualities (including the eight PSDs) of stimulating or restorative design and refers to contact with nature and surrounding life. These are properties that promote stimulation or recovery of the senses and mind, qualities that people desire and prefer to find outdoors. They encourage people to go outdoors, either to find social or physical activities or to find rest, solitude, and peace.

Two projects using evidence-based models to guide the planning, design, and management of urban green spaces

The following two examples illustrate how evidence-based models and tools can be integrated into planning and design processes aiming to create health-promoting outdoor environments. The contexts of the two projects were different, both in terms of planning scale and in terms of targeted users.

Programme to develop a health park corridor

In the first project, a programme for a 'health park corridor in the Swedish municipality of Täby' was created to guide future development of three connected parks (i.e., the parks Åkerbyparken, Byängsparken, and Libbyängen). The development area of these three parks stretches from the Täby city centre to a nearby lake (Rönningesjön; Figure 4.3) and to the city forest (Stolpaskogen) and also connects to green/blue nature-based recreational areas from a newly built residential area ('Täby park').

The programme for the health park corridors is an early-phase planning document that aims to guide the municipality's future development of three connected parks both in terms of design content and of improving accessibility to adjacent natural areas, with the intention of promoting health for Täby's residents. As such, it shows an example of how research evidence on health-promoting environmental qualities can be put into practice in the context of developing public urban green space.

Landscape analysis and user dialogues with a focus on health and well-being

Landscape architects at the city development office in Täby municipality and researchers worked together, using the previously presented evidence-based design models, to map the area's existing health-promoting environmental qualities and to work out proposals for development measures. Landscape architects at Täby municipality carried out resident dialogues to identify local residents' needs from a health and well-being perspective, which, among other things, included questions about environmental qualities for comfortable and stimulating design.

The programme includes proposals for both the overall layout and content of the parks and how they could be interconnected to increase accessibility to green and blue recreational values, as well as for the development of specific content of health-promoting environmental qualities within each park. The information in the programme can also guide the location of activities and functions that are aimed at users who have special needs in relation to the outdoor environment, for example, children and the elderly.

Overall, the programme proposes development for the health park corridor in which stimulating environmental qualities are prioritised in the areas near the centre of Täby. Moving out from the city centre toward connected natural areas, there is a transition toward more and more restorative environmental qualities and experiences of peacefulness and nature. The character of the design follows the same pattern, with an urban and formal design character near the city centre, which gradually transitions into a more natural and informal design character toward the outer parts of the health park corridor, close to adjacent natural areas. The goal is to develop an attractive and safe health park corridor that offers a varied content of health-promoting environmental experiences and connects the centre with recreational areas close to the city.

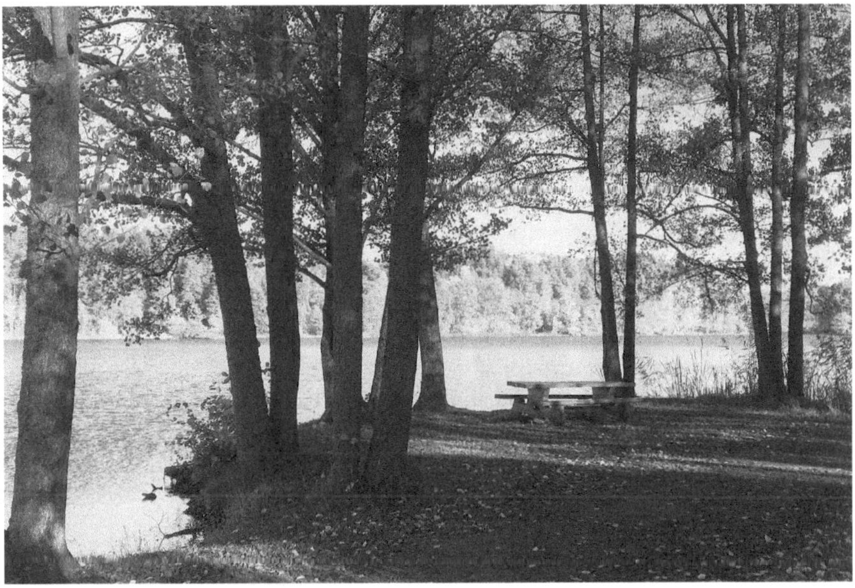

Figure 4.3 Picnic area at Rönningesjön on the edge of the health park corridor, adjacent to green/blue natural recreational areas.

Source: Photo by Anna Åshage.

Green structure plans for three hospitals

The objective of this project was to develop green structure plans for three hospital areas (Ryhov, Värnamo, and Eksjö) in Jönköping County, Sweden. Based on the intention to make use of research-based knowledge from environmental psychology, these green structure plans reveal how research evidence on health-promoting environmental qualities can be put into practice and guide long-term planning and development strategies, with a focus on preserving and developing both social and biological values in hospital contexts.

Implementation

The assignment to draw up green structure plans for Ryhov was a joint collaboration between Region Jönköping County/Regionfastigheter, White arkitekter AB, and researchers from the Swedish University of Agricultural Sciences (SLU) in Alnarp, while the plans for the hospitals in Eksjö and Värnamo were developed in close cooperation between Regionfastigheter[1] in Jönköping County and researchers from SLU in Alnarp.

Existing health-promoting environmental qualities at the hospital sites were inventoried and analysed. Workshops with staff at different care units at the hospitals gave input on how they wished to use the outdoor environments to support patients' use and for their own use. The relationship between the buildings and the outdoor environments was mapped in relation to four zones of contact with the outdoors to identify possibilities for experiencing different qualities from different zones. Values and deficiencies from a health-promoting perspective were then weighed against values and deficiencies from biological, cultural, and historical perspectives to formulate visions and goals for managing and developing health-promoting environmental qualities and experiences. Figure 4.4 shows an example of the outcome at the Värnamo hospital.

In line with the region's sustainability programme and development strategy, the green structure plans specify an overall direction of intent for the long-term development of the green structure on a strategic level, formulating strategic goals, to create a purposeful and functioning whole over time. The plans also provide concrete action proposals and guide prioritisation for ongoing development and management projects. Based on current research in environmental psychology, the plans have a particular focus on identifying the health-promoting qualities of the outdoor environment and its vegetation and propose how such qualities can be preserved and developed to constitute a health-promoting resource for patients, staff, and visitors.

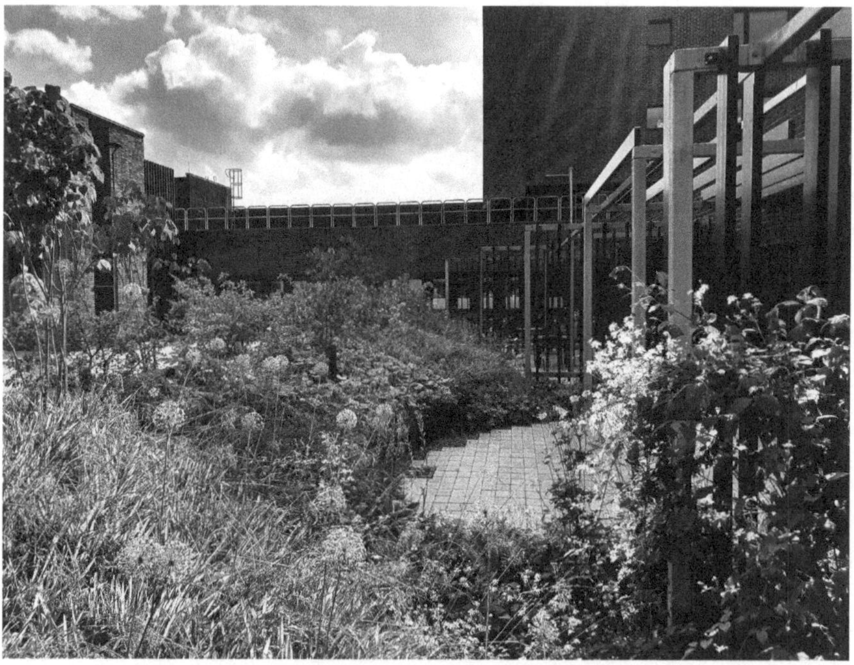

Figure 4.4 Outdoor area for patients at the intensive care unit at the Värnamo hospital. Varied vegetation outside the patients' rooms offers positive distracting views and gives the opportunity to rest outdoors, embedded in greenery.

Source: Photo by Anna Åshage.

The goals and visions formulated in these plans strive to form and maintain environments with content and experiential values that support and stimulate activities and care and where social, biological, and ecological values are protected, developed, and supplemented. For each new project, the green structure plan must therefore be included as a basis for decisions. Preserving values, such as the ones mentioned earlier, must be prioritised, and if this is not possible, the values must be compensated. The outdoor environment must be for everyone: patients, staff, and visitors, as well as passers-by. A variety of experiential values in safe and comfortable environments should promote outdoor activities, physical activity, faster recovery, and greater well-being. Great variety in nature types and biotopes should attract new animal and plant species and promote biological diversity (Egerer & Marselle, this volume, Chapter 8).

Conclusion and transferability

This chapter advocates the use of evidence-based models in the development of health-promoting green areas. The models are built upon research on how green space design may influence people in different zones of contact with the outdoor environment in their living environments. The models also include knowledge on specific environmental qualities within a green space which promote comfortable outdoor living, physical activity, social interaction, and recovery (van den Bosch & Jarvis, this volume, Chapter 6).

Based on our work on different projects (Bengtsson et al., 2024), we have found that the models are useful for projects of varying scales and contexts, projects focusing on different target groups, and projects related to different overarching political goals. Furthermore, practitioners found their own creative ways of working with the models as well as presenting their results visually.

We have also learned that the design process is hardly a linear one. However, to strive for transferability from evidence to practice, we propose four overarching phases for an evidence-based working method for practitioners who want to complement and support established practice with an evidence-based approach specifically focusing on health and well-being. For those who are interested in a more detailed description of the approach, it can be found in a chapter by Bengtsson et al. (2024) in the handbook *Green and healthy Nordic cities: How to plan, design, and manage health-promoting urban green space.*

Phase 1: Identification of existing zones and environmental qualities in and around the green space. In this phase, the zones and the environmental qualities are used to investigate and describe the site as it is today. This phase is important to take advantage of the health-promoting potential of the site, in the site, as well as from different proximities.

Phase 2: Using zones and environmental qualities to identify user perspectives. In Phase 2, the idea is that the practitioners study the needs and preferences of the users in relation to the environmental qualities and in relation to each relevant zone. Useful methods can be interviews, focus groups, surveys, or workshops, which are considered in each unique project.

Phase 3: Using zones and environmental qualities in the design phase. The overall intention of Phase 3 is to use the results of Phase 1 and Phase 2 when working with the programme proposal and the design proposal. To acquire health perspectives in the proposal, designers propose measures for environmental qualities and zones. The proposal can contain plans with overviews of environmental qualities and zones as they appear before and after the design of the green space. The changes can be explained and motivated in relation to the user perspectives identified in Phase 2.

Phase 4: Using zones and environmental qualities in a post-occupancy evaluation. The post-occupancy evaluation is important to learn more about health-promoting environmental qualities and different zones in relation to each unique project. No two projects are the same. The site is always unique, and so is the context, for example, in relation to which zones exist and are relevant to the site and which persons are potential users and recipients of potential health effects. Therefore, there is always much to learn from each project that has applied an evidence-based working process.

Overall, even if the evidence-based models take time to absorb and training is needed to be able to use them in practice, we have found that practitioners perceive both the models and the working process as valuable additions to established practices in green space development. They specifically help highlight people's needs for green space and understand green spaces as health-promoting resources.

Note

1 Unit within the regional administration responsible for the development, management, and operation of properties throughout the county.

References

Akpinar, A. (2017). Urban green spaces for children: A cross-sectional study of associations with distance, physical activity, screen time, general health, and overweight. *Urban Forestry & Urban Greening*, *25*, 66–73.

An, C., Liu, J., Liu, Q., Liu, Y., Fan, X., & Hu, Y. (2022). How perceived sensory dimensions of forest park are associated with stress restoration in Beijing? *International Journal of Environmental Research and Public Health*, *19*(2), 883. https://doi.org/10.3390/ijerph19020883

Artmann, M., Inostroza, L., & Fan, P. (2019). Urban sprawl, compact urban development and green cities. How much do we know, how much do we agree? *Ecological Indicators*, *96*, 3–9.

Astell-Burt, T., Hartig, T., Putra, I. G. N. E., Walsan, R., Dendup, T., & Feng, X. (2022). Green space and loneliness: A systematic review with theoretical and methodological guidance for future research. *Science of the Total Environment*, *847*, 157521. https://doi.org/10.1016/j.scitotenv.2022.157521

Ayala-Azcárraga, C., Diaz, D., & Zambrano, L. (2019). Characteristics of urban parks and their relation to user well-being. *Landscape and Urban Planning*, *189*, 27–35.

Bengtsson, A. (2015). *From experiences of the outdoors to the design of healthcare environments* [Doctoral dissertation, Swedish University of Agricultural Sciences]. Acta Universitatis Agriculurae Sueciae.

Bengtsson, A., Åshage, A., Andersson, M., Dybkjær, E., & Grahn, P. (2024). Improving green space design based on health design theory and environmental psychology. In L. A. Borges, L. Rohrer, & K. Nilsson (Eds.), *Green and healthy Nordic cities: How to plan, design, and manage health-promoting urban green space* (pp. 79–101). Nordregio.

Bengtsson, A., & Grahn, P. (2014). Outdoor environments in healthcare settings: A quality evaluation tool for use in designing healthcare gardens. *Urban Forestry & Urban Greening, 13*(4), 878–891.

Blakemore, R. L., Neveu, R., & Vuilleumier, P. (2017). How emotion context modulates unconscious goal activation during motor force exertion. *NeuroImage, 146*, 904–917.

Buemann, B., & Uvnäs-Moberg, K. (2020). Oxytocin may have a therapeutical potential against cardiovascular disease. Possible pharmaceutical and behavioral approaches. *Medical Hypotheses, 138*, 109597. https://doi.org/10.1016/j.mehy.2020.109597

Cannon, W. B. (1929). *Bodily changes in pain, hunger, fear and rage.* D Appleton & Company.

Chen, H., Qiu, L., & Gao, T. (2019). Application of the eight perceived sensory dimensions as a tool for urban green space assessment and planning in China. *Urban Forestry & Urban Greening, 40*, 224–235.

Chen, X., Hu, J., & Sun, A. (2018). The beneficial effect of enriched environment on pathogenesis of Alzheimer's disease. *Yangtze Medicine, 2*, 225–243.

Clemenson, G. D., Deng, W., & Gage, F. H. (2015). Environmental enrichment and neurogenesis: From mice to humans. *Current Opinion in Behavioral Sciences, 4*, 56–62.

Collins, R. M., Smith, D., Ogutu, B. O., Brown, K. A., Eigenbrod, F., & Spake, R. (2023). The relative effects of access to public greenspace and private gardens on mental health. *Landscape and Urban Planning, 240*, 104902. https://doi.org/10.1016/j.landurbplan.2023.104902

de Bell, S., White, M., Griffiths, A., Darlow, A., Taylor, T., Wheeler, B., & Lovell, R. (2020). Spending time in the garden is positively associated with health and wellbeing: Results from a national survey in England. *Landscape and Urban Planning, 200*, 103836. https://doi.org/10.1016/j.landurbplan.2020.103836

Dijksterhuis, A. (2004). Think different: The merits of unconscious thought in preference development and decision making. *Journal of Personality and Social Psychology, 87*(5), 586–598.

Ekelund, U., Steene-Johannessen, J., Brown, W. J., Fagerland, M. W., Owen, N., Powell, K. E., Bauman, A., & Lee, I.-M. (2016). Does physical activity attenuate, or even eliminate, the detrimental association of sitting time with mortality? A harmonised meta-analysis of data from more than 1 million men and women. *The Lancet, 388*(10051), 1302–1310.

Ekkel, E. D., & de Vries, S. (2017). Nearby green space and human health: Evaluating accessibility metrics. *Landscape and Urban Planning, 157*, 214–220.

Evensen, K. H., Hemsett, G., & Nordh, H. (2021). Developing a place-sensitive tool for park-safety management experiences from green-space managers and female park users in Oslo. *Urban Forestry & Urban Greening, 60*, 127057. https://doi.org/10.1016/j.ufug.2021.127057

Fan, P., Xu, L., Yue, W., & Chen, J. (2017). Accessibility of public urban green space in an urban periphery: The case of Shanghai. *Landscape and Urban Planning, 165*, 177–192.

Farioli-Vecchioli, S., Ricci, V., & Middei, S. (2022). Adult hippocampal neurogenesis in Alzheimer's disease: An overview of human and animal studies with implications for therapeutic perspectives aimed at memory recovery. *Neural Plasticity, 2022*, 9959044. https://doi.org/10.1155/2022/9959044

Fink, G. (2017). Stress: Concepts, definition and history. In J. Stein (Ed.), *Reference module in neuroscience and biobehavioral psychology*. Elsevier. https://doi.org/10.1016/B978-0-12-809324-5.02208-2

Gomes-Leal, W. (2021). Adult hippocampal neurogenesis and affective disorders: New neurons for psychic well-being. *Frontiers in Neuroscience, 15*, 594448. https://doi.org/10.3389/fnins.2021.594448

Gozalo, G. R., Morillas, J. M. B., & González, D. M. (2019). Perceptions and use of urban green spaces on the basis of size. *Urban Forestry & Urban Greening, 46*, 126470. https://doi.org/10.1016/j.ufug.2019.126470

Grahn, P. (1991). The importance of a garden or a yard of your own. In P. Grahn (Ed.), *Om parkers betydelse* (pp. 184–216). The Swedish University of Agricultural Sciences.

Grahn, P. (2007). Barnet och naturen [The child and nature]. In L.-O. Dahlgren, S. Sjölander, J.-P. Strid, & A. Szczepanski (Eds.), *Utomhuspedagogik som kunskapskälla* (pp. 55–104). Studentlitteratur.

Grahn, P., Ottosson, J., & Uvnäs-Moberg, K. (2021). The oxytocinergic system as a mediator of anti-stress and instorative effects induced by nature: The calm and connection theory. *Frontiers in Psychology, 12*, 617814. https://doi.org/10.3389/fpsyg.2021.617814

Grahn, P., & Stigsdotter, U. A. (2003). Landscape planning and stress. *Urban Forestry & Urban Greening, 2*(1), 1–18. https://doi.org/10.1078/1618-8667-00019

Grahn, P., & Stigsdotter, U. K. (2010). The relation between perceived sensory dimensions of urban green space and stress restoration. *Landscape and Urban Planning, 94*(3–4), 264–275.

Grahn, P., & Stoltz, J. (2021). *Urbana grönområden – Indikatorer för hälsa och välbefinnande* [Urban green areas: Indicators for health and well-being]. Movium.

Grahn, P., & Stoltz, J. (2022). *Indikatorer för hälsopromoverande urbana grönområden: Kunskapssammanställning* [Indicators for health-promoting urban green spaces: Knowledge synthesis]. Naturvårdsverket, Stockholm. https://naturvardsverket.diva-portal.org/smash/get/diva2:1665178/FULLTEXT01.pdf

Grahn, P., Stoltz, J., & Bengtsson, A. (2022). The Alnarp method: An interdisciplinary-based design of holistic healing gardens derived from research and development in Alnarp rehabilitation garden. In K. Bishop & L. Corkery (Eds.), *Routledge handbook of urban landscape research* (pp. 299–317). Routledge.

Grahn, P., Stoltz, J., Skärbäck, E., & Bengtsson, A. (2023). Health-promoting nature-based paradigms in urban planning. *Encyclopedia, 3*(4), 1419–1438.

Grońska-Pęski, M., Gonçalves, J. T., & Hébert, J. M. (2021). Enriched environment promotes adult hippocampal neurogenesis through FGFRs. *Journal of Neuroscience, 41*(13), 2899–2910.

Hellier, J. L. (2017). *The five senses and beyond: The encyclopedia of perception*. Greenwood Publishing.

Hentschel, U., Kiessling, M., & Hosemann, A. (2004). Adaptation to boredom and stress. *Advances in Psychology, 136*, 303–323.

Holick, M. F. (2016). Biological effects of sunlight, ultraviolet radiation, visible light, infrared radiation and vitamin D for health. *Anticancer Research, 36*, 1345–1356.

Honold, J., Lakes, T., Beyer, R., & van der Meer, E. (2016). Restoration in urban spaces: Nature views from home, greenways, and public parks. *Environment and Behavior, 48*(6), 796–825.

Hooper, P., Boruff, B., Beesley, B., Badland, H., & Giles-Corti, B. (2018). Testing spatial measures of public open space planning standards with walking and physical activity health outcomes: Findings from the Australian national liveability study. *Landscape and Urban Planning, 171*, 57–67.

Högberg, B., & Strandh, M. (in press). Temporal trends and inequalities in school-related stress in three cohorts in compulsory school in Sweden. *Scandinavian Journal of Educational Research*. https://doi.org/10.1080/00313831.2024.2330932

Jamalishahni, T., Turrell, G., Foster, S., Davern, M., & Villanueva, K. (2023). Neighbourhood socio-economic disadvantage and loneliness: The contribution of green space quantity and quality. *BMC Public Health, 23*(1), 598. https://doi.org/10.1186/s12889-023-15433-0

Jimenez, M. P., DeVille, N. V., Elliott, E. G., Schiff, J. E., Wilt, G. E., Hart, J. E., & James, P. (2021). Associations between nature exposure and health: A review of the evidence. *International Journal of Environmental Research and Public Health, 18*(9), 4790. https://doi.org/10.3390%2Fijerph18094790

Kellmann, M., & Beckmann, J. (Eds.). (2024). *Fostering recovery and well-being in a healthy lifestyle: Psychological, somatic, and organizational prevention approaches*. Routledge.

Kempermann, G. (2019). Environmental enrichment, new neurons and the neurobiology of individuality. *Nature Reviews Neuroscience, 20*, 235–245.

Kempermann, G. (2022). What is adult hippocampal neurogenesis good for? *Frontiers in Neuroscience, 16*, 852680. https://doi.org/10.3389/fnins.2022.852680

Korpela, K., de Bloom, J., & Kinnunen, U. (2015). From restorative environments to restoration in work. *Intelligent Buildings International*, 7(4), 215–223.

Krekel, C., Kolbe, J., & Wüstemann, H. (2016). The greener, the happier? The effects of urban land use on residential well-being. *Ecological Economics, 121*, 117–127.

Kühn, S., Düzel, S., Eibich, P., Krekel, C., Wüstemann, H., Kolbe, J., Martensson, J., Goebel, J., Gallinat, J., Wagner, G. G., & Lindenberger, U. (2017). In search of features that constitute an "enriched environment" in humans: Associations between geographical properties and brain structure. *Scientific Reports*, 7(1), 11920. https://doi.org/10.1038/s41598-017-12046-7

Kühn, S., Forlim, C. G., Lender, A., Wirtz, J., & Gallinat, J. (2021). Brain functional connectivity differs when viewing pictures from natural and built environments using fMRI resting state analysis. *Scientific Reports, 11*(1), 4110. https://doi.org/10.1038/s41598-021-83246-5

Kumar, J., Iwabuchi, S. J., Völlm, B. A., & Palaniyappan, L. (2020). Oxytocin modulates the effective connectivity between the precuneus and the dorsolateral prefrontal cortex. *European Archives of Psychiatry and Clinical Neuroscience, 270*(5), 567–576.

Labib, S. M., Lindley, S., & Huck, J. J. (2020). Spatial dimensions of the influence of urban green-blue spaces on human health: A systematic review. *Environmental Research, 180*, 108869. https://doi.org/10.1016/j.envres.2019.108869

Lambert, K., Eisch, A. J., Galea, L. A. M., Kempermann, G., & Merzenich, M. (2019). Optimizing brain performance: Identifying mechanisms of adaptive neurobiological plasticity. *Neuroscience & Biobehavioral Reviews, 105*, 60–71.

Lenaerts, A., Heyman, S., de Decker, A., Lauwers, L., Sterckx, A., Remmen, R., Bastiaens, H., & Keune, H. (2021). Vitamin nature: How coronavirus disease 2019 has highlighted factors contributing to the frequency of nature visits in Flanders, Belgium. *Frontiers in Public Health, 9*, 646568. https://doi.org/10.3389/fpubh.2021.646568

Li, D., & Sullivan, W. C. (2016). Impact of views to school landscapes on recovery from stress and mental fatigue. *Landscape and Urban Planning, 148*, 149–158.

Liebowitz, J. (2020). *Developing informed intuition for decision-making*. CRC Press.

Lottrup, L., Grahn, P., & Stigsdotter, U. K. (2013). Workplace greenery and perceived level of stress: Benefits of access to a green outdoor environment at the workplace. *Landscape and Urban Planning, 110*, 5–11.

Love, T. M. (2014). Oxytocin, motivation and the role of dopamine. *Pharmacology Biochemistry and Behavior, 119*, 49–60.

Mårtensson, F., Boldemann, C., Söderström, M., Blennow, M., Englund, J.-E., & Grahn, P. (2009). Outdoor environmental assessment of attention promoting settings for preschool children. *Health & Place, 15*(4), 1149–1157.

Memari, S., Pazhouhanfar, M., & Grahn, P. (2021). Perceived sensory dimensions of green areas: An experimental study on stress recovery. *Sustainability, 13*(10), 5419. https://doi.org/10.3390/su13105419

Mohd Sahini, S. N., Mohd Nor Hazalin, N. A., Srikumar, B. N., Jayasingh Chellammal, H. S., & Surindar Singh, G. K. (2024). Environmental enrichment improves cognitive function, learning, memory and anxiety-related behaviours in rodent models of dementia: Implications for future study. *Neurobiology of Learning and Memory, 208*, 107880. https://doi.org/10.1016/j.nlm.2023.107880

Neville, J. J., Palmieri, T., & Young, A. R. (2021). Physical determinants of vitamin D photosynthesis: A review. *JBMR Plus, 5*(1), e10460. https://doi.org/10.1002/jbm4.10460

Nicolaides, N. C., Kyratzi, E., Lamprokostopoulou, A., Chrousos, G. P., & Charmandari, E. (2014). Stress, the stress system and the role of glucocorticoids. *Neuroimmunomodulation, 22*(1–2), 6–19.

Nilsson, K., Bentsen, P., Grahn, P., & Mygind, L. (2019). De quelles preuves scientifiques disposons-nous concernant les effets des forêts et des arbres sur la santé et le bien-être humains? [What is the scientific evidence with regard to the effects of forests, trees on human health and well-being?]. *Santé Publique, 1*, 219–240.

Nowzari, Z., Armitage, R., & Tilaki, M. J. M. (2023). How does the residential complex regulate residents' behaviour? An empirical study to identify influential components of human territoriality on social interaction. *Sustainability, 15*(14), 11276. https://doi.org/10.3390/su151411276

Nutsford, D., Pearson, A. L., & Kingham, S. (2013). An ecological study investigating the association between access to urban green space and mental health. *Public Health, 127*(11), 1005–1011.

Ostfeld, A. M., & D'Atri, D. A. (1975). Psychophysiological responses to the urban environment. *The International Journal of Psychiatry in Medicine, 6*(1–2), 15–28.

Ottosson, J. (2007). *The importance of nature in coping* [Doctoral dissertation, Swedish University of Agricultural Sciences]. Acta Universitatis Agriculurae Sueciae. https://citeseerx.ist.psu.edu/document?repid=rep1&type=pdf&doi=a6164d503cbdb6623a035be10b3a828b72c0f408

Ottosson, J., & Grahn, P. (2008). The role of natural settings in crisis rehabilitation: How does the level of crisis influence the response to experiences of nature with regard to measures of rehabilitation? *Landscape Research, 33*(1), 51–70.

Pálsdóttir, A. M., Persson, D., Persson, B., & Grahn, P. (2014). The journey of recovery and empowerment embraced by nature – clients' perspectives on nature-based rehabilitation in relation to the role of the natural environment. *International Journal of Environmental Research and Public Health, 11*(7), 7094–7115.

Paquet, C., Orschulok, T. P., Coffee, N. T., Howard, N. J., Hugo, G., Taylor, A. W., Adams, R. J., & Daniel, M. (2013). Are accessibility and characteristics of public open spaces associated with a better cardiometabolic health? *Landscape and Urban Planning, 118*, 70–78.

Pelczynski, J., & Tomkowicz, B. (2019). Densification of cities as a method of sustainable development. *Earth and Environmental Science, 362*(1), 012106. https://doi.org/10.1088/1755-1315/362/1/012106

Pont, M. B., Haupt, P., Berg, P., Alstäde, V., & Heyman, A. (2021). Systematic review and comparison of densification effects and planning motivations. *Buildings & Cities, 2*(1), 378–401.

Poortinga, W., Bird, N., Hallingberg, B., Phillips, R., & Williams, D. (2021). The role of perceived public and private green space in subjective health and wellbeing during and after the first peak of the COVID-19 outbreak. *Landscape and Urban Planning, 211*, 104092. https://doi.org/10.1016/j.landurbplan.2021.104092

Pretty, J., Peacock, J., Sellens, M., & Griffin, M. (2005). The mental and physical health outcomes of green exercise. *International Journal of Environmental Health Research, 15*(5), 319–337.

Qiu, L., & Nielsen, A. B. (2015). Are perceived sensory dimensions a reliable tool for urban green space assessment and planning? *Landscape Research, 40*(7), 834–854.

Rigney, N., de Vries, G. J., Petrulis, A., & Young, L. J. (2022). Oxytocin, vasopressin, and social behavior: From neural circuits to clinical opportunities. *Endocrinology, 163*(9), bqac111. https://doi.org/10.1210/endocr/bqac11

Rojas-Rueda, D., Nieuwenhuijsen, M. J., Gascon, M., Perez-Leon, D., & Mudu, P. (2019). Green spaces and mortality: A systematic review and meta-analysis of cohort studies. *The Lancet Planetary Health, 3*(11), e469–e477.

Russell, G., & Lightman, S. (2019). The human stress response. *Nature Reviews Endocrinology, 15*, 525–534.

Selye, H. (1936). A syndrome produced by diverse nocuous agents. *Nature, 138*, 32.

Staats, H., Collado, S., & Sorrel, M. A. (2024). Understimulation resembles overstimulation. *Journal of Environmental Psychology, 95*, 102280. https://doi.org/10.1016/j.jenvp.2024.102280

Stigsdotter, U. A., & Grahn, P. (2004a). A garden at your doorstep may reduce stress – private gardens as restorative environments in the city. In P. Aspinall, S. Bell, & C. Ward Thompson (Eds.), *Proceedings of the open space: People space. An international conference on inclusive environments* (pp. 1–6). Open space, Edinburgh College of Art Edinburgh, Scotland.

Stigsdotter, U. A., & Grahn, P. (2004b). A garden at your workplace may reduce stress. In A. Dilani (Ed.), *Design and health III – health promotion through environmental design* (pp. 147–157). Research Centre for Design and health, Stockholm.

Stoltz, J., & Grahn, P. (2021a). Perceived sensory dimensions: An evidence-based approach to greenspace aesthetics. *Urban Forestry & Urban Greening, 59*, 126989. https://doi.org/10.1016/j.ufug.2021.126989

Stoltz, J., & Grahn, P. (2021b). Perceived sensory dimensions: Key aesthetic qualities for health-promoting urban green spaces. *Journal of Biomed Research, 2*, 22–29.

Teller, J. (2021). Regulating urban densification: What factors should be used? *Buildings & Cities, 2*(1), 302–317.

Triguero-Mas, M., Dadvand, P., Cirach, M., Martinez, D., Medina, A., Mompart, A., Basagaña, X., Gražulevičienė, R., & Nieuwenhuijsen, M. J. (2015). Natural outdoor environments and mental and physical health: Relationships and mechanisms. *Environment International*, 77, 35–41.

Ulrich, R. S. (1984). View through a window may influence recovery from surgery. *Science*, *224*(4647), 420–421.

Uvnäs-Moberg, K., Handlin, L., & Petersson, M. (2015). Self-soothing behaviors with particular reference to oxytocin release induced by non-noxious sensory stimulation. *Frontiers in Psychology*, *5*, 1529. https://doi.org/10.3389%2Ffpsyg.2014.01529

Uvnäs-Moberg, K., & Petersson, M. (2022). Physiological effects induced by stimulation of cutaneous sensory nerves, with a focus on oxytocin. *Current Opinion in Behavioral Sciences*, *43*, 159–166.

Wang, H., Dai, X., Wu, J., Wu, X., & Nie, X. (2019). Influence of urban green open space on residents' physical activity in China. *BMC Public Health*, *19*, 1093. https://doi.org/10.1186/s12889-019-7416-7

Wang, S., & Li, A. (2024). Identify the significant landscape characteristics for the perceived restorativeness of 8 perceived sensory dimensions in urban green space. *Heliyon*, *10*(7), e27925. https://doi.org/10.1016/j.heliyon.2024.e27925

World Health Organization. (2016). *Urban green spaces and health*. Retrieved July 7, 2024 from https://iris.who.int/bitstream/handle/10665/345751/WHO-EURO-2016-3352-43111-60341-eng.pdf?sequence=3

Williams, T. G., Logan, T. M., Zuo, C. T., Liberman, K. D., & Guikema, S. D. (2020). Parks and safety: A comparative study of green space access and inequity in five US cities. *Landscape and Urban Planning*, *201*, 103841. https://doi.org/10.1016/j.landurbplan.2020.103841

Wilson, T. D. (2004). *Strangers to ourselves: Discovering the adaptive unconscious*. Harvard University Press.

Wood, L., Hooper, P., Foster, S., & Bull, F. (2017). Public green spaces and positive mental health – investigating the relationship between access, quantity and types of parks and mental wellbeing. *Health & Place*, *48*, 63–71.

Zeev-Wolf, M., Levy, J., Ebstein, R. P., & Feldman, R. (2020). Cumulative risk on oxytocin-pathway genes impairs default mode network connectivity in trauma-exposed youth. *Frontiers in Endocrinology*, *11*, 335. https://doi.org/10.3389/fendo.2020.00335

Zheng, S., Liang, Z., Qu, Y., Wu, Q., Wu, H., & Liu, Q. (2022). Kuramoto model-based analysis reveals oxytocin effects on brain network dynamics. *International Journal of Neural Systems*, *32*(2), 2250002. https://doi.org/10.1142/S0129065722500022

Part II

Designing home, private, and working environments for recovery

5 Built recovery

New perspectives on designing office and hospital work environments

Gemma Koppen, Mark N. Phillips, Claudia Iovița, and Tanja C. Vollmer

Introduction

Increased digitalisation, mobility, demographic, economic, and environmental changes are only some of the factors leading to societal adjustments that are also influencing and questioning the current culture of the work environment. The Covid-19 pandemic has further accelerated these changes, particularly in Germany, but also worldwide. For many large companies and public institutions, working from home was still unthinkable until 2019. Online team meetings, which are not tied to a fixed workplace, are now part of everyday working life for people in a wide range of sectors and functions.

The mentioned changes highlight the need not only for reinterpretation of the spatial structure and organisation but also for addressing the emotional and physical health of the employees, which are related to these. Recent decades have seen increasing interest in studying the impact of the office environment on health-related outcomes (Clements-Croome, 2018; Jensen & van der Voordt, 2019). However, recent literature reviews (Colenberg et al., 2021; Groen et al., 2018; Jensen & van der Voordt, 2019) show that most studies focus on alleviating the negative effects on employees, while the health-promoting potential of office environments is overlooked. This is a fatal conclusion, as the increased working demand and fast pace are already challenging the resilience of employees and their life domain balance (Beckmann & Kellmann, 2024). In this chapter, we therefore present two architectural concepts that have employee recovery as a target variable in the design of work environments. Describing those, we understand recovery as "an inter- and intraindividual multilevel (e.g., psychological, physiological, social) process in time for the re-establishment of personal resources and their full functional capacity" (Kallus, 2016, p. 42).

In 2020, 44.6% of EU workers reported facing risk factors for their mental well-being at work (Eurostat, 2020). Time pressure related to work overload; dealing with difficult customers, patients, pupils, etc.; and job insecurity were

Koppen, G., Phillips, M. N., Iovița, C., & Vollmer, T. C. (2025). Built recovery: New perspectives on designing office and hospital work environments. In S. Pauleit, M. Kellmann, & J. Beckmann (Eds.), *Creating Urban and Workplace Environments for Recovery and Well-being* (pp. 85–112). Routledge.

DOI: 10.4324/9781003435471-7

said to be the top three risk factors for mental well-being. Simultaneously, society is evolving rapidly from an industrial to a knowledge-based society, moving away from traditional top-down, hierarchical, and rigid working structures and thus changing the concept of work (Bèoschen & Schulz-Schaeffer, 2003). As an outcome of this development, the New Work concept, first introduced in the 1980s by Frithjof Bergmann (2019), reacts to the needs and changes of the current working culture.

New Work, a holistic concept of creating a work environment where people are placed at the centre of the system, is influenced by numerous technological and societal changes (Antonelli, 2001; Bergmann, 2019; Newport, 2016). Bergmann initiated it as a response to the traditional, rigid Industrial Revolution working culture, where the worker was transformed into a tool for the machines rather than the opposite. He proposed using technological advancement as an instrument to facilitate and ease the work overload, supporting autonomous and self-sufficient living, and as an alternative to the then-existing job system. "The work we do should not drain and exhaust us, it should give us more strength and more energy, it should develop us into fuller human beings" (Bergmann, 2019, p. 4). He established the centre for New Work with the task to support and assist people in finding their talents and skills and desirable work that would also bring them material independence. Bergmann can accept a repetitive and mundane activity if "there is meaning, there is goal, a purpose to what one does" (Bergmann, 2019, p. 10). Nowadays, digitalisation, connectivity, globalisation, demographic change, and health crises (such as Covid-19) are reshaping the New Work concept, creating opportunities to identify and implement alternative ways of organising work (Wendt, 2023). Alongside the principles originally attributed to the holistic concept of New Work, it supports greater task autonomy, decentralisation, less-rigid management structures, and alternative spatial solutions (Bouncken et al., 2023; Valenduc, 2018). As the changes previously listed also come with challenges (Niebuhr et al., 2022), it is important to see New Work as a health-supportive tool to address the resilience, recovery, and well-being of employees (López-Cabarcos et al., 2020; Starker et al., 2022). In overarching evidence-based design models, the design of work environments which facilitate these goals is classified as preventive and rehabilitative architectural intervention (Koppen et al., 2021; Vollmer et al., 2020). In recent years, New Work has taken hold of the entire field of knowledge work; hardly any company or institution can afford not to think about how and where work is being performed.

For more than 30 years, knowledge work has been shifting away from one singular workplace to the use of different workplaces. While the traditional office workplace before Covid-19 was mostly dominated by basic workstations and meeting rooms, including little space for retreat, co-creation, and community activities, the current so-called multi-space office already has a balanced distribution of different areas. In the 'post-Covid-19 workplace', basic desks and meeting rooms have been enormously reduced as they lose their relevance with the growth of, for example, home office and videoconferencing. The new workplace is oriented towards focus zones, co-creation, and informal meetings. Interventions like a shared desk or hot desk (instead of a fixed workplace), the change of the office landscape, or the use of the multi-space (different places to work with changing qualities) are facilitating a more autonomous and diverse working process (Becker et al., 2022; Wohlers & Hertel, 2016) linked to increased workspace satisfaction and promoting recovery from workload (Lusa et al., 2019). These interventions can support the New Work principle of autonomy and independence of the employees. Together with the home office and coworking, these interventions have fundamentally extended the workplace beyond the office building (Bouncken, 2023). However, the classic office concept was already dead, as it could not stand up to the economic arguments for open office plans and flexible workplaces. Providing fewer square metres for one employee or even using them twice meant lower rental, heating, and construction costs (Gerlitz & Hülsbeck, 2024).

Only valid studies on the psychosocial and mental stress of employees were able to stop the trend of completely destroying the classic office and provide a starting point for thinking about new, hybrid solutions that no longer focus only on efficiency but also on the recovery and well-being of the employees (Brennan et al., 2002; Brookes & Kaplan, 1972; Hedge, 1982; Sander et al., 2021). In a case study, Forooraghi et al. (2024) investigated the long-term effects of relocating from a cellular office to a combi office (a mix of cellular and open-plan offices). They evaluated how employees' perception of the environment was related to their sense of coherence and the individual's ability to cope effectively with stressors. The data was collected in semi-structured interviews and structured observations (N = 17) after the relocation in two waves (six months and two years post-relocation). Participants' positive perceptions of the office environment degraded from wave 1 to wave 2, whereas most of the negative perceptions remained the same. However, the availability and accessibility of meeting rooms and breakout rooms were long-lasting positive influences. Contrasting to that, participants stated that they had fewer opportunities for social interactions because of an abundance of different spaces and the limited capacities of most breakout areas. This led to a feeling of isolation and increased stress.

In many companies, some principles of New Work that touch on digitalisation and enhanced autonomy of the employees are implemented through measures such as home office or teleworking, mobile technology, and flexible hours (Bloom et al., 2015; Meinel et al., 2017). Adopting such strategies has proved to have positive effects on workers' mental and physical health, satisfaction, and productivity (Giannikis & Mihail, 2011; Kinsman et al., 2024; Knight & Haslam, 2010; Robelski et al., 2019). On the European Union level, the percentage of people working from home has risen from 5.4% in 2019, with a peak in 2022 of 13.4%, and 10.1% in 2023 (Eurostat, 2024). With the fast pace of technological advancement, the globalisation of the job market, and the clear change caused by the Covid-19 pandemic, digitalisation is becoming essential to the survival and resilience of companies. Therefore, investing in employees' abilities, such as adaptability and agility, critical thinking, intercultural awareness (soft skills), and computer literacy, certification and licenses, languages, technical skills (hard skills), as well as their physical and emotional well-being, is becoming part of the new working culture (Helmond, 2021).

While the advantages of remote work, such as the economy of travel time (Elfering & Huber, this volume, Chapter 2) and travel expenses, and the freedom to organise the work process are strong arguments, some downsides come with the new working culture. In a study on distance work environment in Latvia, Simenenko and Lentjushenkova (2021) found that employees are affected by the lack of environmental change, work–life balance, face-to-face communication with other employees, and inspiring working atmosphere, and then difficulty to stop working in the evening. Some of the variables such as the feeling of loneliness and blurred boundaries are more common for female employees than for male, while the management control factor is considered both an advantage by some and as a disadvantage by others. Reducing the physical mediums in which employees interact with each other might serve as a factor in increasing the silo mentality, reducing knowledge exchange, and losing creativity which, in turn, can influence productivity and innovation (Yang et al., 2022). In their study on remote workers' recovery strategies, Pensar and Mäkelä (2023) identified several psychological detachment strategies that the Finish corporate office workers applied in order to cope with the challenges of remote work. Cognitive controlling as a detachment strategy that involved conscious thought management, physical disconnection from work, time-bound routines, and engagement in non-work activities were found to be actively produced habits that enhanced employees' well-being and recovery processes (Pensar & Mäkelä, 2023). Nevertheless, the need for change is undeniable, and with it the search for tools and strategies that better support the concept of a new work environment for knowledge workers.

Even healthcare facilities, such as hospitals, are not exempted from the need for change in designing their work environments. In Germany, especially, the shortages of skilled workers and the different lifestyles of the new generation of professionals have encouraged the New Work concept to enter the hospital work environment (Altgeld, 2022; Starker et al., 2022). While office and hospital workers have many needs and work-related processes in common, they also differ in intensity and challenges. Besides their communication with clients and collaboration with colleagues, the hospital personnel deal with an extra and unique layer of responsibilities toward a major actor in the work environment: the patient. Therefore, hospitals are not only places of work but also places of dignity for both medical staff and patients. With the need for medical assistance around the clock, their lives are stronger than others defined by their work situations (Vollmer, Koppen, et al., 2024). Besides the focused work on the patients, the healthcare system relies on the cooperation and exchange between different specialists. Therefore, the design of the New Work type of hospital needs to reflect these aspects in innovative solutions, providing a much more human-centred spatial design with solutions for both patients' and medical staff's needs. Due to the increasing working demand, intense mental and physical work, and the boundaryless aspect of the job, the New Work hospital model is arguing for integrating principles of psychological empowerment (Starker et al., 2022) as described by Thomas and Velthouse (1990) as well as Spreitzer (1995), such as experiencing competence, meaningfulness, self-determination, and impact. Implementing them in the hospital work environment, together with spatial interventions, contributes to the mental recovery and resilience of hospital employees to deal with stress and exhaustion at work (Haraldsson et al., 2024), as well as with the dilation of the hospital hierarchy and borders between professional groups.

The present chapter introduces two distinct work environments where the principles of the New Work concept are applied and translated into specific architectural concepts: the knowledge work office and the hospital work environment. While classical office spaces suffer from a rigid structure that prevents employees from recovering and stimulating their well-being (Engelen et al., 2018; Sliter & Yuan, 2014), the New Work architectural concept for the knowledge office presented here contains two health-supportive factors: 1) stimulation through environmental variety (Appel-Meulenbroek & Danivska, 2021; Miller et al., 2014; Thoring, 2019), and 2) interaction through coincident encounters (Meinel et al., 2017; Phillips, 2017). This concept focuses on places that "exist outside the home and beyond the 'work lots' of modern economic production" (Oldenburg & Brissett, 1982, p. 269) and is described in the term *Third Place* (Oldenburg & Brissett, 1982). For the hospital work environment, we introduce a future-orientated architectural concept, which directly responds to the psycho-emotional distress and cognitive demands of hospital employees. This concept defines five environmental categories which restructure the environment along task- and contact-orientated categories: (H) *hands on*, (E) *eyes on*, (M_{on}) *mind on*, (M_{off}) *mind off*, (I) *interact*. The so-called HEMI concept was developed in a nationwide observational study in Dutch children's hospitals and applied to the architectural design of the work environments in the newly built University Children's and Youth's Hospital in Freiburg, Germany (Koppen & Vollmer, 2014; Vollmer & Koppen, 2015, 2022).

In both cases – knowledge work environments and hospitals –, interventions in the spatial design are an important tool for supporting and strengthening the mental well-being and recovery of employees from various fields, while the work environments respond to technological and societal changes. However, it has become increasingly clear that efforts to improve the physical environment alone are not likely to help an organisation achieve its goals without a complementary shift in work culture and work practices.

A new perspective on designing office work environments: Third Places

Many office spaces are a result of mobility (due to digitalisation and flexible work processes) and economic rationality, which often lead to universal designs with no spatial character. In consequence, a purely functional, non-appealing environment is affecting the employees' productivity and satisfaction (Foroor-aghi et al., 2024). The high pace and the stress of everyday tasks are multiplying its effects resulting in anxiety, depression, anger, bullying, loneliness, and boredom, overshadowing the quality of life (Teunen, 2021). Considering these challenges, studying the effects of the office environment and the possible impacts of different physical aspects on health-related outcomes becomes increasingly important (Jensen & van der Voordt, 2019; Vollmer & Koppen, 2022). Already in 1968, in his study on knowledge work processes, Propst (1968) concluded that the typical office tends to inhibit the motivation of workers, chokes off liveliness, and prevents recognition. Based on these insights, he developed the *Action Office*, a modular office furniture system that allows flexible configurations as well as the possibility of switching between being more private or more public (von Vegesack & Eisenbrand, 2008). Almost two decades later, architect Luchetti developed a system with different locations that employees could go to for different activities. In doing so, he laid the foundation for what we understand today as activity-based work (Branzi et al., 1994). Both the Action Office as a furniture concept and the principle of activity-based work were intended to change the rigid working conditions at a desk in the workplace but ultimately failed like many other systems. Space is not a neutral system. It is full of meaning and emotional intelligence, full of possibilities. According to the research of Sailer (2020), whether a workplace concept makes people lonely or promotes cohesion always depends on the spatial conditions, the organisational culture, identification with it, and the access people have to it. Furthermore, aspects such as indoor air quality, comfortable physical and thermal conditions, natural light access, ergonomic design, good acoustics, and the incorporation of biophilic elements influence employees' well-being (Hamadah et al., 2023).

Modern knowledge workers find a higher degree of variation in their work environment as they can choose between working indoors at home (first place), in meetings at the office (second place), on the road, and in so-called 'Third Places'. The 'Third Place for Work' is a term created in the figurative sense from 'First Place', 'Second Place', and 'Third Place' in Oldenburg's (1999) *The great good place*. As a sociologist, Oldenburg defined all places apart from home and the office as Third Place. In a world of hybrid working, many places such as airport lounges, hotel lobbies, or libraries can function as Third Places for work. Coworking spaces are such Third Places by definition. More and more companies and corporations are using them to be able to offer their employees an increased number of decentralised possibilities for working. One relatively new area of research is how Third Place offices, such as coworking, can contribute to the way hybrid working is performed (Bouncken, 2023). Coworking spaces, like any other Third Places for work, provide support for informal interaction, which contributes to the individual's well-being and even promote the intuitive systems of human beings. In doing so, these spaces and places can contribute significantly to corporate office concepts and the way multilocal working is defined.

With such new findings, an indoor work environment like coworking and other modern Third Places that are situated inside but also beyond the classic office building are developing an increasing social and scientific relevance. A study done by Gerdenitsch et al. (2016) found that coworking spaces can provide social support for independent professionals. They coded interviews of people working in coworking spaces and distinguished four different categories of social interactions: informal social interactions, exchange of information, instrumental support, and collaboration. Instrumental support and exchange of information represent aspects of direct social support (Gerdenitsch et al., 2016). Social support can work as a buffer for the negative effect of stress on one's well-being (Cohen & Wills, 1985). Therefore, it could be possible that working in a coworking space leads to increased well-being in stressful periods, since the social support experienced in the coworking space could have a buffering effect on stress. Oldenburg (1999) argued that Third Places can enhance one's quality of life due to their characteristics, like being neutral spaces; acting as levellers (meeting people with different backgrounds); being sociable, accessible, accommodating, and playful (the less-official environment makes one relax, converse, and be friendly); serving as places of work, leisure, and socialisation altogether. Also, experts in the field of labour market research currently claim that Third Places provide mental recovery, community, and social connections, with a positive impact on employees' well-being (Gaskell, 2023; Mimoun & Gruen, 2021). For example, to transform coffee shops into Third Places – where socialisation and work come together – some studies indicate that ergonomic seating for short-term meetings, small tables, power outlets and online access, discreet acoustical atmosphere, warmer and dimmer environments, and diverse spatial layouts are important design features to consider (Curaoğlu et al., 2023). In Third Places, physical proximity, which is created by people coming together, can increase interaction and communication between knowledge workers as well as the visibility of leadership roles. Moreover, the spatial design of physical spaces can have an influence on creativity (Meinel et al., 2017; Phillips, 2017). It stimulates movement and then offers a supporting spatial structure for coincident encounters. After all, physical encounters and the resulting social interaction are the driving forces behind a resilient and supportive environment, and spaces designed for that will become increasingly important. In the study of Waber et al. (2014), it was possible to observe that performance was improved when chance encounters were created for employees both inside and outside of the organisation. Sociometric track-and-trace badges that capture interaction, communication, and location information were assigned to 50 executives of a pharmaceutical company and allowed data collection for several weeks. In the attempt to understand what behaviour of salespersons relates to their performance, the results showed that the person who increased interactions (by 10%) with coworkers from other teams also increased their sales numbers (by 10%). These areas, where unplanned and informal encounters take place, so-called 'places for collision' (Waber et al., 2014), are not restricted to the built environment. Examples of places for informal communication are smoking areas, elevators, vending and coffee machines, the bus to the office, the toilet, and the cafeteria. These areas can function as thresholds or transition spaces and can be important for interior planning as they offer great potential for informal and random encounters.

In recent years, well-designed architecture projects have already included places for unplanned meetings in the spatial programme or have already implemented them in the form of wide staircases for lounging, extensions of corridor zones, flexible and homely furniture in lobbies and lounges, etc. There are already good examples and products for all three places of knowledge work: the home office, the corporate headquarters, and coworking spaces functioning as a Third Place. However, planned workplaces and planned learning spaces that promote creativity, recovery, and well-being through unplanned exchange are usually found in the Second and Third Places, and it is precisely there where they only function if they have been designed to avoid disruption as much as possible. A good example is the Rolex Learning Center for Ecole Polytechnique de Lausanne – an undulating space built in 2010 by SAANA Architects, the Japanese office that won the Pritzker Prize in Architecture the same year (EPFL, n.d.). The project was designed to promote cooperation between disciplines, blurring the physical boundaries. At the same time, it serves as a melting pot for scientists, students, and the public. Through the connection of indoor and outdoor with roof-to-bottom glass walls, it allows visual contact with nature and outdoor conditions. This visual contact with nature and other positive distractions provide mini mental breaks (Ulrich, 1999) and support well-being and recovery from stress (Brown et al., 2013; Jo et al., 2019). However, the results of studies on the impact of spatial openness and transparency on recovery through communication and collaboration are mixed (Colenberg et al., 2021; de Croon et al., 2005; Engelen et al., 2018). Among longitudinal studies, the findings are also inconsistent. While Gerdenitsch et al. (2018) show that improvements in communication remained stable between the first and second measurement, the study of Forooraghi et al. (2024) confirms the findings from Haapakangas et al. (2019) that report a decrease in satisfaction with communication and the sense of belonging, three and twelve months post-relocation.

Almost as a matter of course, within the group of knowledge workers, creative people need a particular space for social interaction, concentration, relaxation, as well as recovery. How can they be encouraged and inspired to be creative and to interact with others? In the study of Weinberger et al. (2018), it was found that the creativity of entrepreneurs was influenced by processes and activities of off-work recovery (de Jonge & Taris, 2024) from stress, both physiological and mental. Including recovery practices during and after working hours increased their resilience in the face of stressful jobs, enhanced their well-being, and maintained physical health. Therefore, the space should not only provide stimulation and interaction but must also provide facilities for recovery, concentration, and exchange, as "good architecture extends and enhances human capacities" (Clements-Croome, 2006, p. 27). Of all these offers and interventions, which are slightly being proven to be helpful, the aspect of autonomy is the most interesting from the viewpoint of architectural psychology to explain the effects on recovery and well-being (Vollmer, 2023a, 2023b): the feeling of being able to freely choose one's workplace – one of the core demands of the New Work movement – seems to be playing an ever-greater role in mental health in our increasingly individualised society. Although earlier studies have also linked autonomy with a positive influence on well-being, job satisfaction, and work motivation (Deci & Ryan, 2008; Gagné et al., 1997; Ilardi et al., 1993), this aspect is currently not investigated in evidence-based design research on work environments.

A new perspective on designing hospital work environments: The HEMI architectural concept

While in many office environments, areas with and without customer contact can be clearly distinguished from each other in terms of function, atmosphere, and quality, the work environments in hospitals merge in many places (Lepik & Vollmer, 2023; van der Zwart & Pilosof, 2020). Areas accessible to patients and relatives and areas accessible to medical staff are neither structurally nor architecturally differentiated from one another, which causes medication communication process problems and affects patient safety (Liu et al., 2014). Undisturbed retreat areas are not present in the hospital architecture anymore, except for senior manager functions, while quick access to the outside space is scarce. This outlines an additional, hierarchical problem in hospitals: the lower the professional rank, the less space is available to the individual for recovery and concentrated work (Koppen & Vollmer, 2014, 2022; Peavey & Cai, 2018). The consequences are measurable in work-related burnout rates and decreased well-being (Haraldsson et al., 2024).

Long working hours (Kallus, this volume, Chapter 3; Wong et al., 2019), time pressure (Gohar et al., 2020), intense mental activity, work with patients and their families (Guo et al., 2021), responsibility for patient recovery and lives (Nazarov et al., 2024), as well as many other situational constraints define the job stressors in the hospital work environment (Rollin et al., 2022) and negatively affect employee health (Dall'Ora et al., 2020). The increasing financial needs of the hospital institution have increased pressure on the medical staff's performance, shifting the focus from health to productivity, a problem often discussed in the New Work movement (Starker et al., 2022) as well as in the earlier literature on evidence-based healthcare design (Ulrich et al., 2004, 2008). Work in hospitals is no longer limited to two professional groups of doctors and nurses. Scientists, study nurses, quality managers, psychologists, psychotherapists, and other therapeutic professionals now have a say in the interdisciplinary work environment in the hospital. The larger the hospital and the range of care offered, the more complex the collaboration and communication (Behrendt et al., 2009; Peavey & Cai, 2018). The interdisciplinary cooperation as well as the increasing quality and patient requirements, complexity of medical treatment processes, and clinical imagery are the characteristic challenges of hospital work systems (Fagerdal et al., 2023; Jelen et al., 2024). These challenges are increasingly becoming a burden for clinical staff, resulting in staff shortages and sickness-related absences from work (Bauer & Groneberg, 2013; Dall'Ora et al., 2020; Tamata & Mohammadnezhad, 2022).

To this day, healthcare work environments have been organised to support the individual work efforts of practitioners in various roles and disciplines who work primarily in their areas of expertise and attempt to coordinate with others by orders, notes, phone calls, pages, and other methods of individual communication. In contrast, a growing body of evidence demonstrates that healthcare work happens most effectively when practitioners work highly interdependently in well-functioning teams (for an overview, see Constable & Russell, 1986; Halawa et al., 2020). There is evidence that a team-supportive physical work environment, along with other factors, such as high autonomy, low work pressure, and supervisor support, positively impacts job satisfaction and burnout among nurses (Mroczek et al., 2005; Tyson et al., 2002). In a national study conducted on a large sample of US physicians, symptoms of burnout have been found to be 37.9% compared to 27.8% in the control population, with family medicine, general internal medicine, and emergency medicine professionals at greater risk (de Hert, 2020). Although systemic review reveals substantial variability in the prevalence estimation of burnout among physicians, ranging from 0% to 80% (Rotenstein et al., 2018), studies indicate that doctors who are mentally stressed or ill rarely seek help (Beschoner et al., 2019), although it has been proven that both their health is seriously at risk and the quality of patient care can be jeopardised (Wallace et al., 2009). There are four areas identified to cause stress in healthcare workers: work organisation, gratification crises, lack of social and professional support from colleagues and superiors, and misguided problem-solving strategies (Bauer & Groneberg, 2013). Systematic review revealed high levels of burnout, especially among nurses, and its negative association with poor quality of life (Dall'Ora et al., 2020; Khatatbeh et al., 2021).

To deal with the new and existing challenges, health economists as well as professional health and hospital associations have been calling for a change process in hospitals, focused on employee health and well-being, to begin (Halawa et al., 2020; Tomo & de Simone, 2017; Vollmer et al., 2023). There is evidence to support workplace interventions (reducing workload, enhancing teamwork and leadership, changing work schedules, clinical supervision) to reduce stress, distress, and burnout in physicians and nurses in hospital settings (Busireddy et al., 2017; de Simone et al., 2019; Panagioti et al., 2017; Romppanen & Häggman-Laitila, 2016; Ruotsalainen et al., 2014). Some of the evidence reinforces the idea of a participatory approach to improve nurse work conditions, such as tailoring interventions to the organisation and implementing iterative processes as intervention strategies (Paguio et al., 2020). Otherwise, there is a lack of evidence to benefit the work environment in hospital settings – especially when it comes to architectural interventions and workplace design (Haraldsson et al., 2024; Koppen & Vollmer, 2022). The majority of methodologically acceptable studies currently relate to selective, ergonomic interventions, such as the height of operating tables (Lee et al., 2014) or nurse station counters (Chanchai et al., 2016). Adjustments of this kind lead to significantly increased comfort and well-being, as well as better physical health (Chanchai et al., 2016; Lee et al., 2014). Only a few studies have shown a relationship between hospital work environment and staff outcomes (for a review, see Chaudhury et al., 2009; Halawa et al., 2020). For instance, Shepley et al. (2008) found that staff members working in single-family rooms of neonatal intensive care units were more satisfied with the physical environment, had higher job satisfaction, and had lower stress than those staff members working in an open-bay unit. Andrade et al. (2013) showed that healthcare professionals working in hospitals with better physical conditions feel more satisfied with their jobs and perceive the care unit as closer to the ideal, although no differences were found regarding stress levels in this study. One can assume that a good physical workplace might support healthcare professionals' health, recovery, and well-being, but it could also directly facilitate increased job performance. Furthermore, a positive physical environment for staff satisfaction will, in turn, positively affect their ability to respond to patients' needs (Tanja-Dijkstra & Andrade, 2018). Studies have shown that nurses spend less than half their time delivering direct patient care and a lot of their time searching for other staff, materials, missing meds, and supplies and also are frequently interrupted during their work to address these problems (Tucker & Spear, 2006). In one study, a hospital nurse was interrupted 43 times during a 10-hour period, including ten instances when the necessary materials, equipment, and personnel were unavailable (Potter et al., 2004). Nurses spend a lot of time walking to locate and gather supplies and equipment, almost 28.9% (Burgio et al., 1990). This came second only to patient-care activities, which accounted for 56.9% of observed behaviour in this study. Studies showed that time saved walking was translated into more time spent on patient-care activities and interaction with family members (Shepley, 2002; Shepley & Davies, 2003). Shepley and Davies (2003) also found that the subjective well-being of nursing staff increased in correlation with higher contact rates with patients.

In 2010, Koppen and Vollmer conducted a nationwide observational study in Dutch children's hospitals (commissioned by the Dutch Society of Paediatric Oncology) to identify criteria and properties that the hospital environment should have to support the health and well-being of patients and family, but also of staff members (Koppen & Vollmer, 2010; Vollmer & Koppen, 2021). A total of 200 doctors, nurses, and psychologists were asked in a structured online survey about their experience of stress in relation to architectural design features (layout, atmosphere, transparency). To date, the results have only been published in the mentioned Dutch research report. The results showed that the design quality of the hospital architecture always plays a major role in the experience of stress when two factors are experienced as particularly challenging: 1) proximity and contact intensity to the patient, and 2) interaction with other colleagues. Based on these findings, Koppen and Vollmer developed a new approach to the work environment in hospitals: the HEMI architectural concept. This concept defines five environmental categories which restructure the environment along task- and contact-orientated categories: (H) *hands on*, (E) *eyes on*, (M_{on}) *mind on*, (M_{off}) *mind off*, (I) *interact*. In 2014, the concept was adapted to the architectural design of the work environments in the new University Children's and Youth's Hospital in Freiburg, Germany (Koppen & Vollmer, 2014; Vollmer & Koppen, 2015, 2022). The five categories of the HEMI concept enable a profession-independent, needs-oriented categorisation of the entire work environment in future hospitals and directly respond to the psycho-emotional distress and cognitive demands on hospital employees:

Category 1: *Hands on* (H). Work involving patients in direct patient contact. This includes examinations, discussions with patients and parents, administration of therapies, care, and counselling activities.

Category 2: *Eyes on* (E). Work close to the patient, or 'keeping an eye on the patient'. This includes handovers, ward meetings, activities within the research framework (monitoring), and behavioural observations.

Category 3: *Mind on* (M_{on}). Work with a high level of concentration without the need for direct patient contact (but with the patient in mind). This includes case discussions, diagnosis, conferences, further training, documentation, leadership and management tasks, supervision, research, and teaching.

Category 4: *Mind off* (M_{off}). Recreational activities. These include informal conversations, withdrawal, the processing of difficult situations and feelings that arise, for example, when bad news must be delivered, as well as breaks from work, recovering exercises, walks through the park.

Category 5: *Interact* (I). Describes the activities within categories 1–4 that are performed either by an individual or in contact with colleagues. Strictly speaking, it is an additive category that differentiates the four previously named categories into work with or without interaction with colleagues and moderates the stress level.

Figure 5.1a shows the possible (re)combinations of the individual categories identified in the HEMI concept. The pie chart provides information on the contact-related demands of employees working in one of the four categories. The fuller the individual circle of the pie chart, the higher the contact-related stress. This means that while working in the *hands on* (H) and *eyes on* (E) areas the work is carried out in direct contact with the patient and is therefore ad hoc, the employees in the *mind on* (M_{on}) areas have the opportunity to reflect undisturbed on situations and cases and work on them in a concentrated manner. In the *hands on* (H) areas, all parts of the single circle are switched *on*. Here, the employee works with the patient, keeps an eye on them, and works in a concentrated manner. In the *eyes on* (E) areas, on the other hand, the third circle of hands is empty, that is, switched *off*. Here, as shown in the diagram, the level of stress decreases as there is no direct patient contact. In the *mind on* areas, (H) and (E) are correspondingly empty, that is, switched *off*, and in the *mind off* areas, (M) is also empty, that is, switched *off*. All patient contact–related stresses are eliminated here.

a) contact-related stress

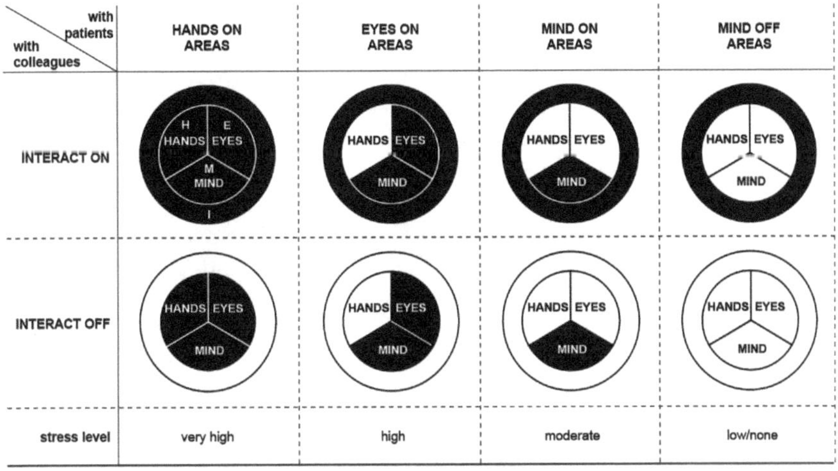

b)

spatial qualities	- closed - maximum privacy for patients - maximum efficiency for care and treatment processes - daylight - noise-insulated	- semi-open - immediate proximity (visual distance) to the *hands on* areas - maximum efficiency for other activities - indirect daylight - noise-reduced	- closed as individual or open as group workstations - 2 minutes walking distance to *hands on* areas - privacy between and for employees - maximum efficiency for concentrated work - direct or indirect daylight - noise-insulated or noise-reduced	- open - low-threshold, inviting - stimulation of dialogue and encounters or individual recovery - indirect daylight - noise-insulated - access to the outside
area and room allocation	- emergency room - treatment and examination rooms of the outpatient clinics - functional diagnostics - endoscopy - patient rooms (with restrictions) - day clinic	- nurses' station: front office - nurses' station: back office - waiting areas	- individual and group workstations - meeting, conference, and seminar rooms - doctor's office - service rooms of the outpatient clinics - back offices on the wards - training rooms - research areas, laboratories	- cafeteria - break rooms - informal meeting spaces such as bicycle garages, smoking areas, circulation areas, anteroom secretariat, lockers, changing rooms - - - - - - - - - - - - - - - - relaxation room "room of silence" porch garden, outdoor space

Figure 5.1 a) Schematic representation of the five categories of occupation-independent, needs-oriented work in the hospital ([H], [E], [M_{on}], [M_{off}], [I]) and their recombination (*hands on/off, eyes on/off, mind on, mind off,* and *interact on/off*). The white field describes the absence of the respective requirement (off); the black field, the presence (on). The cognitive and psycho-emotional demands increase from left to right, while the degree of interaction decreases from top to bottom.

Source: Modified after Vollmer and Koppen (2022).

b) Allocation of individual spatial qualities and spatial functions.

Source: Modified after Vollmer and Koppen (2022).

Focus group analysis ($n = 12$ nurses, psychologists, pedagogues, and physicians), as well as an online survey ($n = 354$ physicians between the ages of 30 and 60 years) of Vollmer and Koppen (2022), showed that room qualities and functions (room assignments) that address the cognitive and psycho-emotional stress and the interaction of employees can be easily assigned to the HEMI architectural concept (Figure 5.1b). Furthermore, there was no gender difference regarding the acceptance of the HEMI architectural concept. The specifically designed questionnaire based on Venkatesh and Bala's (2008) 'Recording the Acceptance of Technical Innovations' showed comparatively high acceptance values in three dimensions of the used acceptance scale: 'comprehensibility', 'willingness to use', and 'expectation of results'. The 'willingness to use' dimension was primarily attributable to the group of younger participants (YG), aged 30–45 years. For the 'usefulness' and 'relevance to everyday life' scales, the mean values for acceptance tended to be in the middle range.

In September 2024, the new University Children's and Youth's Hospital in Freiburg (Germany) was opened and became the first hospital to apply the HEMI architectural concept to its work environments. In a far-reaching study on the impact of architecture on social interaction and the well-being of children, parents, and staff, the German Federal Institute for Research on Building, Urban Affairs, and Spatial Development (BBSR) has been funding the scientific evaluation of the Freiburg concepts as part of a pre- and post-controlled trial. Since 2022, the baseline evaluation in the old hospital and the reference clinic in Munich are taking place (Vollmer, Deubzer, et al., 2024). The publication of the results of the rigorous evidence-based design research is expected in 2026. Figures 5.2 and 5.3 represent the innovative inpatient work environment of the Freiburg pilot as a result of the application of the HEMI architectural concept. In the schematic floor plan, a clear zoning of the inpatient work environment is created by clustering the nursing and medical *hands off* areas. In the inner, central part of the ward, direct work processes and short distances architecturally support team building between disciplines on the ward. As described earlier, numerous studies show that interdisciplinary teamwork contributes to the well-being of employees. A Norwegian case study even describes the formation of team relationships as one of four key factors in being able to adapt to highly stressful work situations in terms of maintaining mental health (Fagerdal et al., 2023). In addition, in the HEMI concept, each professional group is given its own service areas following their tasks, which are either *hands on* or *eyes on* areas and provide maximum support for concentration on the respective activity. The individual service areas are connected within a short distance (maximum walking distance of half a minute) and stimulate mutual exchange. The aforementioned walking distances and amounts are significantly related to nurses' burnout and, conclusively, to their well-being. The transition between the closed service areas to the open ones, shown in Figure 5.2, creates informal meeting spaces that also encourage dialogue and coincident encounters. The staff lounge forms the heart of the inter-professional encounter and is, at the same time, the common retreat from the *hands on* area. Being accessible from two sides, the arrangement guarantees equal use as well as maintaining contact with what is happening on the ward. All service areas receive direct or indirect daylight. Medical staff also has access to the outdoor area, enabling ad hoc retreat and recovery. A recent review of nine studies identified a selection of biophilic parameters specifically relevant to the building typology of healthcare environments. For staff's physical

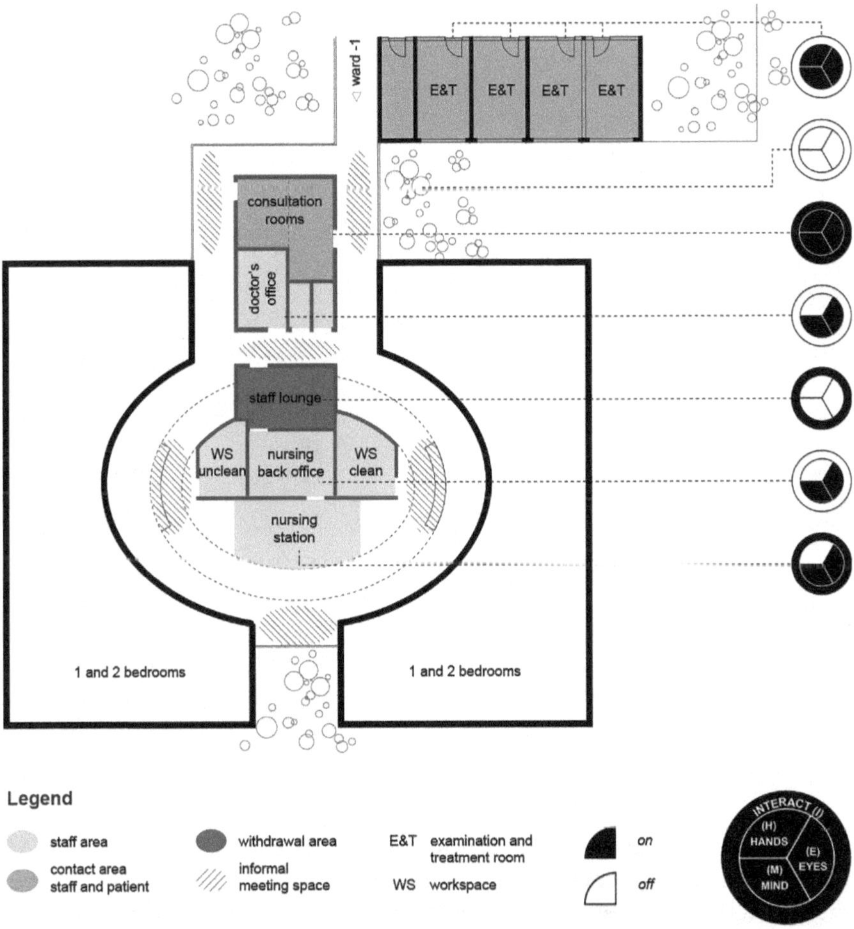

Figure 5.2 The application of the HEMI architectural concept to the ward design of the new University Children's and Youth's Hospital in Freiburg, Germany: an innovative inpatient work environment.

Source: Adapted from Vollmer and Koppen (2022); © Kopvol architecture and psychology.

and psychological well-being, outdoor privacy refuge and quietness were recognised as most critical (Tekin et al., 2023). Access to the care support point (*eyes on*) is separated for team colleagues and patients. This clear division of circulation flows structures and disciplines the communication and meeting processes. The hypothesis is that this architectural intervention in particular will make the complex work environment in the hospital less complicated and reduce staff stress.

Answering the needs of employees through architectural design and depictions makes it possible to reduce the scientifically well-documented high level

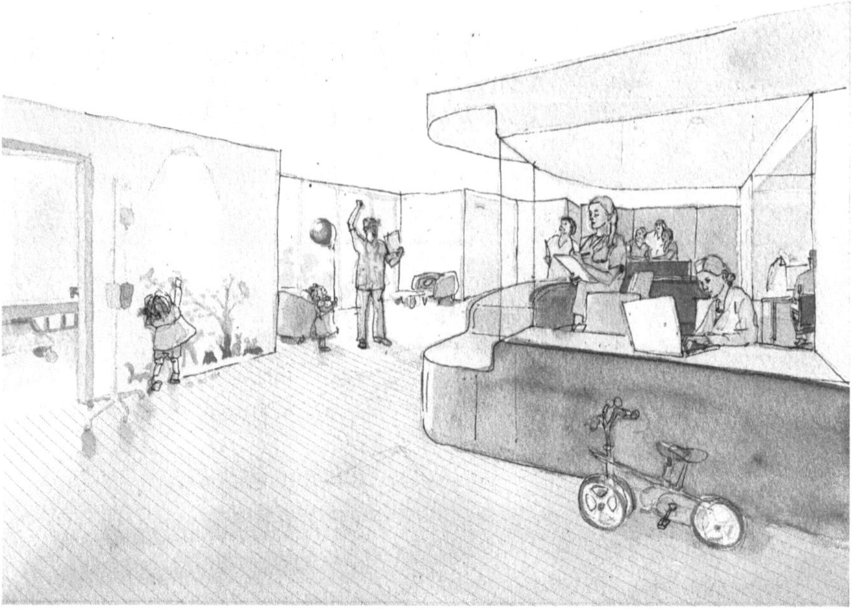

Figure 5.3 Impression of the application of the HEMI architectural concept to the ward design of the new University Children's and Youth's Hospital in Freiburg, Germany: an innovative inpatient work environment.

Source: From Koppen and Vollmer (2014); © Kopvol architecture and psychology.

of stress among medical staff linked to their working conditions. The HEMI architectural concept considers the degree of cognitive strain, emotional stress, and interaction with colleagues and patients when structuring the work process, allowing for recovery. It promotes social support both within and between professional groups through clearly demarcated structures. Studies have shown that the demarcation of care and other work areas supports the structuring of activities and contributes significantly to job satisfaction, productivity, and employee health (Mourshed & Zhao, 2012). Also, if there is a lack of opportunities for retreat and separately designated meeting areas, conflicts arise, commitment decreases, and the risk of overload increases (Leiter & Maslach, 1988; Shepley et al., 2017). The dual use of meeting room, break room, and workroom has been shown to lead to ineffective communication and constant interruptions to important work and decision-making processes in the long term (Chaudhury et al., 2009). The consequences are a lack of concentration, treatment errors, and excessive demands (Parker & Coiera, 2000). If, as envisaged in the HEMI architectural concept, separate work and compensation areas are planned, these also help avoid errors and exhaustion. In the compensation area, the employees who are very much involved in *hands on* activities are provided with sufficient space for concentration and retreat. These spatial attributes support spiritual and psycho-emotional recovery, a need particularly emphasised in hospitals where delivering bad news is also part of the daily work and routine for many. Because the HEMI concept provides for close links between the individual work categories and thus creates short walking distances, it supports the autonomy of employees. As a nurse or doctor, it is not usually possible to decide for yourself where to work at any given time. The unexpected urgency and requirement for constant emergency presence prevent this. HEMI-adapted workplaces, on the other hand, make autonomy possible and have a high potential to support employee relaxation in the future. We have already addressed this particularly interesting causal relationship from the point of view of architectural psychology in the previous section (Third Places).

Since 1970 to the present day, hospital architecture has primarily been geared towards supporting and increasing effective and flexible work processes (Hofrichter, 2019; Koppen & Vollmer, 2022). As part of this development, the needs of employees have increasingly faded into the background, while increasing demands and stress levels have been insufficiently addressed (Bräutigam et al., 2014; Simonsen et al., 2022; Tanja-Dijkstra & Andrade, 2018). Although evidence-based design that is based on robust studies is still in its infancy, we can no longer ignore the fact that the built environment in hospitals has an impact on employee health. That is why Kempny and Breimann (2020), Koppen and Vollmer (2014, 2023a), as well as other experts in this field call for a well-structured, pro-active, and balancing work environment, so that the multitasking required of many professional groups in everyday hospital life does not take place to the disadvantage of the actual care mission. It also gives architecture an active role in the process of improving and maintaining employee's health and well-being. The HEMI architectural concept offers an employee-centred solution aligning itself with the New Work values, as it supports the well-being of hospital workers with the need for interaction on one hand and recovery on the other. Above all, it brings out the maximum possible self-determination in a strongly regulated and operationally dictated hospital work environment.

Conclusion

The built environment is an important key to human health. It affects us through the perception and satisfaction of needs, for example, for relationships, safety, and autonomy, along with stimulation and regeneration (Koppen & Vollmer, 2022, 2023b; Vollmer et al., 2020). The effect of the built environment is particularly strong when we spend many hours in one place, as is usually the case at our workplace. Although the number of reliable studies on the interaction of workplace design and well-being – as part of the research field of evidence-based design – is still comparatively small, there are indications that certain architectural design features influence whether employees feel comfortable or stressed. These include spatial and design features for individual retreat and, at the same time, for chance encounters with colleagues or other work disciplines. Stepping out of rigid spatial structures and getting into contact with natural elements or nature itself also support relaxation and well-being. How these factors are to be translated into specific spatial and architectural solutions when designing work environments must be decided based on the specific work fields. Each field of work has its challenges that are linked to the stress experienced by employees and thus to their well-being and need for recovery.

In this chapter, two fields of work and new perspectives on their design were presented: the knowledge worker in the office, and the health worker in the hospital. For the office environment, the so-called Third Places, which have long been described, are being rediscovered. Third Places offer the opportunity to improve the recovery and well-being of employees, as they motivate people to change locations and allow them to choose their place of work and atmosphere. The resulting variance can help temporarily escape the feeling of being externally determined, controlled, restricted, still-standing, or rushed. In addition to this effect, which is more associated with withdrawal or escape from one space to another, contact with other people can be sought and established. Libraries, coworking spaces, cafés, airport lounges, and hotel lobbies are examples of Third Places. Their most important design characteristic is neutrality, that is, the built environment is not primarily occupied with thoughts of one's work. The perception of the architecture is not associated with the actual work task but with a place that is freed from this. They are low-threshold, are easily accessible, and have an atmosphere reminiscent of leisure activities: *everything can – nothing has to*. The latter is expressed in the lighting, the room climate, the furnishings, as well as the room layout, proportions, and individual decorations. At the same time, it must be ensured that technical requirements for modern, digital working, such as Wi-Fi, are met. However, Third Places do not necessarily have to be located a long way from the actual workplace but can also be realised in a specially designed area of an office building.

For the working environment in hospitals, the HEMI architectural concept offers an innovative approach, actively utilising the built environment to increase well-being and maintain the health of employees. The eponymous categories (H) *hands on*, (E) *eyes on*, (M) *mind on*, and (I) *interact*, according to which the work environment is reorganised, are derived from a nationwide observational study in the Netherlands. It found that task-bound proximity to the patient had an influence on whether, and to what extent, design features of the work environment were experienced as pleasant or unpleasant, and the work as stressful or relaxed. In addition, the effect was moderated when the doctors, nurses, and psychologists surveyed carried out their work alone or in contact with colleagues. From these initial observations, the researchers derived a concept in which the workplace designs are not based on who is doing or what is being done but on whether this must be done in direct, intimate contact with patients and colleagues. The more direct the contact with the patient and thus the experience of stress, the more closed, private, efficient, less-stimulating, and daylight-intensive the work environment must be to contribute to stress reduction and the well-being of employees. The more indirect the patient contact is, for example, during dictation, sorting, or typing work, the more open, stimulating, and interactive the work environment can be designed to positively influence stress and well-being. In line with the HEMI concept, there is already evidence that recovery and well-being are particularly supported when areas are available in which 'all categories are turned *off*'. This means that relaxation and rooms of silence, porches, or gardens should be accessible and can be reached within a short walking distance from patients. These spaces need to have a high design quality that is clearly different from that of a traditional hospital (white walls, institutionally closed facades, dark hallways, sterile interiors, etc.). The HEMI architectural concept was first applied to the design of the work environment in the new University Children's and Youth's Hospital in Freiburg.

In this chapter, we explained the resulting ward floor plan and its hypothesised impact on employees' stress perception. As the overworking of hospital workers has become apparent since the Covid-19 pandemic, at the latest, but has long since been proven in studies on burnout rates and nursing shortages, sustainable and reliable interventions are needed to counteract this situation. Including the built environment as an important component of workers' health is new and promising. However, this approach, which is being driven by the New Work movement, requires further in-depth studies. The German Federal Building Research Institute has therefore decided to support the scientific evaluation of the Freiburg pilot from 2021 to 2026.

Digitalisation processes, health crises, and demographic, economic, and ecological changes are not only affecting the current work environment in offices and hospitals but also, to a large extent, across the board, thus posing a challenge to the resilience and well-being of the entire society. Responding to these challenges with architectural design and actively contributing to the preservation of health, well-being, and recovery should be the most important future goal of the disciplines concerned. However, for the success of achieving measurable effectiveness of spatial-architectural interventions, it is crucial that designing workplace environments be based on scientific evidence.

References

Altgeld, T. (2022). New Work im Gesundheitswesen [New work in health care]. *Impulse für Gesundheitsförderung*, *177*(4). https://www.gesundheit-nds-hb.de/fileadmin/Publikationen/Impulse/impulse-nr117-web.pdf

Andrade, C. C., Hernández-Fernaud, E., & Lima, M. L. (2013). A better physical environment in the workplace means higher well-being? A study with healthcare professionals. *Psyecology*, *4*(1), 89–110.

Antonelli, P. (2001). *Workspheres: Design and contemporary work styles*. ABRAMS.

Appel-Meulenbroek, R., & Danivska, V. (2021). *A handbook of theories on designing alignment between people and the office environment*. Routledge.

Bauer, J., & Groneberg, D. A. (2013). Perception of stress-related working conditions in hospitals (iCept-study): A comparison between physicians and medical students. *Journal of Occupational Medicine and Toxicology*, *8*(1), 3. https://doi.org/10.1186/1745-6673-8-3

Becker, C., Soucek, R., & Göritz, A. S. (2022). Activity-based working: How the use of available workplace options increases perceived autonomy in the workplace. *Work – a Journal of Prevention Assessment & Rehabilitation*, *73*(4), 1325–1336.

Beckmann, J., & Kellmann, M. (2024). Fostering recovery and well-being in a healthy lifestyle: A concluding summary. In M. Kellmann & J. Beckmann (Eds.), *Fostering recovery and well-being in a healthy lifestyle: Psychological, somatic, and organizational prevention approaches* (pp. 218–222). Routledge.

Behrendt, I., König, H.-J., & Krystek, U. (Eds.). (2009). *Zukunftsorientierter Wandel im Krankenhausmanagement: Outsourcing, IT-Nutzenpotenziale, Kooperationsformen, Changemanagement* [Future-oriented change in hospital management: Outsourcing, IT benefit potential, forms of co-operation, change management]. Springer.

Bèoschen, S., & Schulz-Schaeffer, I. (2003). *Wissenschaft in der Wissensgesellschaft* [Science in the knowledge society]. VS Verlag.

Bergmann, F. (2019). *New work new culture: Work we want and a culture that strengthens us*. John Hunt Publishing.

Beschoner, P., Limbrecht-Ecklundt, K., & Jerg-Bretzke, L. (2019). Psychische Gesundheit von Ärzten [Mental health of doctors]. *Der Nervenarzt*, *90*(9), 961–974.

Bloom, N., Liang, J., Roberts, J., & Ying, Z. J. (2015). Does working from home work? Evidence from a Chinese experiment. *The Quarterly Journal of Economics*, *130*(1), 165–218.

Bouncken, R. B. (2023). *Awakening the management of coworking spaces*. Emerald Publishing Limited.

Bouncken, R. B., Aslam, M. M., Gantert, T. M., & Kallmuenzer, A. (2023). New work design for knowledge creation and sustainability: An empirical study of coworking-spaces. *Journal of Business Research*, *154*, 113337. https://doi.org/10.1016/j.jbusres.2022.113337

Branzi, A., DeLucci, M., & Sottsass, E. (1994). *Citizen Office: Ideen und Notizen zu einer neuen Bürowelt* [Citizen office: Ideas and notes on a new office world]. Steidl.

Bräutigam, C., Evans, M., Hilbert, J., & Öz, F. (2014). *Arbeitsreport Krankenhaus: Eine Online-Befragung von Beschäftigten deutscher Krankenhäuser* [Hospital labour report: An online survey of employees in German hospitals]. Hans Böckler Stiftung. Retrieved January 15, 2022 from https://www.boeckler.de/pdf/p_arbp_306.pdf

Brennan, A., Chugh, J. S., & Kline, T. (2002). Traditional versus open office design: A longitudinal field study. *Environment and Behavior*, *34*(3), 279–299.

Brookes, M. J., & Kaplan, A. (1972). The office environment: Space planning and affective behavior. *Human Factors*, *14*(5), 373–391.

Brown, D. K., Barton, J. L., & Gladwell, V. F. (2013). Viewing nature scenes positively affects recovery of autonomic function following acute mental stress. *Environmental Science & Technology*, *47*(11), 5562–5569.

Burgio, L. D., Engel, B. T., Hawkins, A., McCormick, K., & Scheve, A. (1990). A descriptive analysis of nursing staff behaviors in a teaching nursing home: Differences among NAs, LPNs, and RNs. *The Gerontologist*, *30*(1), 107–112.

Busireddy, K. R., Miller, J., Ellison, K., Ren, V., Qayyum, R., & Panda, M. (2017). Efficacy of interventions to reduce resident physician burnout: A systematic review. *Journal of Graduate Medical Education*, *9*(3), 294–301.

Chanchai, W., Songkham, W., Ketsomporn, P., Sappakitchanchai, P., Siriwong, W., & Robson, M. G. (2016). The impact of an ergonomics intervention on psychosocial factors and musculoskeletal symptoms among Thai hospital orderlies. *International Journal of Environmental Research and Public Health*, *13*(5), 464. https://doi.org/10.3390/ijerph13050464

Chaudhury, H., Mahmood, A., & Valente, M. (2009). The effect of environmental design on reducing nursing errors and increasing efficiency in acute care settings. *Environment and Behavior, 41*(6), 755–786.

Clements-Croome, D. (2006). Indoor environment and productivity. In D. Clements-Croome (Ed.), *Creating the productive workplace* (2nd ed., pp. 25–54). Taylor & Francis.

Clements-Croome, D. (2018). Effects of the built environment on health and wellbeing. In D. Clements-Croome (Ed.), *Creating productive workplace* (3rd ed., pp. 3–40). Routledge.

Cohen, S., & Wills, T. A. (1985). Stress, social support, and the buffering hypothesis. *Psychological Bulletin, 98*(2), 310–357.

Colenberg, S., Jylhä, T., & Arkesteijn, M. (2021). The relationship between interior office space and employee health and well-being – a literature review. *Building Research & Information, 49*(3), 352–366.

Constable, J. F., & Russell, D. W. (1986). The effect of social support and the work environment upon burnout among nurses. *Journal of Human Stress, 12*(1), 20–26.

Curaoğlu, F., Çobanlar, G. A., & Koyuncu, Ş. (2023). Interior design codes of coffee shops as the Third Place during COVID-19 pandemic: Z-generation and distance concept. *Sanat Ve Tasarım Dergisi, 13*(2), 350–367.

Dall'Ora, C., Ball, J., Reinius, M., & Griffiths, P. (2020). Burnout in nursing: A theoretical review. *Human Resources for Health, 18*(1), 41. https://doi.org/10.1186/s12960-020-00469-9

de Croon, E., Sluiter, J., Kuijer, P. P., & Frings-Dresen, M. (2005). The effect of office concepts on worker health and performance: A systematic review of the literature. *Ergonomics, 48*(2), 119–134.

de Hert, S. (2020). Burnout in healthcare workers: Prevalence, impact and preventative strategies. *Local and Regional Anesthesia, 13*, 171–183.

de Jonge, J., & Taris, T. W. (2024). Off-job and on-job recovery as predictors of employee health. In M. Kellmann & J. Beckmann (Eds.), *Fostering recovery and well-being in a healthy lifestyle: Psychological, somatic, and organizational prevention approaches* (pp. 24–37). Routledge.

de Simone, S., Vargas, M., & Servillo, G. (2019). Organizational strategies to reduce physician burnout: A systematic review and meta-analysis. *Aging Clinical and Experimental Research, 33*(4), 883–894.

Deci, E. L., & Ryan, R. M. (2008). Self-determination theory: A macrotheory of human motivation, development, and health. *Canadian Psychology, 49*(3), 182–185.

Engelen, L., Chau, J., Young, S., Mackey, M., Jeyapalan, D., & Bauman, A. (2018). Is activity-based working impacting health, work performance and perceptions? A systematic review. *Building Research & Information, 47*(4), 468–479.

EPFL. (n.d.). *The Rolex learning center.* EPFL. Retrieved February 1, 2024 from https://www.epfl.ch/campus/visitors/buildings/rolex-learning-center/

Eurostat. (2020). *Self-reported work-related health problems and risk factors – key statistics.* Retrieved February 1, 2024 from https://ec.europa.eu/eurostat/statistics-explained/index.php?title=Self-reported_work-related_health_problems_and_risk_factors_-_key_statistics

Eurostat. (2024). *Employed persons working from home as a percentage of the total employment, by sex, age and professional status (%).* Retrieved March 26, 2024 from https://ec.europa.eu/eurostat/databrowser/view/lfsa_ehomp$defaultview/default/table?lang=en

Fagerdal, B., Lyng, H. B., Guise, V., Anderson, J., & Wiig, S. (2023). No size fits all – a qualitative study of factors that enable adaptive capacity in diverse hospital teams. *Frontiers in Psychology, 14*, 1142286. https://doi.org/10.3389/fpsyg.2023.1142286

Forooraghi, M., Cobaleda-Cordero, A., & Chafi, M. B. (2024). Exploring the concept of a healthy office and healthy employees. In S. Emmitt (Ed.), *Building health and well-being* (pp. 5–30). Routledge.

Gagné, M., Senécal, C. B., & Koestner, R. (1997). Proximal job characteristics, feelings of empowerment, and intrinsic motivation: A multidimensional model. *Journal of Applied Social Psychology, 27*(14), 1222–1240.

Gaskell, A. (2023). Is 2023 the year of "third place" working? *Forbes*. Retrieved February 1, 2024 from https://www.forbes.com/sites/adigaskell/2023/03/16/is-2023-the-year-of-third-space-working/?sh=3cc742674778

Gerdenitsch, C., Korunka, C., & Hertel, G. (2018). Need-supply fit in an activity-based flexible office: A longitudinal study during relocation. *Environment and Behavior, 50*(3), 273–297.

Gerdenitsch, C., Scheel, T., Andorfer, J., & Korunka, C. (2016). Coworking spaces: A source of social support for independent professionals. *Frontiers in Psychology*, 7, 581. https://doi.org/10.3389/fpsyg.2016.00581

Gerlitz, A., & Hülsbeck, M. (2024). The productivity tax of new office concepts: A comparative review of open-plan offices, activity-based working, and single-office concepts. *Management Review Quarterly, 74*, 745–775.

Giannikis, S. K., & Mihail, D. M. (2011). Flexible work arrangements in Greece: A study of employee perceptions. *International Journal of Human Resource Management, 22*(2), 417–432.

Gohar, B., Larivière, M., & Nowrouzi-Kia, B. (2020). Sickness absence in healthcare workers during the COVID-19 pandemic. *Occupational Medicine, 70*(5), 338–342.

Groen, B. H., Jylhä, T., & van Sprang, H. (2018, September 19–21). *Healthy offices: An evidence-based trend in facility management?* [Conference paper]. Transdisciplinary Workplace Research Conference, Tampere, Finland. http://www.twrnetwork.org/wp-content/uploads/2018/10/TWR2018-Proceedings.pdf

Guo, Y., Hu, S., & Liang, F. (2021). The prevalence and stressors of job burnout among medical staff in Liaoning, China: A cross-section study. *BMC Public Health, 21*(1), 777. https://doi.org/10.1186/s12889-021-10535-z

Haapakangas, A., Hallman, D. M., Mathiassen, S. E., & Jahncke, H. (2019). The effects of moving into an activity-based office on communication, social relations and work demands – a controlled intervention with repeated follow-up. *Journal of Environmental Psychology, 66*, 101341. https://doi.org/10.1016/j.jenvp.2019.101341

Halawa, F., Madathil, S. C., Gittler, A., & Khasawneh, M. T. (2020). Advancing evidence-based healthcare facility design: A systematic literature review. *Health Care Management Science, 23*(3), 453–480.

Hamadah, M., Elseragy, A., & Eldeeb, S. (2023). Well-being as a tool to improve productivity in existing office space: Case study in Alexandria, Egypt. *F1000Research, 12*, 639. https://doi.org/10.12688/f1000research.133199.2

Haraldsson, P., Nylander, E., Jonker, D., Ros, A., & Josefsson, K. A. (2024). Workplace interventions focusing on how to plan, organize and design the work environment in hospital settings: A systematic review. *Work, 78*(2), 331–348.

Hedge, A. (1982). The open-plan office: A systematic investigation of employee reactions to their work environment. *Environment and Behavior, 14*(5), 519–542.

Helmond, M. (2021). *New work, transformational and virtual leadership: Lessons from COVID-19 and other crises*. Springer.

Hofrichter, L. (2019). Krankenhausarchitektur: Gestaltungsqualität und die Berücksichtigung medizinischer Ablaufprozesse sind [Hospital architecture: Design quality and the consideration of medical processes are]. In H. Stockhorst, L. Hofrichter, & A. Franke (Eds.), *Krankenhausbau: Architektur und Planung, bauliche Umsetzung, Projekt- und Betriebsorganisation* (pp. 137–154). Medizinisch Wissenschaftliche Verlagsgesellschaft.

Ilardi, B. C., Leone, D., Kasser, T., & Ryan, R. M. (1993). Employee and supervisor ratings of motivation: Main effects and discrepancies associated with job satisfaction and adjustment in a factory setting. *Journal of Applied Social Psychology, 23*(21), 1789–1805.

Jelen, A., Goldfarb, R., Rosart, J., Graham, L., & Rubin, B. B. (2024). A qualitative co-design-based approach to identify sources of workplace-related distress and develop well-being strategies for cardiovascular nurses, allied health professionals, and physicians. *BMC Health Services Research, 24*(1), 246. https://doi.org/10.1186/s12913-024-10669-x

Jensen, P. A., & van der Voordt, T. (2019). Healthy workplaces: What we know and what else we need to know. *Journal of Corporate Real Estate, 22*(2), 95–112.

Jo, H., Song, C., & Miyazaki, Y. (2019). Physiological benefits of viewing nature: A systematic review of indoor experiments. *International Journal of Environmental Research and Public Health, 16*(23), 4739. https://doi.org/10.3390/ijerph16234739

Kallus, K. W. (2016). Stress and recovery: An overview. In K. W. Kallus & M. Kellmann (Eds.), *The Recovery-Stress Questionnaires: User manual* (pp. 27–48). Pearson Assessment.

Kempny, C., & Breimann, C. (2020). Retention Management im Krankenhaus – Arbeiten im Spannungsfeld der Gesundheitsversorgung [Retention management in hospitals – working in the field of tension in healthcare]. *Gruppe. Interaktion. Organisation, 51*, 235–248.

Khatatbeh, H., Pakai, A., Al-Dwaikat, T., Onchonga, D., Amer, F., Prémusz, V., & Oláh, A. (2021). Nurses' burnout and quality of life: A systematic review and critical analysis of measures used. *Nursing Open, 9*(3), 1564–1574.

Kinsman, N., Marris, N., & Oakman, J. (2024). The impact of coworking spaces on workers' performance, mental and physical health: A scoping review. *Work*, 77(1), 61–75.

Knight, C., & Haslam, S. A. (2010). The relative merits of lean, enriched, and empowered offices: An experimental examination of the impact of workspace management strategies on well-being and productivity. *Journal of Experimental Psychology: Applied, 16*(2), 158–172.

Koppen, G., & Vollmer, T. C. (2010). *The child development supportive building: Design criteria for the Princess Máxima Center for Pediatric Oncology. Report.* Bilthoven.

Koppen, G., & Vollmer, T. C. (2014). Weil Experten Menschen sind! – Qualitatives Raumkonzept, Arbeits- und Ausbildungsbereiche: Neubauprojekt ‚Unsere Kinder- und Jugendklinik Freiburg' [Because experts are humans! – qualitative architectural concept, work and training areas: New building project 'Our Children's Hospital Freiburg']. In T. C. Vollmer & G. Koppen (Eds.), *Unsere Kinder- und Jugendklinik Freiburg. Klinik für Zukunft!* INITIATIVE.

Koppen, G., & Vollmer, T. C. (2022). *Architektur als zweiter Körper: Eine Entwurfslehre für den evidenzbasierten Gesundheitsbau* [Architecture as a second body: A design manual for evidence-based healthcare architecture]. Gebrüder Mann Verlag.

Koppen, G., & Vollmer, T. C. (2023a). The healing seven: Key variables of an evidence-based hospital architecture. In T. C. Vollmer, A. Lepik, & L. Luksch (Eds.), *Building to heal: New architecture for hospitals* (pp. 120–133). ArchiTangle.

Koppen, G., & Vollmer, T. C. (2023b). *Der Mensch als Maßstable. Architektur und psychosoziale Gesundheit im bezahlbaren Wohnungsbau. Bedürfnisse, Analysen, Konzepte* [The human scale. Architecture and psychosozial health in affordable housing. Needs, analyses, concepts]. Pabst Science Publisher.

Koppen, G., Vollmer, T. C., & Kohler, K. (2021). Designing urban health: The PAKARA Model. In ANCB The Aedes Metropolitan Laboratory (Ed.), *Human scale remeasured. New spatial requirements, societal demands and economic values in architecture* (pp. 172–174). AEDES Publisher.

Lee, H. C., Yun, M., Hwang, J., Na, H., Kim, D., & Park, J. (2014). Higher operating tables provide better laryngeal views for tracheal intubation. *British Journal of Anaesthesia, 112*(4), 749–755.

Leiter, M. P., & Maslach, C. (1988). The impact of interpersonal environment on burnout and organizational commitment. *Journal of Organizational Behavior, 9*(4), 297–308.

Lepik, A., & Vollmer, T. C. (2023). Hospitals as indicators of socially responsible policy. In T. C. Vollmer, A. Lepik, & L. Luksch (Eds.), *Building to heal: New architecture for hospitals* (pp. 8–13). Architangle.

Liu, W., Manias, E., & Gerdtz, M. (2014). The effects of physical environments in medical wards on medication communication processes affecting patient safety. *Health & Place, 26*, 188–198.

López-Cabarcos, M. Á., López-Carballeira, A., & Ferro-Soto, C. (2020). New ways of working and public healthcare professionals' well-being: The response to face the COVID-19 pandemic. *Sustainability, 12*(19), 8087. https://doi.org/10.3390/su12198087

Lusa, S., Käpykangas, S., Ansio, H., Houni, P., & Uitti, J. (2019). Employee satisfaction with working space and its association with well-being – a cross-sectional study in a multi-space office. *Frontiers in Public Health*, 7, 358. https://doi.org/10.3389/fpubh.2019.00358

Meinel, M., Maier, L., Wagner, T., & Voigt, K.-I. (2017). Designing creativity-enhancing workspaces: A critical look at empirical evidence. *Journal of Technology and Innovation Management, 1*(1), 1–12. https://ssrn.com/abstract=3051058

Miller, R., Casey, M., & Konchar, M. (2014). *Change your space, change your culture: How engaging workspaces lead to transformation and growth* (1st ed.). John Wiley & Sons.

Mimoun, L., & Gruen, A. (2021). Customer work practices and the productive third place. *Journal of Service Research, 24*(4), 563–581.

Mourshed, M., & Zhao, Y. (2012). Healthcare providers' perception of design factors related to physical environments in hospitals. *Journal of Environmental Psychology, 32*(4), 362–370.

Mroczek, J., Mikitarian, G., Vieira, E. K., & Rotarius, T. (2005). Hospital design and staff perceptions: An exploratory analysis. *The Health Care Manager, 24*(3), 233–244.

Nazarov, A., Forchuk, C., Houle, S. A., Hansen, K. T., Plouffe, R. A., Liu, J. J. W., Dempster, K. S., Le, T., Kocha, I., Hosseiny, F., Heesters, A., & Richardson, J. D. (2024). Exposure to moral stressors and associated outcomes in healthcare workers: Prevalence, correlates, and impact on job attrition. *European Journal of Psychotraumatology, 15*(1), 2306102. https://doi.org/10.1080/20008066.2024.2306102

Newport, C. (2016). *Deep work: Rules for focused success in a distracted world.* Piatkus Books.

Niebuhr, F., Steckhan, G. M., & Voelter-Mahlknecht, S. (2022). New work poses new challenges – the importance of work design competencies revealed in cluster analysis. *International Journal of Environmental Research and Public Health, 19*(21), 14107. https://doi.org/10.3390/ijerph192114107

Oldenburg, R. (1999). *The great good place: Cafes, coffee shops, bookstores, bars, hair salons, and other hangouts at the heart of a community*. Da Capo Press.

Oldenburg, R., & Brissett, D. (1982). The third place. *Qualitative Sociology, 5*(4), 265–284.

Paguio, J. T., Yu, D. S., & Su, J. J. (2020). Systematic review of interventions to improve nurses' work environments. *Journal of Advanced Nursing, 76*(10), 2471–2493.

Panagioti, M., Panagopoulou, E., Bower, P., Lewith, G., Kontopantelis, E., Chew-Graham, C. A., Dawson, S., Van Marwijk, H., Geraghty, K., & Esmail, A. (2017). Controlled interventions to reduce burnout in physicians. *Journal of the American Medical Association Internal Medicine, 177*(2), 195. https://doi.org/10.1001/jamainternmed.2016.7674

Parker, J., & Coiera, E. (2000). Improving clinical communication. A view from psychology. *Journal of the American Medical Informatics Association, 7*(5), 453–461.

Peavey, E., & Cai, H. (2018). A systems framework for understanding the environment's relation to clinical teamwork: A systematic literature review of empirical studies. *Environment and Behavior, 52*(7), 726–760.

Pensar, H., & Mäkelä, L. (2023). Roads to recovery in remote working. Exploration of the perceptions of energy-consuming elements of remote work and self-promoted strategies toward psychological detachment. *Employee Relations, 45*(7), 140–161.

Phillips, M. N. (2017). *Collisions: Room for creativity and innovation in the office* (Vol. 9). Cuvillier Verlag.

Potter, P., Boxerman, S., Wolf, L., Marshall, J., Grayson, D., Sledge, J., & Evanoff, B. (2004). Mapping the nursing process: A new approach for understanding the work of nursing. *The Journal of Nursing Administration, 34*(2), 101–109.

Propst, R. (1968). *The office. A facility based on change.* Herman Miller Research Corporation.

Robelski, S., Keller, H. R., Harth, V., & Mache, S. (2019). Coworking spaces: The better home office? A psychosocial and health-related perspective on an emerging work environment. *International Journal of Environmental Research and Public Health, 16*(13), 2379. https://doi.org/10.3390/ijerph16132379

Rollin, L., Géhanno, J., & Leroyer, A. (2022). Occupational stressors in healthcare workers in France. *Revue D'épidémiologie et de Santé Publique, 70*(2), 59–65.

Romppanen, J., & Häggman-Laitila, A. (2016). Interventions for nurses' well-being at work: A quantitative systematic review. *Journal of Advanced Nursing, 73*(7), 1555–1569.

Rotenstein, L. S., Torre, M., Ramos, M. A., Rosales, R. C., Guille, C., Sen, S., & Mata, D. A. (2018). Prevalence of burnout among physicians: A systematic review. *Journal of the American Medical Association, 320*(11), 1131–1150.

Ruotsalainen, J. H., Verbeek, J. H., Mariné, A., & Serra, C. (2014). Preventing occupational stress in healthcare workers. *The Cochrane Database of Systematic Reviews, 12*, CD002892. https://doi.org/10.1002/14651858.CD002892.pub4

Sailer, K. (2020). Covid will force us to reimagine the office: Let's get it right this time. *The Guardian*. Retrieved February 1, 2024 from https://www.theguardian.com/commentisfree/2020/aug/04/covid-reimagine-office-workplace-cubicles-hotdesking

Sander, E. J., Marques, C., Birt, J. R., Stead, M., & Baumann, O. (2021). Open-plan office noise is stressful: Multimodal stress detection in a simulated work environment. *Journal of Management & Organization, 27*(6), 1021–1037.

Shepley, M. M. (2002). Predesign and post occupancy analysis of staff behavior in a neonatal intensive care unit. *Children's Health Care, 31*(3), 237–253.

Shepley, M. M., & Davies, K. (2003). Nursing unit configuration and its relationship to noise and nurse walking behavior: An AIDS/HIV unit case study. *AIA Academy Journal, 6*, 12–14.

Shepley, M. M., Harris, D., & White, R. D. (2008). Open-bay and single-family room neonatal intensive care units. *Environment and Behavior, 40*(2), 249–268.

Shepley, M. M., Watson, A., Pitts, F., Garrity, A., Spelman, E., Fronsman, A., & Kelkar, J. (2017). Mental and behavioral health settings: Importance & effectiveness of environmental qualities & features as perceived by staff. *Journal of Environmental Psychology, 50*, 37–50.

Simenenko, O., & Lentjushenkova, O. (2021, September 16). *Advantages and disadvantages of distance working* [Conference presentation]. 18th International Conference: Perspectives of Business and Entrepreneurship Development, Brno, Czech Republic.

Simonsen, T., Sturge, J., & Duff, C. (2022). Healing architecture in healthcare: A scoping review. *HERD, 15*(3), 315–328.

Sliter, M., & Yuan, Z. (2014). Workout at work: Laboratory test of psychological and performance outcomes of active workstations. *Journal of Occupational Health Psychology, 20*(2), 259–271.

Spreitzer, G. M. (1995). Psychological empowerment in the workplace: Dimensions, measurement and validation. *Academy of Management Journal, 38*(5), 1442–1465.

Starker, V., Thies, D. R., & Frommelt, M. (2022). *New Work in der Medizin: Wie uns die Utopie gelingen kann!* [New work in medicine: How we can achieve utopia!]. Rossberg Verlag.

Tamata, A. T., & Mohammadnezhad, M. (2022). A systematic review study on the factors affecting shortage of nursing workforce in the hospitals. *Nursing Open, 10*(3), 1247–1257.

Tanja-Dijkstra, K., & Andrade, C. C. (2018). Healthcare settings. In A. S. Devlin (Ed.), *Environmental psychology and human well-being: Effects of built and natural settings* (pp. 313–334). Elsevier Academic Press.

Tekin, B. H., Corcoran, R., & Gutiérrez, R. U. (2023). A systematic review and conceptual framework of biophilic design parameters in clinical environments. *HERD, 16*(1), 233–250.

Teunen, J. (2021). Die Drehung zum Ursprung [Turning to the origin]. In C. Kohlert (Ed.), *Das menschliche Büro – The human(e) office* (pp. 21–26). Springer.

Thomas, K. W., & Velthouse, B. A. (1990). Cognitive elements of empowerment: An "interpretive" model of intrinsic task motivation. *The Academy of Management Review, 15*(4), 666–681.

Thoring, K. (2019). *Designing creative space: A systemic view on workspace design and its impact on the creative process* [Dissertation (TU Delft), Delft University of Technology]. https://doi.org/10.4233/uuid:77070b57-9493-4aa6-a9a5-7fed52e45973

Tomo, A., & de Simone, S. (2017). Exploring factors that affect the well-being of healthcare workers. *International Journal of Business and Management, 12*(6), 49–61.

Tucker, A. L., & Spear, S. J. (2006). Operational failures and interruptions in hospital nursing. *Health Services Research, 41*(3 Pt 1), 643–662.

Tyson, G., Lambert, G., & Beattie, L. (2002). The impact of ward design on the behaviour, occupational satisfaction and well-being of psychiatric nurses. *International Journal of Mental Health Nursing, 11*(2), 94–102.

Ulrich, R. (1999). Effects of gardens on health outcomes: Theory and research. In C. C. Marcus & M. Barnes (Eds.), *Healing gardens: Therapeutic benefits and design recommendations* (pp. 27–86). John Wiley.

Ulrich, R., Quan, X., Zimring, C., Joseph, A., & Choudhary, R. (2008). A review of literature on evidence-based healthcare design (Part 1). *HERD, 1*, 27–38.

Ulrich, R., Zimring, C., Joseph, A., Quan, X., & Choudhary, R. (2004). *The role of the physical environment in the hospital of the 21st century: A once-in-a-lifetime opportunity*. The Center for Health Design.

Valenduc, G. (2018). New forms of work and employment in the digital economy. In A. Serrano-Pascual & M. Jepsen (Eds.), *The deconstruction of employment as a political question: 'Employment' as a floating signifier* (pp. 63–80). Springer.

van der Zwart, J., & Pilosof, N. P. (2020). Evidence-based design for healthcare work environments. In L. Tevik Løvseth & A. de Lange (Eds.), *Integrating the organization of health services, worker wellbeing and quality of care* (pp. 245–262). Springer Nature.

Venkatesh, V., & Bala, H. (2008). Technology acceptance model 3 and a research agenda on interventions. *Decision Sciences, 39*(2), 273–315.

Vollmer, T. C. (Ed.). (2023a). *Architekturpsychologie Perspektiven. Band 1 Forschung und Lehre* [Architectural psychology perspectives. Vol. 1 Research and teaching]. Springer Vieweg.

Vollmer, T. C. (2023b). Withdrawal and privacy: In conversation with Beate Rössler. In T. C. Vollmer, A. Lepik, & L. Luksch (Eds.), *Building to heal: New architecture for hospitals* (pp. 186–191). Architangle.

Vollmer, T. C., Deubzer, H., Koppen, G., Kere, F., Niemeyer, C., Vraetz, T., Iovita, C., Kohler, K., Bauer, M., & Eggers, I. (2024). *Ren(n) wenn du kannst. Architektur und psychosoziale Gesundheit schwerkranker Kinder und Jugendlicher sowie ihrer Eltern im Krankenhaus* [Run if you can. Architecture and psychosocial health of severely ill children and adolescents and their co-admitted parents]. BBSR-Online-Publikation, 76. Retrieved September 18, 2024 from https://www.bbsr.bund.de/BBSR/DE/veroeffentlichungen/bbsr-online/2024/bbsr-online-76-2024-dl.pdf;jsessionid=F8720142A567FD4FDAA9C8CD81326CA6.live11291?__blob=publicationFile&v=2

Vollmer, T. C., & Koppen, G. (2015). *Unsere Kinder- und Jugendklinik Freiburg: Ein Krankenhaus für die Region, eine Klinik für die ganze Welt!* [Our children's and youth hospital Freiburg: A hospital for the region, a clinic for the entire world!]. INITIATIVE.

Vollmer, T. C., & Koppen, G. (2021). The parent-child patient unit (PCPU): Evidence-based patient room design and parental distress in pediatric cancer centers. *International Journal of Environmental Research and Public Health, 18*(19), 9993. https://doi.org/10.3390/ijerph18199993

Vollmer, T. C., & Koppen, G. (2022). Bedürfnisorientierte Arbeitswelten im Krankenhaus: Entwicklung und Akzeptanz des HEMI-Architekturkonzepts [Needs-orientated work environments in hospitals: Development and acceptance of the HEMI architectural concept]. *Gruppe. Interaktion. Organisation. Zeitschrift für Angewandte Organisationspsychologie, 53*(2), 225–240.

Vollmer, T. C., Koppen, G., Iovița, C., & Schießl, L. (2024). Therapeutic architecture and temporality: Evidence-based design for long-stay facilities for individuals with severe intellectual disabilities and challenging behaviour. *Architecture, 4*, 541–570.

Vollmer, T. C., Koppen, G., & Kohler, K. (2020). Wie Stadtarchitektur die Gesundheit beeinflusst: Das PAKARA-Modell [How urban architecture influences health: The PAKARA model]. *Bundesgesundheitsblatt-Gesundheitsforschung-Gesundheitsschutz, 63*(8), 972–978.

Vollmer, T. C., Lepik, A., & Luksch, L. (2023). *Building to heal: New architecture for hospitals.* Architangle.

von Vegesack, A., & Eisenbrand, J. (2008). *George Nelson: Architekt, Autor, Designer, Lehrer* [George Nelson: Architect, author, designer, teacher]. Vitra Design Museum.

Waber, B., Magnolfi, J., & Lindsay, G. (2014). Workspaces that move people. *Harvard Business Review, 92*(10), 68–77.

Wallace, J. E., Lemaire, J. B., & Ghali, W. A. (2009). Physician wellness: A missing quality indicator. *The Lancet, 374*(9702), 1714–1721.

Weinberger, E., Wach, D., Stephan, U., & Wegge, J. (2018). Having a creative day: Understanding entrepreneurs' daily idea generation through a recovery lens. *Journal of Business Venturing, 33*(1), 1–19.

Wendt, T. (2023). Sinn als Grundbegriff der Managementlehre. Die Neuerfindung organisationaler Beweglichkeit durch New Work, Purpose und Humanocracy [Meaning as a basic concept of management theory. The reinvention of organisational agility through new work, purpose and humanocracy]. *Gruppe. Interaktion. Organisation. Zeitschrift für Angewandte Organisationspsychologie, 54*(4), 557–567.

Wohlers, C., & Hertel, G. (2016). Choosing where to work at work – towards a theoretical model of benefits and risks of activity-based flexible offices. *Ergonomics, 60*(4), 467–486.

Wong, K., Chan, A. H. S., & Ngan, S. (2019). The effect of long working hours and overtime on occupational health: A meta-analysis of evidence from 1998 to 2018. *International Journal of Environmental Research and Public Health, 16*(12), 2102. https://doi.org/10.3390/ijerph16122102

Yang, L., Holtz, D., Jaffe, S., Suri, S., Sinha, S., Weston, J., Joyce, C., Shah, N., Sherman, K., Hecht, B., & Teevan, J. (2022). The effects of remote work on collaboration among information workers. *Nature Human Behaviour, 6*(1), 43–54.

6 Natural spaces for recovery from stress and for mental well-being across the life course

Matilda van den Bosch and Ingrid Jarvis

Introduction

Mental illness contributes significantly to the global burden of disease (Arias et al., 2022). The symptoms and consequences of poor mental health vary at different stages of life, presenting distinct challenges and opportunities for intervention and support activities (Dijk & Mierau, 2023). In this chapter, we will introduce challenges and environmental recovery and resilience processes, as they may vary across life stages, but also address the more general associations on a population level.

Childhood is a sensitive period when genetic and environmental factors can interact to shape mental health outcomes, such as Attention Deficit Hyperactivity Disorder (ADHD) or Autism Spectrum Disorders (ASD), but also the risk of mental illness later in life (Persson Waye et al., 2023). Early intervention and support are critical to mitigating the long-term consequences of mental health challenges in children. Supportive environments, such as green areas for free play, promote childhood mental health and development and can increase mental resilience across the life course (Hanson & Gluckman, 2014).

The transition to adulthood marks a critical life phase, characterised by increased independence and new responsibilities, in combination with hormonal changes. Young adults may be genetically vulnerable and face challenges like mood disorders, anxiety, or substance abuse, and environmental factors, such as air pollution, can impact the young, still-developing brain, resulting in impaired mental health (van den Bosch & Meyer-Lindenberg, 2019). An all-inclusive perspective is needed when planning settings where young people live to address the specific challenges related to a sometimes turbulent and stressful life period.

As individuals progress through midlife and into older age, mental health issues take on new dimensions. The *cumulative* effects of environmental exposures and life experiences, stressors, and chronic health conditions can contribute

van den Bosch, M., & Jarvis, I. (2025). Natural spaces for recovery from stress and for mental well-being across the life course. In S. Pauleit, M. Kellmann, & J. Beckmann (Eds.), *Creating Urban and Workplace Environments for Recovery and Well-being* (pp. 113–134). Routledge.

DOI: 10.4324/9781003435471-8

to distinct mental health challenges. In addition, factors such as social isolation, physical health issues, or the loss of loved ones may contribute to increased risk of depression and anxiety (Singh & Misra, 2009). Cognitive disorders, like dementia, are also becoming more common, and environmental factors can either increase the risk (Peters et al., 2019) or be protective (Paul et al., 2020). People suffering from dementia may be in particular need of recognisable, natural environments, potentially with connection to their childhood landscapes (Marshall & Gilliard, 2014).

Addressing the global burden of mental illness requires a comprehensive and integrated approach that considers the multifaceted nature of mental health and how it can be supported throughout life. In the following, we will discuss how the interplay between chronic stress, mental illness, and living environments can determine mental well-being. We will particularly address how contact with nature can be an important, protective factor, increasing resilience among individuals and communities and improving the capacity for recovery and thereby promoting mental health.

Stress, resilience, and mental illness

Stress can be described as a state where an organism's equilibrium, homeostasis, is disrupted. This occurs when available resources of an individual are insufficient to meet situational demands (McEwen & Stellar, 1993). The concept of stress was introduced by Selye (1936, p. 32) as a "syndrome produced by diverse nocuous agents". Sources of stress include environmental (e.g., noise), social (e.g., interpersonal conflicts), and individual (e.g., divorce) stressors. Understanding basic stress physiology is fundamental to unravelling the intricate relationship between stress, resilience, and mental health, as well as the relation to nature in this context.

Stress is a natural response to challenging situations and has been a necessary bodily reaction throughout evolution. The body's stress response system is primarily governed by the hypothalamus-pituitary-adrenal (HPA) axis and the sympathetic nervous system, which, when faced with a stressor, respectively trigger the release of cortisol and, as initially described by Cannon (1929), the fight-or-flight response through the release of adrenaline and noradrenaline (Kudielka & Kirschbaum, 2005). These physiological changes prepare the body to cope with the stressor by enhancing alertness, energy, and other adaptive responses, such as recovery (McEwen, 2007).

While the stress response is a vital survival mechanism, chronic stress can lead to dysregulation of the stress system, contributing to mental illness (Chrousos & Gold, 1992; Lupien et al., 2009). In early life, adverse experiences, such as childhood trauma or environmental stressors, can influence the developing stress response system, leading to long-lasting alterations in stress reactivity (Suzuki et al., 2014). In adolescence, when the brain is still maturing, chronic stress can impact the development of brain regions implicated in emotional regulation and cognitive functions (Eiland & Romeo, 2013). During adulthood, persistent stressors can contribute to mental health disorders, including anxiety and depression, by dysregulating the HPA axis and the sympathetic nervous system (Iob et al., 2020).

Since stressors are ubiquitous in every society, humans need to be able to adapt to various circumstances to avoid harmful consequences. An important factor here is how natural environments can help individuals recover from stress and also build and maintain resilience to various stressors (Wells, 2021; White et al., 2023). Resilience represents the capacity to adapt positively to stress, adversity, or trauma (McEwen, 2019) and is strongly associated with good mental health and well-being (Davydov et al., 2010). In the following, we will describe how nature can contribute to mental health by reducing stress and promoting recovery and resilience.

Theories of the association between nature, stress, recovery, resilience, and mental health

Natural environments are important spaces for mental well-being, potentially because of their role in the interplay between stress, resilience, and mental health (Figure 6.1).

The scientific exploration of the health benefits derived from nature arose within the environmental psychology discipline, and several prominent theories have been presented to explain the relation, several referring to stress and recovery from stress.

The concept of biophilia, initially coined by the American biologist Wilson (1984), describes how the human being is evolutionary-wired towards an emotional connection with the natural world. This connection means that humans are dependent on nature, not only for material and physical sustenance, but also for our intellectual, cognitive, and emotional well-being (Kellert & Wilson, 1995). This partly genetic attraction to nature would explain the universal appreciation of natural shapes, forms, and patterns (Kellert & Wilson, 1995).

The *Attention Restoration Theory* (ART; Kaplan & Kaplan, 1989) and the *Stress Recovery Theory* (SRT; Ulrich, 1986) stand out as foundational frameworks that collectively contributed to our initial understanding of the multifaceted relationship between nature, stress, and health through empirical studies starting in the late 20th century. It should be noted that this research was conducted in a Western science framework; within traditional ecological knowledge, the interdependence between nature and human health has been well understood for millennia (Finn et al., 2017).

The ART, proposed by psychologists Rachel and Stephen Kaplan, posits that nature offers a unique restorative experience, allowing individuals to replenish their directed attention capacities (Kaplan & Kaplan, 1989). According to ART, urban living and modern lifestyles often deplete our cognitive resources as we engage in sustained, directed attention, leading to cognitive fatigue and reduced performance in tasks requiring focus. Natural spaces, characterised by soft fascination and a more effortless form of attention, provide a restorative contrast

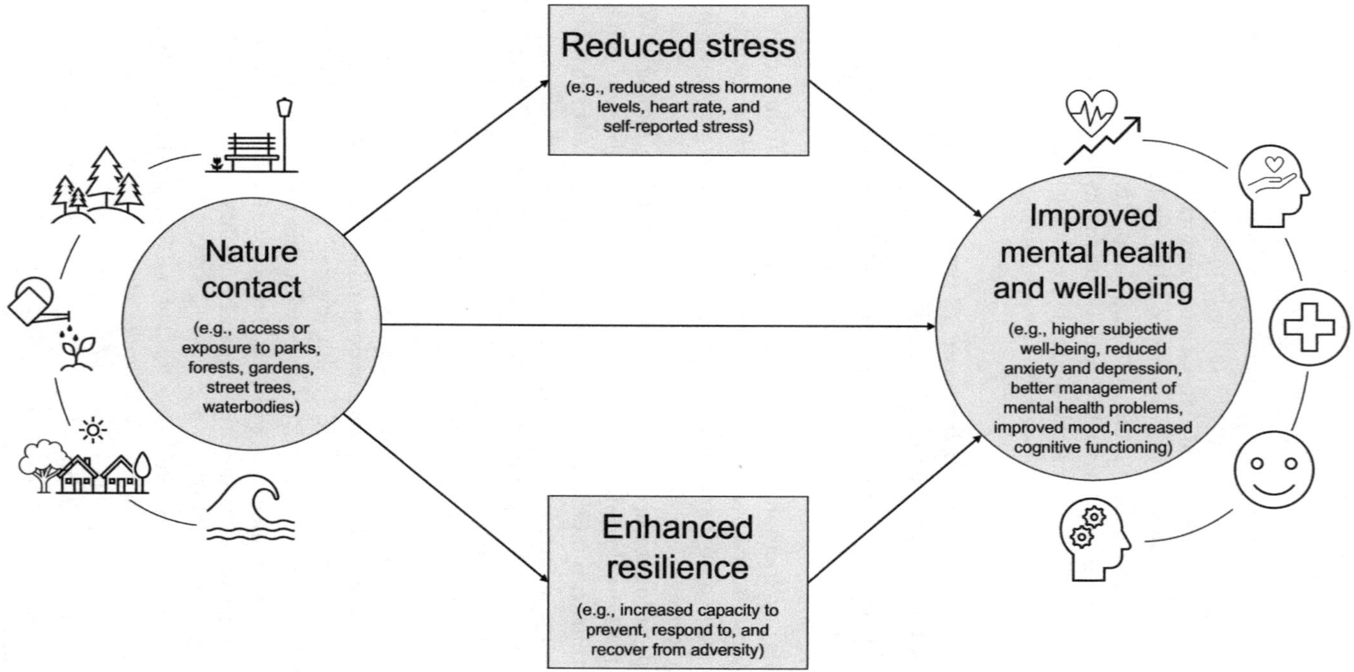

Figure 6.1 Conceptual model of the interplay between nature contact, stress reduction, resilience, and mental health. Various forms of direct or indirect nature contacts contribute to improved mental health and well-being. This improved health status may be mediated through, for example, reduced stress and/or enhanced resilience and recovery.

to the demands of urban life. Pioneering studies supporting ART found that individuals who spent time in nature exhibited enhanced cognitive function and increased attentional capacities compared to those in urban settings (Berman et al., 2008, 2012). Further research based on the ART demonstrated that individuals with depression reported improved mood following interaction with nature (Berman et al., 2012). Research following Kaplan's work also emphasises the importance of the perceived restorativeness of an environment (Grahn, 1991; Grahn & Stigsdotter, 2003), underscoring that individuals' subjective experiences play a crucial role in the restorative effects of nature.

The SRT, proposed by Ulrich (1986), builds upon the idea that nature has a stress-reducing influence on individuals. The theory partly refers to the biophilia concept and suggests that due to our evolutionary origin, exposure to natural environments can elicit immediate and automatic physiological and psychological responses that counteract the effects of stress. Ulrich's seminal study in 1984, which examined the recovery of surgical patients with views of nature versus those with views of a brick wall, revealed that patients with nature views experienced less postoperative stress, required fewer pain medications, and had shorter hospital stays. Subsequent research has reinforced the evidence for the stress-buffering effects of nature contact, demonstrating reductions in cortisol levels, heart rate, and subjective feelings of stress in natural spaces compared to urban environments (Kohlleppel et al., 2002; Parsons et al., 1998; van den Berg & Custers, 2011).

The *Biopsychosocial Resilience Theory* (BRT; White et al., 2023) is a recently proposed theory and framework that aims to integrate the concept of resilience even further into the nature and health nexus, emphasising the interconnectedness of biological, psychological, and social factors and how it shapes our responses to various stressors. Within this framework, the natural world is considered in terms of ecosystems, settings, and affordances, all of which affect an individual's contact with nature. The theory suggests that contact with nature influences resilience across multiple dimensions – biological, psychological, and social. This means that through nature's impact on, for example, the immune system (Roslund et al., 2022), our biological resilience increases, and nature contact can also enhance psychological and social resilience by, for example, strengthened happiness (MacKerron & Mourato, 2013) and altruism (Zhang et al., 2014). By building their stock of resilience resources through nature contact, humans can draw upon them at different phases in the cycle of stress response and recovery to help 1) prevent or reduce the risk of a stressor (*preventive resilience*), 2) reduce the initial impact of a stressor (*response resilience*), and 3) recover towards a new equilibrium (*recovery resilience*) (White et al., 2023).

An important aspect of the BRT is its consideration of feedback loops, meaning, that contact with nature can contribute to biopsychosocial resilience resources directly by, for instance, building new coping strategies, such as increased self-esteem (Marselle et al., 2019), but also indirectly by, for instance, leading to greater support for nature protection and more contact experiences.

This could potentially have important consequences for nature connectedness and how we relate to the natural world as a society (Alcock et al., 2020). The framework also highlights the potential synergies with nature-based solutions and the promotion of social-ecological resilience that can be deployed to mitigate climate change–related and other environmental stressors (*preventive resilience*) (Ferreira et al., 2022).

Evidence on human health benefits of nature

The research on human health benefits of nature contact has seen a significant rise since 2014 (Zhang et al., 2022). The literature indicates that natural spaces are perceived as more restorative than urban, built environments (e.g., busy streets, city centres; Menardo et al., 2021), and that nature exposure is associated with improved physical, social, and mental health across the life course (Yang et al., 2021). Within most research, nature has been understood as settings that contain green space (e.g., forests, street trees, gardens, parks) and/or blue space (e.g., ponds, lakes, rivers, coastal waters).

Researchers have demonstrated a beneficial association between nature contact and reduced stress (Kondo et al., 2018; Yao et al., 2021). A recent meta-analysis found that direct experiences from walking and sitting in and/or viewing natural settings (e.g., forests, urban parks, tree-lined streets) can lead to stress reduction, as indicated by, for example, decreased levels of stress hormones, blood pressure, heart rate, and self-reported stress (Yao et al., 2021). These findings complement scientific exploration of the stress reduction potential of *shinrin yoku* (i.e., forest bathing), which involves intentional immersion in forested settings for physical and psychological healing (Siah et al., 2023). Research examining virtual reality as a proxy for real immersion in nature further demonstrates that exposure to images and videos of natural spaces may reduce stress levels and increase restoration and positive affect (Frost et al., 2022). In addition to direct nature contact, observational studies using population data in combination with geospatial data indicate that higher availability of residential green space is associated with reduced stress compared to areas with lower availability. For example, a higher neighbourhood park area has been associated with reduced perceived stress among residents compared to those living with less surrounding park area (Feda et al., 2015), while a high residential tree cover has been associated with reduced allostatic load, a composite biomarker for chronic stress (Egorov et al., 2020). Nearby nature may further help buffer or dampen the adverse effects of stress on mental health and well-being and build resilience (Wells, 2021).

Likewise, green space is associated with improved mental health (Gascon et al., 2015; Houlden et al., 2018; Li et al., 2021). Research indicates that time spent in and interacting with green space through nature walks lowers anxiety and depressive symptoms (Kotera et al., 2021). Using brain imaging techniques, research has linked brief green space experiences to more stable (Joung et al., 2015) or even reduced activity (Bratman et al., 2015) in parts of the prefrontal cortex which are associated with greater relaxation and less rumination, respectively. Many population-based studies demonstrate that green space exposure is associated with reduced risk of depression and anxiety, as well as improved mental well-being, mood, and cognitive capacity (Li et al., 2021). Research also suggests that green space exposure, as measured by the availability, accessibility, and usage of green space, is associated with reduced prescription rates and healthcare expenditures for mental health conditions (Patwary et al., 2024). While most evidence comes from cross-sectional studies, a few longitudinal studies have confirmed a protective effect of living in areas with more green space on mental health (Alcock et al., 2014; Annerstedt et al., 2012). Studies employing a life course approach have further indicated that children who grow up in areas with high levels of overall green space availability are less likely to develop a range of psychiatric disorders in adulthood, including schizophrenia, mood disorder, and depression (Engemann et al., 2019). Similar positive effects of childhood green space exposure, as measured by neighbourhood park provision, have been found for cognitive functioning in adulthood (Cherrie et al., 2018). Finally, research has highlighted the health-promoting role of green space during the Covid-19 pandemic, with some studies reporting that green space exposure through, for example, residential surrounding nature, nature views, nature visits, and gardening was important for alleviating stress, depression, anxiety, and loneliness while improving mental health and well-being (Labib et al., 2022).

While research has revealed the health benefits of green space, what remains unclear are the differences in associations based on green space type and quality and form of exposure. Prior studies comparing the health associations of distinct vegetation types have generally reported more consistent health benefits for exposure to tree cover compared to grass cover, though findings are mixed and too few studies have compared the health associations of multiple vegetation types to make conclusive generalisations (Nguyen et al., 2021). Within our own work in Canada, we found that higher residential surrounding shrub and grass cover were associated with lower odds of poor mental health and self-reported common mental disorders, respectively, though tree cover was not associated with any health outcome (Jarvis, Koehoorn, et al., 2020). Conversely, we observed that higher early-life residential surrounding tree cover was more strongly associated with childhood developmental outcomes relative to grass cover (Jarvis et al., 2022). Beneficial health associations have been reported for green space accessibility (e.g., proximity to parks) and availability (e.g., quantity of vegetation in an area), though few studies have compared the relative importance of these distinct forms of exposure (Jarvis, Gergel, et al., 2020). In general, a limited number of prior studies comparing the health associations of these exposure measures have reported more consistent mental health benefits for residential availability of green space than accessibility to nearby green space (Amoly et al., 2014; Jarvis, Koehoorn, et al., 2020; Triguero-Mas et al., 2015).

While less abundant relative to research on green space, there is observational evidence linking blue space accessibility to improved mental health and reduced risk of stress, depression, and anxiety (Smith et al., 2021). Studies have demonstrated lower risk of poor mental health and depression among adults with higher levels of blue space visibility (Dempsey et al., 2018; Nutsford et al., 2016). Likewise, the quantity and proximity of neighbourhood blue space may be related to lower antidepressant prescription prevalence (McDougall et al., 2021). Compared to other settings, blue spaces are associated with greater perceived restoration and positive affect (White et al., 2013), though maintenance of good-quality blue space may be important for restorative quality. Furthermore, intentional visits to blue spaces for recreation have been associated with higher subjective well-being (Garrett et al., 2019).

Most research on the health associations of nature contact have focused on adult populations, while less is known about the influence on children, adolescents, and older adults. Among children, studies have reported that residential green space exposure is associated with improved well-being, better emotional, behavioural, and cognitive functioning, and reduced risk of ASD and ADHD and symptom severity (Davis et al., 2021). For instance, in our own research, we found that increased availability of early-life residential green space, particularly tree cover, was associated with improved childhood development in kindergarten children in Canada, including dimensions of social competence, emotional maturity, language and cognitive development, and communication skills (Jarvis et al., 2021, 2022). In addition, we found that prenatal residential green space exposure was associated with lower odds of ASD in childhood (Pagalan et al., 2022), and that children living in residential environments with high green space and low air pollution exposure had lower incidence of ADHD (Yuchi et al., 2022). Among adolescents, research suggests associations between green space exposure and reduced stress and depressive symptoms and improved positive mood and emotions (Zhang et al., 2020). Likewise, research has linked the amount of residential blue space to positive emotional well-being in children and adolescents (Huynh et al., 2013) and time spent in blue space to fewer emotional problems and more pro-social behaviours in children (Amoly et al., 2014). Studies indicate that nature exposure in schools, a setting in which young people spend a considerable proportion of their daily time outside of the home, may be associated with improved well-being, cognitive performance, and behaviour among both children and adolescents (Díaz-Martínez et al., 2023).

Research focused on older adulthood indicates that green space exposure, including gardening and park visits, may be linked to improved mental well-being and lower risk of stress, depression, anxiety, and cognitive decline and dementia (de Keijzer et al., 2020). Mental health benefits among older adults have further been shown for home and street views of blue space (Dempsey et al., 2018; Garrett et al., 2019). Nature views may be particularly important among older adults, given emerging mobility issues in late adulthood, and limited research suggests that nature-based virtual reality experiences may promote relaxation, positive affect, and social engagement (Sadowski & Khoury, 2022).

Several pathways have been proposed to link nature contact with improved health outcomes (Markevych et al., 2017). These pathways may be understood as mediators, which are intermediate variables that help explain how or why nature is related to human health. For instance, contact with nature may increase levels of physical activity and social engagement and reduce levels of stress and harmful environmental exposures (e.g., air pollution, noise, heat), leading to better overall mental health. Prior research has identified stress reduction as an underlying pathway linking streetscape greenery to mental health (de Vries et al., 2013). Studies have also indicated a mediating effect of stress reduction and restoration on the association between residential green space exposure and anxiety and depression (Dzhambov et al., 2019; Liu et al., 2019). Weeland and colleagues (2019) investigated the association of residential green space exposure on externalising behaviours in childhood but found no evidence of mediation via stress reduction. Beyond green space, restoration and stress reduction have been found to mediate links between blue space exposure and mental well-being (Dzhambov, 2018; Triguero-Mas et al., 2017).

There is a growing body of research on the association between nature and human health (Zhang et al., 2022). In general, the available evidence converges to indicate that exposure to nature, particularly green and blue spaces, is associated with reduced stress and improved mental health across the life course. These findings support the incorporation of nature in urban planning to create living environments that promote recovery and improved mental health for residents across all life stages.

Policy and practice

Urban planners have long recognised the role of urban nature for human health, with considerations of human well-being having motivated prominent developments, such as the Garden City movement promoted by Ebenezer Howard in the 20th century. As an alternative to the overcrowding and deteriorating conditions of industrialised cities, Garden Cities were small cities that planned for accessible nature within the city centre and limited surrounding expansion via a protected rural green belt (Howard, 1902). In recent decades, a growth of scientific evidence supporting a relationship between nature contact and human health has prompted renewed interest in the planning and management of urban nature to support public health (UNICEF, 2021; World Health Organization, 2017). Urban design approaches that focus on maximising the quantity, quality, and accessibility of natural settings have the potential to facilitate population-wide health improvements. Urban nature interventions, often called nature-based solutions, also provide social, economic, and environmental co-benefits, such as reduced crime and violence (Kondo et al., 2017), improved temperature regulation and reduced energy costs (Gill et al., 2007), maintained urban biodiversity and wildlife habitat (Nielsen et al., 2014), and increased carbon sequestration (Nowak & Crane, 2002). Many of these nature-based solutions result in human health co-benefits (van den Bosch et al., 2024), such as opportunities for recreation and physical activity, which prevent much morbidity related to sedentary lifestyles.

Roe and McCay (2021) describe key characteristics of green and blue spaces that should be considered when designing urban environments for optimal mental health and well-being. Their recommendations stem from characteristics of nature that may modify exposure opportunities and mental health impacts, including the amount, accessibility, type, visibility, perceived quality, biodiversity, and usage patterns of natural settings (Roe & McCay, 2021). Findings from our own research in Canada indicate that nature–health associations vary according to vegetation type, though there are no clear trends regarding which vegetation type is most consistently associated with health benefits (Jarvis, Koehoorn, et al., 2020; Jarvis et al., 2022). The heterogeneity in findings may suggest that a variety of vegetation types may be needed to suit the different needs of residents to support improved health. Our own work further indicates that the overall availability of nature in residential settings is more consistently associated with improved mental health outcomes than accessibility to nearby parks (Jarvis, Koehoorn, et al., 2020). This suggests that planning strategies should aim towards increasing the availability and connectivity of natural settings in residential environments for daily exposure opportunities, in addition to maintaining accessible public natural spaces. Cities can utilise this information to alter nature characteristics through the management of existing, and the creation of new, natural spaces. These planning strategies may include, for example, increasing tree canopy cover, greening vacant lots and schoolyards, establishing community gardens, greening grey areas, ensuring accessible transport to parks, and addressing aesthetic, cleanliness, and safety concerns. It is, however, difficult to provide specific design recommendations because of multiple and diverse needs depending on health state (Bengtsson & Grahn, 2014), but also on demographic characteristics, like age and cultural context and background. In addition, local ecosystem functionality must be acknowledged, and trade-offs between people's preferences and environmental conditions may occur.

Investments should increase urban nature across the urban landscape, with specific focus on design features for children, youth, older adults, and marginalised communities. Creating supportive environments for optimal development in childhood and adolescence is important for lifelong health trajectories, while age-friendly community designs help improve the health and quality of life of aging populations (Beckmann et al., 2024; Chu et al., 2023). Prior research indicates that the protective health effects of nature may be pronounced among lower socioeconomic groups (Rigolon et al., 2021), who are more likely to suffer poor health outcomes and have lower availability of neighbourhood nature compared to more privileged populations (OECD, 2019; Rigolon, 2016). Urban nature interventions may be directed towards marginalised communities while keeping the risks of green gentrification in mind, whereby an increase in nature provision may cause displacement of marginalised populations (Quinton et al., 2022). Interventions that are accompanied by policies that prevent socioenvironmental injustices, promote community engagement, and are tailored to local needs may help alleviate potential gentrification and optimise mental health impacts.

Examples of efforts by planning and policymakers to create and manage urban nature for both humans and ecosystems can be found across the world. In 2013, the city of Barcelona, Spain, introduced the *Superilla* (i.e., superblocks) project to improve the living conditions of urban residents by closing clusters of streets to vehicle traffic and providing public space for people to recover and socialise (Rueda, 2019; Figure 6.2). The superblock model explicitly addresses public health and sustainability and aims to achieve these goals by reducing motorised transport, reclaiming public open space for people, promoting sustainable mobility and active lifestyles, providing urban green spaces, and mitigating the effects of climate change (Mueller et al., 2020). As part of the superblock model, the local government has proposed the *Eixos Verds Plan* (i.e., *Green Axis Plan*; Ajuntament de Barcelona, 2021). The *Green Axis Plan* intends to increase street greening across the city to increase biodiversity and climate resiliency, provide ecosystem services, augment aesthetics, and reduce levels of harmful environmental exposures (e.g., air pollution, noise, heat). A recent health impact study evaluating the potential mental health benefits of the *Green Axis Plan* found that, if fully implemented, the intervention would reduce visits to mental health specialists by 13% and prevent 14% of self-perceived poor mental health, 13% of cases of antidepressant use, and 8% of cases of sedative use (Vidal Yañez et al., 2023). These numbers were obtained by comparing the green space baseline situation with the counterfactual *Green Axis Plan* scenario as of the Urban and Transport Planning Health Impact Assessment (UTOPHIA) methodology, which is based on a comparative risk assessment framework (Mueller et al., 2017; Murray et al., 2003).

In addition to landscape changes to increase the availability of urban nature, which are likely to reduce the risk of stressors and promote resilience and recovery, it is likewise important to consider interventions that encourage engagement with natural environments for stress-related and mental health benefits. Cities can support mental health, increase happiness, and cultivate thriving communities in numerous ways by promoting nature engagement. There are various examples from across the world, including Singapore, which has incorporated therapeutic gardens into its urban landscape, including spaces like the Healing Garden within the Singapore Botanic Gardens. These gardens feature carefully curated plantings and tranquil settings aimed at promoting relaxation and stress reduction (Singapore Botanic Gardens, n.d.). Another example is Portland, Oregon, USA, which is known for its community-focused approach to urban gardening and green spaces. The city's numerous community gardens provide opportunities for residents to connect with nature, grow their own food, and participate in communal activities, fostering social cohesion and mental well-being (City of Portland, n.d.). In Canada, the non-profit organisation Tree Canada is greening schoolyards across the country to facilitate connections with nature, enhance learning, and improve mental health among students (Tree Canada, n.d.). A final example is the concept of 'pocket parks' as implemented in Melbourne, Australia, with small urban green spaces scattered throughout the city. These pocket parks provide accessible opportunities for residents to connect with nature close to home, promoting mental health and community engagement (Victoria State Government, 2024). While these are just a few examples,

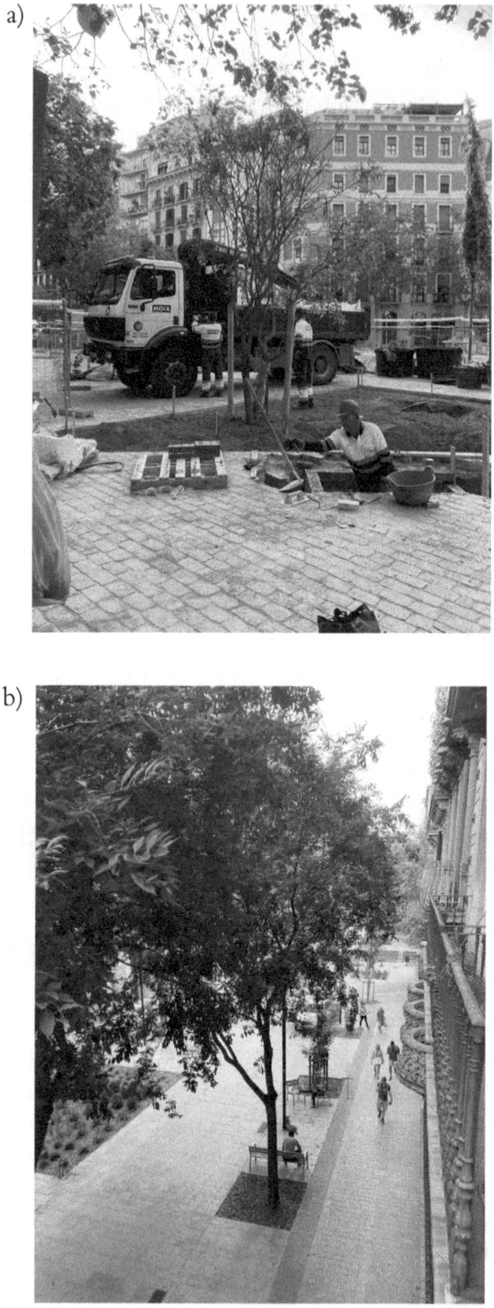

Figure 6.2 a) Construction of a *Superilla* (superblock) in central Barcelona, with greening of a previously busy street. b) People walking and socialising on a newly established *Superilla*. The street was previously busy with traffic, emitting air pollution, and opportunities for recovery and social interactions were non-existent.

Source: Photos by Matilda van den Bosch.

they provide inspiration for how green elements can be incorporated also in dense cities for sustainable and healthy urban landscapes.

Finally, nature can also work directly as an intervention and promote recovery from disease. There is growing interest around the world in nature-assisted therapy, nature prescription programmes, and green care (in short, nature-based therapies; NbTs) as a public health intervention that supplements conventional healthcare practices. NbTs aim to put people in contact with nature for improved health and well-being or treatment of disease and typically include planned therapeutic activities performed in natural spaces (Segal et al., 2021). There are a number of different types of NbTs, including therapeutic horticulture, conservation activities, nature walks, nature play, and social activities. The natural setting and activities of NbTs are modified to suit the abilities and needs of the patient or client. A recent systematic review with meta-analysis reported that NbTs are effective for various age groups, including children and older adults, and can lead to reductions in systolic and diastolic blood pressure, depression, and anxiety (Nguyen et al., 2023). Other systematic reviews have similarly reported improved mental health outcomes among NbT participants, including decreased stress, depression, and anxiety and improved well-being (Britton et al., 2020; Coventry et al., 2021).

With the introduction of new programmes and increasing uptake of existing programmes, an understanding of the evidence level for various health impacts of NbTs should grow. This will help in mainstreaming these kinds of initiatives as a critical complement to an often-strained mental healthcare system and increase the general awareness of the potential importance of NbTs to improve mental health and well-being.

Conclusion

Poor mental health is one of the largest contemporary public health crises, and mental disorders constitute more than 30% of the global burden of disease (Vigo et al., 2016). The aetiology of mental illness is complex, but we know that urban living (Peen et al., 2007) and chronic stress are major risk factors. By designing cities that promote recovery from stress and build resilience, we can therefore contribute to counteracting the worldwide epidemic of mental illness. While an accumulating body of research demonstrates the beneficial role of nature in creating healthy urban environments, we still need to know more about the specific components and elements that may be most beneficial for mental health. For this, longitudinal studies and experimental research are required, including analyses of structural and functional neurological reactions to natural features to assess the relative impact on mental health. Available evidence from brain imaging studies support a positive impact on brain function and a reduction of activity in stress-related brain structures following nature exposure (Bratman et al., 2015; Sudimac et al., 2022), but such studies need to be replicated in diverse settings, and more specific natural elements (e.g., vegetation structure and composition, biodiversity, quality, and usage patterns) should be studied to guide urban planning.

Studies should also analyse associations between specific nature characteristics and mental health across different life stages, since current knowledge is limited, in spite of the distinct mental health challenges across different age groups. In addition, research has primarily focused on high-income countries, and there is a need for more studies in low- and middle-income countries, especially since the Global South is where urbanisation is currently increasing the most, and we can expect a mental health crisis to further unfold in these areas of the world (Limenih et al., 2023). Addressing these limitations will be important for advancing scientific knowledge of linkages between nature contact, stress, recovery, and mental health, as well as contributing clear recommendations for policy and practice across different contexts and settings.

While a number of urban nature planning initiatives exist, policy and practice recommendations should even further address social, environmental, and health inequalities and target marginalised communities when implementing nature-based solutions, such as urban green initiatives or nature-based therapies. Through evidence-based planning of natural spaces, substantial mental health and well-being benefits can be obtained across generations now and in the future through recovery and resilience processes supported by healthy urban environments.

References

Ajuntament de Barcelona. (2021). *Mesura de govern Superilla Barcelona per regenerar Barcelona i el seus barris* [Superilla Barcelona government measure to regenerate Barcelona and its neighbourhoods]. Retrieved February 14, 2024 from https://bcnroc.ajuntament.barcelona.cat/jspui/bitstream/11703/123221/1/Llibret_SUPERILLA_MdG_A4_web.pdf

Alcock, I., White, M. P., Pahl, S., Duarte-Davidson, R., & Fleming, L. E. (2020). Associations between pro-environmental behaviour and neighbourhood nature, nature visit frequency and nature appreciation: Evidence from a nationally representative survey in England. *Environment International*, *136*, 105441. https://doi.org/10.1016/j.envint.2019.105441

Alcock, I., White, M. P., Wheeler, B. W., Fleming, L. E., & Depledge, M. H. (2014). Longitudinal effects on mental health of moving to greener and less green urban areas. *Environmental Science & Technology*, *48*(2), 1247–1255.

Amoly, E., Dadvand, P., Forns, J., López-Vicente, M., Basagaña, X., Julvez, J., Alvarez-Pedrerol, M., Nieuwenhuijsen, M. J., & Sunyer, J. (2014). Green and blue spaces and behavioral development in Barcelona schoolchildren: The BREATHE project. *Environmental Health Perspectives*, *122*(12), 1351–1358.

Annerstedt, M., Östergren, P. O., Björk, J., Grahn, P., Skärbäck, E., & Währborg, P. (2012). Green qualities in the neighbourhood and mental health – results from a longitudinal cohort study in Southern Sweden. *BMC Public Health*, *12*, 337. https://doi.org/10.1186/1471-2458-12-337

Arias, D., Saxena, S., & Verguet, S. (2022). Quantifying the global burden of mental disorders and their economic value. *eClinicalMedicine*, *54*, 101675. https://doi.org/10.1016/j.eclinm.2022.101675

Beckmann, J., Huber, M., & Andonian-Dierks, C. S. (2024). Chronic illness and well-being: Promoting quality of life with broadened concept of recovery. In M. Kellmann & J. Beckmann (Eds.), *Fostering recovery and well-being in a healthy lifestyle: Psychological, somatic, and organizational prevention approaches* (pp. 3–23). Routledge.

Bengtsson, A., & Grahn, P. (2014). Outdoor environments in healthcare settings: A quality evaluation tool for use in designing healthcare gardens. *Urban Forestry & Urban Greening, 13*(4), 878–891.

Berman, M. G., Jonides, J., & Kaplan, S. (2008). The cognitive benefits of interacting with nature. *Psychological Science, 19*(12), 1207–1212.

Berman, M. G., Kross, E., Krpan, K. M., Askren, M. K., Burson, A., Deldin, P. J., Kaplan, S., Sherdell, L., Gotlib, I. H., & Jonides, J. (2012). Interacting with nature improves cognition and affect for individuals with depression. *Journal of Affective Disorders, 140*(3), 300–305.

Bratman, G. N., Hamilton, J. P., Hahn, K. S., Daily, G. C., & Gross, J. J. (2015). Nature experience reduces rumination and subgenual prefrontal cortex activation. *Proceedings of the National Academy of Sciences of the United States of America, 112*(28), 8567–8572.

Britton, E., Kindermann, G., Domegan, C., & Carlin, C. (2020). Blue care: A systematic review of blue space interventions for health and wellbeing. *Health Promotion International, 35*(1), 50–69.

Cannon, W. B. (1929). *Bodily changes in pain, hunger, fear and rage.* D Appleton & Company.

Cherrie, M. P. C., Shortt, N. K., Mitchell, R. J., Taylor, A. M., Redmond, P., Thompson, C. W., Starr, J. M., Deary, I. J., & Pearce, J. R. (2018). Green space and cognitive ageing: A retrospective life course analysis in the Lothian Birth Cohort 1936. *Social Science & Medicine, 196*, 56–65.

Chrousos, G. P., & Gold, P. W. (1992). The concepts of stress and stress system disorders. Overview of physical and behavioral homeostasis. *Journal of the American Medical Association, 267*(9), 1244–1252.

Chu, T. L., Harmison, R. J., & Martin, S. B. (2023). Quality of life and recovery. In M. Kellmann, S. Jakowski, & J. Beckmann (Eds.), *The important of recovery for physical and mental health: Negotiating the effects of underrecovery* (pp. 84–100). Routledge.

City of Portland. (n.d.). *Community gardens.* Retrieved April 10, 2024 from https://www.portland.gov/parks/community-gardens

Coventry, P. A., Brown, J. E., Pervin, J., Brabyn, S., Pateman, R., Breedvelt, J., Gilbody, S., Stancliffe, R., McEachan, R., & White, P. L. (2021). Nature-based outdoor activities for mental and physical health: Systematic review and meta-analysis. *SSM – Population Health, 16*, 100934. https://doi.org/10.1016/j.ssmph.2021.100934

Davis, Z., Guhn, M., Jarvis, I., Jerrett, M., Nesbitt, L., Oberlander, T., Sbihi, H., Su, J., & van den Bosch, M. (2021). The association between natural environments and childhood mental health and development: A systematic review and assessment of different exposure measurements. *International Journal of Hygiene and Environmental Health, 235*, 113767. https://doi.org/10.1016/j.ijheh.2021.113767

Davydov, D. M., Stewart, R., Ritchie, K., & Chaudieu, I. (2010). Resilience and mental health. *Clinical Psychology Review, 30*(5), 479–495.

de Keijzer, C., Bauwelinck, M., & Dadvand, P. (2020). Long-term exposure to residential greenspace and healthy ageing: A systematic review. *Current Environmental Health Reports*, 7(1), 65–88.

de Vries, S., van Dillen, S. M. E., Groenewegen, P. P., & Spreeuwenberg, P. (2013). Streetscape greenery and health: Stress, social cohesion and physical activity as mediators. *Social Science & Medicine, 94*, 26–33.

Dempsey, S., Devine, M. T., Gillespie, T., Lyons, S., & Nolan, A. (2018). Coastal blue space and depression in older adults. *Health & Place, 54*, 110–117.

Díaz-Martínez, F., Sánchez-Sauco, M. F., Cabrera-Rivera, L. T., Sánchez, C. O., Hidalgo-Albadalejo, M. D., Claudio, L., & Ortega-García, J. A. (2023). Systematic review: Neurodevelopmental benefits of active/passive school exposure to green and/or blue spaces in children and adolescents. *International Journal of Environmental Research and Public Health, 20*(5), 3958. https://doi.org/10.3390/IJERPH20053958

Dijk, H., & Mierau, J. (2023). Mental health over the life course: Evidence for a U-shape? *Health Economics, 32*(1), 155–174.

Dzhambov, A. M. (2018). Residential green and blue space associated with better mental health: A pilot follow-up study in university students. *Archives of Industrial Hygiene and Toxicology, 69*(4), 340–349.

Dzhambov, A. M., Hartig, T., Tilov, B., Atanasova, V., Makakova, D. R., & Dimitrova, D. D. (2019). Residential greenspace is associated with mental health via intertwined capacity-building and capacity-restoring pathways. *Environmental Research, 178*, 108708. https://doi.org/10.1016/j.envres.2019.108708

Egorov, A. I., Griffin, S. M., Converse, R. R., Styles, J. N., Klein, E., Scott, J., Sams, E. A., Hudgens, E. E., & Wade, T. J. (2020). Greater tree cover near residence is associated with reduced allostatic load in residents of central North Carolina. *Environmental Research, 186*, 109435. https://doi.org/10.1016/j.envres.2020.109435

Eiland, L., & Romeo, R. D. (2013). Stress and the developing adolescent brain. *Neuroscience, 249*, 162–171.

Engemann, K., Pedersen, C. B., Arge, L., Tsirogiannis, C., Mortensen, P. B., & Svenning, J. C. (2019). Residential green space in childhood is associated with lower risk of psychiatric disorders from adolescence into adulthood. *Proceedings of the National Academy of Sciences of the United States of America, 116*(11), 5188–5193.

Feda, D. M., Seelbinder, A., Baek, S., Raja, S., Yin, L., & Roemmich, J. N. (2015). Neighborhood parks and reduction in stress among adolescents: Results from Buffalo, New York. *Indoor and Built Environment, 24*(5), 631–639.

Ferreira, V., Barreira, A. P., Pinto, P., & Panagopoulos, T. (2022). Understanding attitudes towards the adoption of nature-based solutions and policy priorities shaped by stakeholders' awareness of climate change. *Environmental Science & Policy, 131*, 149–159.

Finn, S., Herne, M., & Castille, D. (2017). The value of traditional ecological knowledge for the environmental health sciences and biomedical research. *Environmental Health Perspectives, 125*(8), 085006. https://doi.org/10.1289/ehp858

Frost, S., Kannis-Dymand, L., Schaffer, V., Millear, P., Allen, A., Stallman, H., Mason, J., Wood, A., & Atkinson-Nolte, J. (2022). Virtual immersion in nature and psychological well-being: A systematic literature review. *Journal of Environmental Psychology, 80*, 101765. https://doi.org/10.1016/j.jenvp.2022.101765

Garrett, J. K., White, M. P., Huang, J., Ng, S., Hui, Z., Leung, C., Tse, L. A., Fung, F., Elliott, L. R., Depledge, M. H., & Wong, M. C. S. (2019). Urban blue space and health and wellbeing in Hong Kong: Results from a survey of older adults. *Health & Place, 55*, 100–110.

Gascon, M., Triguero-Mas, M., Martínez, D., Dadvand, P., Forns, J., Plasència, A., & Nieuwenhuijsen, M. J. (2015). Mental health benefits of long-term exposure to residential green and blue spaces: A systematic review. *International Journal of Environmental Research and Public Health, 12*(4), 4354–4379.

Gill, S. E., Handley, J. F., Ennos, A. R., & Pauleit, S. (2007). Adapting cities for climate change: The role of the green infrastructure. *Built Environment, 33*(1), 115–133.

Grahn, P. (1991). Landscapes in our minds: People's choice of recreative places in towns. *Landscape Research, 16*(1), 11–19.

Grahn, P., & Stigsdotter, U. (2003). Landscape planning and stress. *Urban Forestry & Urban Greening, 2*(1), 1–18.

Hanson, M. A., & Gluckman, P. D. (2014). Early developmental conditioning of later health and disease: Physiology or pathophysiology? *Physiological Reviews, 94*(4), 1027–1076.

Houlden, V., Weich, S., Porto de Albuquerque, J., Jarvis, S., & Rees, K. (2018). The relationship between greenspace and the mental wellbeing of adults: A systematic review. *PLoS One, 13*(9), e0203000. https://doi.org/10.1371/journal.pone.0203000

Howard, E. (1902). *Garden cities of to-morrow*. Swan Sonnenschein & Co.

Huynh, Q., Craig, W., Janssen, I., & Pickett, W. (2013). Exposure to public natural space as a protective factor for emotional well-being among young people in Canada. *BMC Public Health, 13*, 407. https://doi.org/10.1186/1471-2458-13-407

Iob, E., Kirschbaum, C., & Steptoe, A. (2020). Persistent depressive symptoms, HPA-axis hyperactivity, and inflammation: The role of cognitive-affective and somatic symptoms. *Molecular Psychiatry, 25*(5), 1130–1140.

Jarvis, I., Davis, Z., Sbihi, H., Brauer, M., Czekajlo, A., Davies, H. W., Gergel, S. E., Guhn, M., Jerrett, M., Koehoorn, M., Oberlander, T. F., Su, J., & van den Bosch, M. (2021). Assessing the association between lifetime exposure to greenspace and early childhood development and the mediation effects of air pollution and noise in Canada: A population-based birth cohort study. *The Lancet Planetary Health, 5*(10), e709–e717.

Jarvis, I., Gergel, S., Koehoorn, M., & van den Bosch, M. (2020). Greenspace access does not correspond to nature exposure: Measures of urban natural space with implications for health research. *Landscape and Urban Planning, 194*, 103686. https://doi.org/10.1016/j.landurbplan.2019.103686

Jarvis, I., Koehoorn, M., Gergel, S. E., & van den Bosch, M. (2020). Different types of urban natural environments influence various dimensions of self-reported health. *Environmental Research, 186*, 109614. https://doi.org/10.1016/j.envres.2020.109614

Jarvis, I., Sbihi, H., Davis, Z., Brauer, M., Czekajlo, A., Davies, H. W., Gergel, S. E., Guhn, M., Jerrett, M., Koehoorn, M., Nesbitt, L., Oberlander, T. F., Su, J., & van den Bosch, M. (2022). The influence of early-life residential exposure to different vegetation types and paved surfaces on early childhood development: A population-based birth cohort study. *Environment International, 163*, 107196. https://doi.org/10.1016/j.envint.2022.107196

Joung, D., Kim, G., Choi, Y., Lim, H., Park, S., Woo, J. M., & Park, B. J. (2015). The prefrontal cortex activity and psychological effects of viewing forest landscapes in autumn season. *International Journal of Environmental Research and Public Health, 12*(7), 7235–7243.

Kaplan, R., & Kaplan, S. (1989). *The experience of nature: A psychological perspective*. Cambridge University Press.

Kellert, S., & Wilson, E. (1995). *The biophilia hypothesis*. Island Press.

Kohlleppel, T., Bradley, J. C., & Jacob, S. (2002). A walk through the garden: Can a visit to a botanic garden reduce stress? *HortTechnology, 12*(3), 489–492.

Kondo, M. C., Han, S. H., Donovan, G. H., & MacDonald, J. M. (2017). The association between urban trees and crime: Evidence from the spread of the emerald ash borer in Cincinnati. *Landscape and Urban Planning, 157*, 193–199.

Kondo, M. C., Jacoby, S. F., & South, E. C. (2018). Does spending time outdoors reduce stress? A review of real-time stress response to outdoor environments. *Health & Place, 51*, 136–150.

Kotera, Y., Lyons, M., Vione, K. C., & Norton, B. (2021). Effect of nature walks on depression and anxiety: A systematic review. *Sustainability*, *13*(7), 4015. https://doi.org/10.3390/su13074015

Kudielka, B. M., & Kirschbaum, C. (2005). Sex differences in HPA axis responses to stress: A review. *Biological Psychology*, *69*(1), 113–132.

Labib, S. M., Browning, M. H. E. M., Rigolon, A., Helbich, M., & James, P. (2022). Nature's contributions in coping with a pandemic in the 21st century: A narrative review of evidence during COVID-19. *Science of The Total Environment*, *833*, 155095. https://doi.org/10.1016/J.SCITOTENV.2022.155095

Li, D., Menotti, T., Ding, Y., & Wells, N. M. (2021). Life course nature exposure and mental health outcomes: A systematic review and future directions. *International Journal of Environmental Research and Public Health*, *18*(10), 5146. https://doi.org/10.3390/ijerph18105146

Limenih, G., MacDougall, A., Wedlake, M., & Nouvet, E. (2023). Depression and global mental health in the global south: A critical analysis of policy and discourse. *International Journal of Social Determinants of Health and Health Services*, *54*(2), 95–107.

Liu, Y., Wang, R., Xiao, Y., Huang, B., Chen, H., & Li, Z. (2019). Exploring the linkage between greenness exposure and depression among Chinese people: Mediating roles of physical activity, stress and social cohesion and moderating role of urbanicity. *Health & Place*, *58*, 102168. https://doi.org/10.1016/J.HEALTHPLACE.2019.102168

Lupien, S. J., McEwen, B. S., Gunnar, M. R., & Heim, C. (2009). Effects of stress throughout the lifespan on the brain, behaviour and cognition. *Nature Reviews Neuroscience*, *10*(6), 434–445.

MacKerron, G., & Mourato, S. (2013). Happiness is greater in natural environments. *Global Environmental Change*, *23*(5), 992–1000.

Markevych, I., Schoierer, J., Hartig, T., Chudnovsky, A., Hystad, P., Dzhambov, A. M., de Vries, S., Triguero-Mas, M., Brauer, M., Nieuwenhuijsen, M. J., Lupp, G., Richardson, E. A., Astell-Burt, T., Dimitrova, D., Feng, X., Sadeh, M., Standl, M., Heinrich, J., & Fuertes, E. (2017). Exploring pathways linking greenspace to health: Theoretical and methodological guidance. *Environmental Research*, *158*, 301–317.

Marselle, M. R., Warber, S. L., & Irvine, K. N. (2019). Growing resilience through interaction with nature: Can group walks in nature buffer the effects of stressful life events on mental health? *International Journal of Environmental Research and Public Health*, *6*(6), 986. https://doi.org/10.3390/IJERPH16060986

Marshall, M., & Gilliard, J. (2014). *Creating culturally appropriate outside spaces and experiences for people with dementia: Using nature and the outdoors in person-centred care*. Jessica Kingsley Publishers.

McDougall, C. W., Hanley, N., Quilliam, R. S., Bartie, P. J., Robertson, T., Griffiths, M., & Oliver, D. M. (2021). Neighbourhood blue space and mental health: A nationwide ecological study of antidepressant medication prescribed to older adults. *Landscape and Urban Planning*, *214*, 104132. https://doi.org/10.1016/J.LANDURBPLAN.2021.104132

McEwen, B. S. (2007). Physiology and neurobiology of stress and adaptation: Central role of the brain. *Physiological Reviews*, *87*(3), 873–904.

McEwen, B. S. (2019). Resilience of the brain and body. In G. Fink (Ed.), *Stress: Physiology, biochemistry, and pathology* (pp. 19–33). Academic Press.

McEwen, B. S., & Stellar, E. (1993). Stress and the individual. Mechanisms leading to disease. *Archives of Internal Medicine*, *153*(18), 2093–2101.

Menardo, E., Brondino, M., Hall, R., & Pasini, M. (2021). Restorativeness in natural and urban environments: A meta-analysis. *Psychological Reports*, *124*(2), 417–437.

Mueller, N., Rojas-Rueda, D., Basagaña, X., Cirach, M., Cole-Hunter, T., Dadvand, P., Donaire-Gonzalez, D., Foraster, M., Gascon, M., Martinez, D., Tonne, C., Triguero-Mas, M., Valentín, A., & Nieuwenhuijsen, M. (2017). Urban and transport planning related exposures and mortality: A health impact assessment for cities. *Environmental Health Perspectives*, *125*(1), 89–96.

Mueller, N., Rojas-Rueda, D., Khreis, H., Cirach, M., Andrés, D., Ballester, J., Bartoll, X., Daher, C., Deluca, A., Echave, C., Milà, C., Márquez, S., Palou, J., Pérez, K., Tonne, C., Stevenson, M., Rueda, S., & Nieuwenhuijsen, M. (2020). Changing the urban design of cities for health: The superblock model. *Environment International*, *134*, 105132. https://doi.org/10.1016/J.ENVINT.2019.105132

Murray, C. J. L., Ezzati, M., Lopez, A. D., Rodgers, A., & Vander Hoorn, S. (2003). Comparative quantification of health risks conceptual framework and methodological issues. *Population Health Metrics*, *1*(1), 1. https://doi.org/10.1186/1478-7954-1-1

Nguyen, P.-Y., Astell-Burt, T., Rahimi-Ardabili, H., & Feng, X. (2021). Green space quality and health: A systematic review. *International Journal of Environmental Research and Public Health*, *18*(21), 11028. https://doi.org/10.3390/IJERPH182111028

Nguyen, P.-Y., Astell-Burt, T., Rahimi-Ardabili, H., & Feng, X. (2023). Effect of nature prescriptions on cardiometabolic and mental health, and physical activity: A systematic review. *The Lancet Planetary Health*, 7(4), e313–e328.

Nielsen, A. B., van den Bosch, M., Maruthaveeran, S., & van den Bosch, C. K. (2014). Species richness in urban parks and its drivers: A review of empirical evidence. *Urban Ecosystems*, *17*(1), 305–327.

Nowak, D. J., & Crane, D. E. (2002). Carbon storage and sequestration by urban trees in the USA. *Environmental Pollution*, *116*(3), 381–389.

Nutsford, D., Pearson, A. L., Kingham, S., & Reitsma, F. (2016). Residential exposure to visible blue space (but not green space) associated with lower psychological distress in a capital city. *Health & Place*, *39*, 70–78.

OECD. (2019). *Health for everyone? Social inequalities in health and health systems*. Paris, France. Retrieved February 14, 2024 from https://doi.org/10.1787/3c8385d0-en

Pagalan, L., Oberlander, T. F., Hanley, G. E., Rosella, L. C., Bickford, C., Weikum, W., Lanphear, N., Lanphear, B., Brauer, M., & van den Bosch, M. (2022). The association between prenatal greenspace exposure and Autism spectrum disorder, and the potentially mediating role of air pollution reduction: A population-based birth cohort study. *Environment International*, *167*, 107445. https://doi.org/10.1016/j.envint.2022.107445

Parsons, R., Tassinary, L., Ulrich, R., Hebl, M., & Grossman-Alexander, M. (1998). The view from the road: Implications for stress recovery and immunization. *Journal of Environmental Psychology*, *18*(2), 113–140.

Patwary, M. M., Bardhan, M., Browning, M. H. E. M., Astell-Burt, T., van den Bosch, M., Dong, J., Dzhambov, A. M., Dadvand, P., Fasolino, T., Markevych, I., McAnirlin, O., Nieuwenhuijsen, M. J., White, M. P., & Van Den Eeden, S. K. (2024). The economics of nature's healing touch: A systematic review and conceptual framework of green space, pharmaceutical prescriptions, and healthcare expenditure associations. *Science of the Total Environment*, *914*, 169635. https://doi.org/10.1016/J.SCITOTENV.2023.169635

Paul, L. A., Hystad, P., Burnett, R. T., Kwong, J. C., Crouse, D. L., van Donkelaar, A., Tu, K., Lavigne, E., Copes, R., Martin, R. V., & Chen, H. (2020). Urban green space and the risks of dementia and stroke. *Environmental Research, 186*, 109520. https://doi.org/10.1016/J.ENVRES.2020.109520

Peen, J., Dekker, J., Schoevers, R. A., ten Have, M., de Graaf, R., & Beekman, A. T. (2007). Is the prevalence of psychiatric disorders associated with urbanization? *Social Psychiatry and Psychiatric Epidemiology, 42*(12), 984–989.

Persson Waye, K., Löve, J., Lercher, P., Dzhambov, A. M., Klatte, M., Schreckenberg, D., Belke, C., Leist, L., Ristovska, G., Jeram, S., Kanninen, K. M., Selander, J., Arat, A., Lachmann, T., Clark, C., Botteldooren, D., White, K., Julvez, J., Foraster, M., . . . Vincens, N. (2023). Adopting a child perspective for exposome research on mental health and cognitive development – conceptualisation and opportunities. *Environmental Research, 239*, 117279. https://doi.org/10.1016/j.envres.2023.117279

Peters, R., Ee, N., Peters, J., Booth, A., Mudway, I., & Anstey, K. J. (2019). Air pollution and dementia: A systematic review. *Journal of Alzheimer's Disease, 70*(s1), S145–S163.

Quinton, J., Nesbitt, L., & Sax, D. (2022). How well do we know green gentrification? A systematic review of the methods. *Progress in Human Geography, 46*(4), 960–987.

Rigolon, A. (2016). A complex landscape of inequity in access to urban parks: A literature review. *Landscape and Urban Planning, 153*, 160–169.

Rigolon, A., Browning, M. H. E. M., McAnirlin, O., & Yoon, H. (2021). Green space and health equity: A systematic review on the potential of green space to reduce health disparities. *International Journal of Environmental Research and Public Health, 18*(5), 2563. https://doi.org/10.3390/ijerph18052563

Roe, J., & McCay, L. (2021). *Restorative cities: Urban design for mental health and wellbeing. Restorative cities*. Bloomsbury Visual Arts. Retrieved February 14, 2024 from https://doi.org/10.5040/9781350112919

Roslund, M. I., Parajuli, A., Hui, N., Puhakka, R., Grönroos, M., Soininen, L., Nurminen, N., Oikarinen, S., Cinek, O., Kramná, L., Schroderus, A.-M., Laitinen, O. H., Kinnunen, T., Hyöty, H., Sinkkonen, A., Cerrone, D., Grönroos, M., Laitinen, O. H., Luukkonen, A., . . . Sinkkonen, A. (2022). A placebo-controlled double-blinded test of the biodiversity hypothesis of immune-mediated diseases: Environmental microbial diversity elicits changes in cytokines and increase in T regulatory cells in young children. *Ecotoxicology and Environmental Safety, 242*, 113900. https://doi.org/10.1016/j.ecoenv.2022.113900

Rueda, S. (2019). Superblocks for the design of new cities and renovation of existing ones: Barcelona's case. In M. Nieuwenhuijsen & H. Khreis (Eds.), *Integrating human health into urban and transport planning* (pp. 135–153). Springer.

Sadowski, I., & Khoury, B. (2022). Nature-based mindfulness-compassion programs using virtual reality for older adults: A narrative literature review. *Frontiers in Virtual Reality, 3*, 892905. https://doi.org/10.3389/frvir.2022.892905

Segal, D., Harper, N. J., & Rose, K. (2021). *Nature-based therapy*. In N. J. Harper & W. W. Dobud (Eds.), *Outdoor therapies: An introduction to practices, possibilities, and critical perspectives* (pp. 95–107). Routledge.

Selye, H. (1936). A syndrome produced by diverse nocuous agents. *Nature, 138*, 32.

Siah, C. J. R., Goh, Y. S., Lee, J., Poon, S. N., Ow Yong, J. Q. Y., & Tam, W. S. W. (2023). The effects of forest bathing on psychological well-being: A systematic review and meta-analysis. *International Journal of Mental Health Nursing, 32*(4), 1038–1054.

Singapore Botanic Gardens. (n.d.). *Healing garden*. Retrieved April 10, 2024 from https://www.nparks.gov.sg/sbg/our-gardens/nassim-entrance/healing-garden

Singh, A., & Misra, N. (2009). Loneliness, depression and sociability in old age. *Industrial Psychiatry Journal, 18*(1), 51–55.

Smith, N., Georgiou, M., King, A. C., Tieges, Z., Webb, S., & Chastin, S. (2021). Urban blue spaces and human health: A systematic review and meta-analysis of quantitative studies. *Cities, 119*, 103413. https://doi.org/10.1016/j.cities.2021.103413

Sudimac, S., Sale, V., & Kühn, S. (2022). How nature nurtures: Amygdala activity decreases as the result of a one-hour walk in nature. *Molecular Psychiatry, 27*(11), 4446–4452.

Suzuki, A., Poon, L., Papadopoulos, A. S., Kumari, V., & Cleare, A. J. (2014). Long term effects of childhood trauma on cortisol stress reactivity in adulthood and relationship to the occurrence of depression. *Psychoneuroendocrinology, 50*, 289–299.

Tree Canada. (n.d.). *Greening Canada's school grounds*. Retrieved April 12, 2024 from https://treecanada.ca/grants-awards/greening-canadas-school-grounds/

Triguero-Mas, M., Dadvand, P., Cirach, M., Martínez, D., Medina, A., Mompart, A., Basagaña, X., Gražulevičienė, R., & Nieuwenhuijsen, M. J. (2015). Natural outdoor environments and mental and physical health: Relationships and mechanisms. *Environment International*, 77, 35–41.

Triguero-Mas, M., Donaire-Gonzalez, D., Seto, E., Valentín, A., Martínez, D., Smith, G., Hurst, G., Carrasco-Turigas, G., Masterson, D., van den Berg, M., Ambròs, A., Martínez-Íñiguez, T., Dedele, A., Ellis, N., Grazulevicius, T., Voorsmit, M., Cirach, M., Cirac-Claveras, J., Swart, W., . . . Nieuwenhuijsen, M. J. (2017). Natural outdoor environments and mental health: Stress as a possible mechanism. *Environmental Research, 159*, 629–638.

Ulrich, R. S. (1984). View through a window may influence recovery from surgery. *Science, 224*(4647), 420–421.

Ulrich, R. S. (1986). Human responses to vegetation and landscapes. *Landscape and Urban Planning, 13*, 29–44.

UNICEF. (2021). *The necessity of urban green space for children's optimal development*. New York. Retrieved April 10, 2024 from https://www.unicef.org/documents/necessity-urban-green-space-childrens-optimal-development

van den Berg, A. E., & Custers, M. H. G. (2011). Gardening promotes neuroendocrine and affective restoration from stress. *Journal of Health Psychology, 16*(1), 3–11.

van den Bosch, M., Bartolomeu, M. L., Williams, S., Basnou, C., Hamilton, I., Nieuwenhuijsen, M., Pino, J., & Tonne, C. (2024). A scoping review of human health co-benefits of forest-based climate change mitigation in Europe. *Environment International, 186*, 108593. https://doi.org/10.1016/J.ENVINT.2024.108593

van den Bosch, M., & Meyer-Lindenberg, A. (2019). Environmental exposures and depression: Biological mechanisms and epidemiological evidence. *Annual Review of Public Health, 40*(1), 239–259.

Victoria State Government. (2024). *Pocket parks*. Retrieved April 10, 2024 from https://www.exploreoutdoors.vic.gov.au/investing-in-nature/suburban-parks-program/pocket-parks-old

Vidal Yañez, D., Pereira Barboza, E., Cirach, M., Daher, C., Nieuwenhuijsen, M., & Mueller, N. (2023). An urban green space intervention with benefits for mental health: A health impact assessment of the Barcelona "Eixos Verds" Plan. *Environment International, 174*, 107880. https://doi.org/10.1016/J.ENVINT.2023.107880

Vigo, D., Thornicroft, G., & Atun, R. (2016). Estimating the true global burden of mental illness. *The Lancet Psychiatry, 3*(2), 171–178.

Weeland, J., Laceulle, O. M., Nederhof, E., Overbeek, G., & Reijneveld, S. A. (2019). The greener the better? Does neighborhood greenness buffer the effects of stressful life events on externalizing behavior in late adolescence? *Health and Place, 58*, 102163. https://doi.org/10.1016/j.healthplace.2019.102163

Wells, N. M. (2021). The natural environment as a resilience factor: Nature's role as a buffer of the effects of risk and adversity. In A. R. Schutte, J. C. Torquati, & J. R. Stevens (Eds.), *Nature and psychology* (pp. 195–233). Springer.

White, M. P., Hartig, T., Martin, L., Pahl, S., van den Berg, A. E., Wells, N. M., Costongs, C., Dzhambov, A. M., Elliott, L. R., Godfrey, A., Hartl, A., Konijnendijk, C., Litt, J. S., Lovell, R., Lymeus, F., O'Driscoll, C., Pichler, C., Pouso, S., Razani, N., . . . van den Bosch, M. (2023). Nature-based biopsychosocial resilience: An integrative theoretical framework for research on nature and health. *Environment International, 181*, 108234. https://doi.org/10.1016/j.envint.2023.108234

White, M. P., Pahl, S., Ashbullby, K., Herbert, S., & Depledge, M. (2013). Feelings of restoration from recent nature visits. *Journal of Environmental Psychology, 35*, 40–51.

Wilson, E. (1984). *Biophilia: The human bond with other species*. Harvard University Press Cambridge.

World Health Organization. (2017). *Urban green spaces: A brief for action*. Retrieved April 28, 2024 from https://www.who.int/europe/publications/i/item/9789289052498

Yang, B. Y., Zhao, T., Hu, L. X., Browning, M. H. E. M., Heinrich, J., Dharmage, S. C., Jalaludin, B., Knibbs, L. D., Liu, X. X., Luo, Y. N., James, P., Li, S., Huang, W. Z., Chen, G., Zeng, X. W., Hu, L. W., Yu, Y., & Dong, G. H. (2021). Greenspace and human health: An umbrella review. *The Innovation, 2*(4), 100164. https://doi.org/10.1016/J.XINN.2021.100164

Yao, W., Zhang, X., & Gong, Q. (2021). The effect of exposure to the natural environment on stress reduction: A meta-analysis. *Urban Forestry and Urban Greening, 57*, 126932. https://doi.org/10.1016/j.ufug.2020.126932

Yuchi, W., Brauer, M., Czekajlo, A., Davies, H. W., Davis, Z., Guhn, M., Jarvis, I., Jerrett, M., Nesbitt, L., Oberlander, T. F., Sbihi, H., Su, J., & van den Bosch, M. (2022). Neighborhood environmental exposures and incidence of attention deficit/hyperactivity disorder: A population-based cohort study. *Environment International, 161*, 107120. https://doi.org/10.1016/J.ENVINT.2022.107120

Zhang, J. W., Piff, P. K., Iyer, R., Koleva, S., & Keltner, D. (2014). An occasion for unselfing: Beautiful nature leads to prosociality. *Journal of Environmental Psychology, 37*, 61–72.

Zhang, S., Li, X., Chen, Z., & Ouyang, Y. (2022). A bibliometric analysis of the study of urban green spaces and health behaviors. *Frontiers in Public Health, 10*, 1005647. https://doi.org/10.3389/fpubh.2022.1005647

Zhang, Y., Mavoa, S., Zhao, J., Raphael, D., & Smith, M. (2020). The association between green space and adolescents mental well-being: A systematic review. *International Journal of Environmental Research and Public Health*, 17(18), 6640. https://doi.org/10.3390/ijerph17186640

7 Urban densification, access to green space, and well-being

Consequences of not owning private green space and crowded public green spaces

Sjerp de Vries and Lauriane S. Chalmin-Pui

Introduction

To accommodate the demand for dwellings in regions with a growing population, cities within such regions are likely to expand and to densify. In expanding cities, the distance to peri-urban natural areas will increase for at least some of its inhabitants. Visiting such areas will come at higher costs (travel time, financial, etc.; Elfering & Huber, this volume, Chapter 2). Densification can take shape in different ways. One possibility is by way of infill. An area that used to have a non-residential function becomes a residential area. If infill takes place in a former urban green space, the local supply of green space is diminished, and local communities must travel much further to access their closest green space. Empirical data from various cities shows that densification is indeed associated with lowered amounts of green space (Balikçi et al., 2022; Bille et al., 2023; Haaland & van den Bosch, 2015; McDonald et al., 2023). Densification can also occur by building more and/or higher residential apartment buildings. This implies that even if public green spaces are spared in the densification process, the number of citizens that have to be serviced by these spaces will increase. Put differently, the amount of public green space per capita decreases with increasing population density (Sun et al., 2019). Furthermore, increasing the proportion of apartments within a city implies that fewer people will have access to a private green space in the shape of a domestic garden. In addition, the size of parcels for new ground-level homes is likely to decrease, with indoor surface area being prioritised over garden space, which will shrink. Empirical evidence shows that the amount of private green space is indeed smaller in areas with greater dwelling density (Lin et al., 2015; Osborne et al., 2021).

In this chapter, we focus on how urban densification will affect people's access to nearby nature and what this, in turn, implies for their health and well-being.

de Vries, S., & Chalmin-Pui, L. S. (2025). Urban densification, access to green space, and well-being: Consequences of not owning private green space and crowded public green spaces. In S. Pauleit, M. Kellmann, & J. Beckmann (Eds.), *Creating Urban and Workplace Environments for Recovery and Well-being* (pp. 135–150). Routledge.

DOI: 10.4324/9781003435471-9

Spatially, we focus on vegetation in urban residential environments, especially on having a domestic garden or not, and the amount of vegetation in that garden. Although there are multiple intertwined pathways from (private) garden exposure to end-health outcomes, we focus on recovery from stress as a key mechanism by which contact with nature positively impacts mental and physical health. Having said this, access to public green spaces will also be discussed, as well as other pathways linking contact with nature to human health and well-being.

The importance of contact with nature for human well-being

The most straightforward theory with regard to the importance of contact with (living) nature is perhaps the *Biophilia Hypothesis* (Kellert & Wilson, 1993). Its basic idea is that humans have an innate tendency to seek connections with nature and other forms of life. Not being able to fulfil this need will negatively affect our mental well-being (Baxter & Pelletier, 2019; Gillis & Gatersleben, 2015). Associated with this are concerns about the extinction of nature experiences (Gaston & Soga, 2020; Soga & Gaston, 2016). It may be pointed out that (positive) nature experiences are also considered instrumental in establishing or strengthening one's connection with nature, and thereby one's pro-environmental attitudes and behaviour, including support for nature conservation and biodiversity-promoting policies (Martin et al., 2020).

Other theories also focusing on mental well-being are *Stress Reduction Theory* (SRT; Ulrich, 1983) and *Attention Restoration Theory* (ART; Kaplan, 1995). Especially the SRT has a strong psycho-evolutionary basis, implying a virtually universal applicability. Contact with nature is theorised to be conducive to recovering from stress, improving mood, and enhancing the restoration of attentional fatigue. Even without a psycho-evolutionary basis, it can be argued that (for whatever reason) many people prefer residential environments that contain green spaces or other natural elements to those that do not, which is exemplified by their willingness to pay higher housing prices if such spaces and elements are present (Bockarjova et al., 2020; Lin et al., 2024). If so, the presence of nature in the residential environment makes this environment more pleasurable, increasing residential satisfaction and quality of life (improved person–environment fit; Kahana et al., 2003). More specifically, people may use favourite places for emotional self-regulation, with natural environments being strongly represented among favourite places, next to the home itself (Korpela & Ylén, 2007; Korpela et al., 2001).

The presence of and contact with nature are not only relevant for *mental* health and well-being. Numerous epidemiological studies have shown beneficial associations between exposure to nature and *physical* health, ranging from birthweight to longevity. Between birth and death, prevalences of a wide range of health outcomes have shown to be more positive when more greenery is present in the residential environment. This includes the neurological development of children, the cardiometabolic health of adults, and the cognitive functioning of the elderly, besides their mental health and well-being (Dadvand et al., 2023).

The beneficial association for each health outcome could be due to a different pathway or mechanism. However, stress reduction might be a rather central pathway, given its association with several of the aforementioned health outcomes (Juster et al., 2010). This could be due to chronic stress negatively affecting immune system functioning (Padgett & Glaser, 2003). Another potentially central pathway that is currently getting more attention is based on the *Biodiversity Hypothesis* (Haahtela, 2019), which states that contact with nature is likely to positively affect the composition of the human microbiome. Especially the composition of the gut microbiome is relevant for a good functioning of the immune system (Kuo, 2015). Other broad-ranging pathways likely to affect a range of health outcomes, include stimulating physical activity and facilitating (positive) social contacts and social cohesion in the neighbourhood (Hartig et al., 2014). More 'narrow' pathways deal with mitigating environmental stressors, such as heatwaves (especially in cities: urban heat island effect; Bauer et al., this volume, Chapter 9). All in all, there are several plausible mechanisms that can explain why having nature nearby is beneficially associated with human health and well-being, with nature being the driving force (Marselle et al., 2021).

Type of exposure and engagement with nature, and how they are experienced

In the preceding sections, different terms were used in connection to nature: presence, access, contact, experience. Expanding the model developed by Bratman et al. (2019), de Vries (2022) developed a framework that identifies four different 'steps' that may be involved in nature resulting in health benefits, the *Environment for Health Impact Assessment* (E4HIA) framework (Figure 7.1). The first step in this framework is the presence of nearby nature and its characteristics (*Existence*). For some mechanisms, this presence alone may be enough to bring about certain health benefits, for example, by way of increasing thermal comfort within cities. What is present where also greatly influences its accessibility, relevant for the next steps.

Other proposed mechanisms require a second step, actual (sensory) contact (*Exposure*). In that case, the frequency and/or amount of time spent in contact with nature are likely to be relevant, based on the assumption that more contact is better, at least up to a certain point. For example, White et al. (2019) conclude that at least up to two hours in nature per week, the benefits will increase. The third (simultaneous) step is the way one interacts with nature during this contact, the type of contact (*Engagement*). One may just look at nature, perhaps even through a window, be physically present in it, or interact with it directly, as in the case of gardening (Soga & Gaston, 2020, on types of interactions). For physical activity as mediator, the relevance of the type of interaction is self-evident. Chalmin-Pui, Griffiths, et al. (2021) found that gardening on a frequent basis, that is, at least two to three times a week, corresponded with the greatest

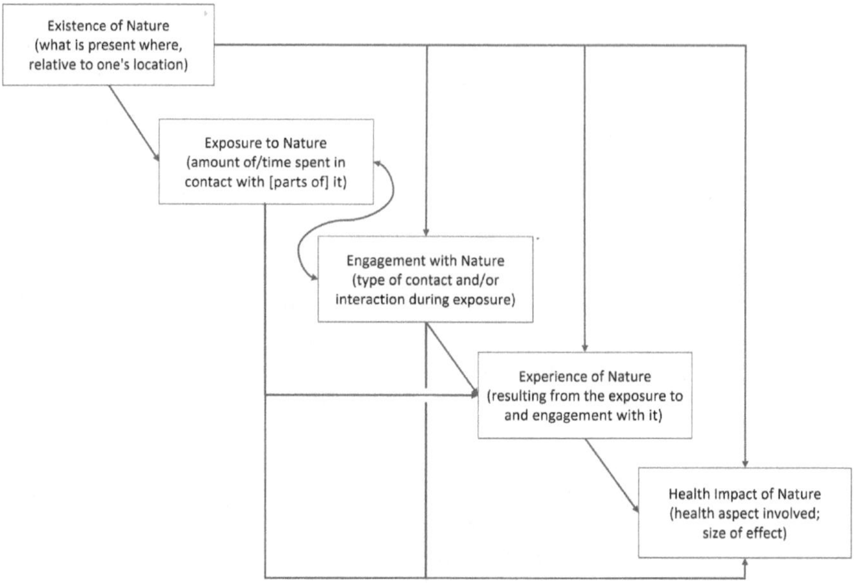

Figure 7.1 The Environment for Health Impact Assessment (E4HIA) framework.

Source: Adapted from de Vries (2022).

perceived health benefits. Also, the level of awareness of the natural environment during the interaction may be relevant for the (mental) well-being effects (Lin et al., 2014; Pasanen et al., 2018).

The fourth step is that the experience resulting from the contact and interaction may be important with regard to impact on the well-being (*Experience*). For example, the perception of safety seems to be a precondition to achieving stress reduction and relaxation by a visit to a green space (Weimann et al., 2017).

The importance of each step is likely to depend on the specific health outcome that one is interested in, and the accompanying relevant mechanism(s). The mechanism, in turn, is likely to determine which characteristics of the nearby nature are important for optimal benefits. Furthermore, favourable characteristics may differ by step. For example, what is good for exposure need not be good for experience as well. A visit to a remote nature area may be more restorative than a visit to a local neighbourhood park. However, the first may occur only four times a year, and the latter weekly. Of course, urban neighbourhood parks themselves may also differ widely in the level of immersiveness that they afford (i.e., level of shielding from the surroundings). This has been shown to affect the expected mental well-being benefits of a visit in terms of enabling rest and recovery (Nordh & Østby, 2013).

As mentioned before, densification is likely to affect *Existence*, in terms of amount and characteristics of nearby nature, directly. As a result, it can indirectly influence the subsequent steps including *Exposure*. Densification may also affect subsequent steps in other ways. For example, densification may lead to increased visitation levels, which are likely to affect the experience when visiting a public green space, an issue that we will turn to later on in this chapter. Indirectly, due to a high use intensity, there may also be less (perceived) avian biodiversity, which is associated with lower perceived well-being (Cameron et al., 2020). With regard to health impact, much of the research to date, especially in the epidemiological literature, is limited to looking at associations between the presence of nearby nature and a variety of health outcomes. Usually, this presence is measured by making use of available land-use or remote-sensing data. Land-use data measurements tend to be limited to green areas of at least a certain size, and oftentimes to public green areas. Remote-sensing data often involves calculating the Normalized Difference Vegetation Index (NDVI; Markevych et al., 2017) – or similar indicators – for the presence or amount of green biomass. Small natural elements, such as street trees and domestic gardens, may also contribute to the NDVI score of an area. Noteworthy is that the term 'exposure' is often used in connection to such measures, without actual contact with nature being measured. We consider the amount of nearby vegetation at best a proxy for actual contact.

One of the reasons that actual contact is often not measured in epidemiological studies is that it is more difficult to measure than presence, especially at a large scale. This is even more so the case when not only visits to green areas during leisure time are considered relevant but also more incidental contacts with nature, for example, while traveling or even when at home. And there are good reasons to do so. For example, at least two studies have shown an association between the density of street trees and the prescription of antidepressants (Marselle et al., 2020; Taylor et al., 2015). Moreover, several studies conducted during the Covid-19 pandemic showed beneficial associations between having a view on nature from one's living room window and mental well-being (Dzhambov et al., 2021; Soga et al., 2021; Zhang, Browning, et al., 2023).

Beute et al. (2023) conclude that, at present, there is no convincing evidence that the type of nature is very important with regard to enhancing mental well-being, partially because of a lack of direct comparisons between different types. Rather than its biophysical characteristics, how the area is perceived may be more relevant. ART specifies four conceptually formulated components that an environment should possess to be restorative: (soft) fascination, being away, extent, and compatibility (with the latter being about a temporal person–environment fit). This theory has inspired a large body of research on the extent to which a natural area possesses each of these four components, thereby leading to perceived restorativeness of the environment and well-being effects (see review by Neilson et al., 2019). To apply the outcomes of this type of research to the planning and design of green spaces requires that users' perceptions be translated into mandating certain (compositions of) (bio)physical features, which may include equipment (e.g., benches). Grahn and Stigsdotter (2010) distinguish eight perceived sensory dimensions that seem more amenable to such a translation. Of these, the most relevant in supporting recovery from stress are how natural, sheltered, serene, and cohesive the area is – elements which are more likely to be perceived in larger green spaces (Stoltz & Grahn, 2021) rather than small and crowded green spaces.

Individual differences in access and beyond

Access to nature depends on where one lives and therefore differs greatly between individuals. In urban areas, people with lower socioeconomic status tend to have poorer access in terms of total amount of nearby nature, distance to the nearest public green space, and quality of that space (de Vries et al., 2020; Hoffimann et al., 2017; Rigolon et al., 2018). Contact with nature has the strongest effect on the most stressed, presumably because they have a higher need for restoration (Meuwese et al., 2021). Lower socioeconomic status and living in a deprived neighbourhood are both associated with higher chronic stress and its physiological pendant, allostatic load (Baum et al., 1999; Ribeiro et al., 2019). Based on their review, Rigolon et al. (2021) conclude that people with a lower socioeconomic position indeed benefit more from nearby nature than their more affluent counterparts. Consequently, improving distributive environmental justice with regard to access to nature may help reduce socioeconomic health disparities (Wang et al., 2022).

Of course, besides one's socioeconomic position, other individual characteristics may influence the nature–health connection. Gender, for example, may affect how safe one feels going to an urban park by oneself (Ceccato, this volume, Chapter 10; Jorgensen et al., 2013), and thereby the level of exposure. This is also true for age, with frail people also being concerned about falling (Plaut et al., 2021). For unsupervised outdoor play by young children, it is important that not only the child itself perceive the green play area as safe (and attractive) but that its parents do so too (Loebach et al., 2021). Martin et al. (2020) show that nature connectedness, as a trait, may increase the well-being benefits of contact with nature. In general, the characteristics of the natural environment that are - directly or indirectly - important for exposure, engagement, experience, and well-being may differ for each pathway and for each individual (Pauleit et al., this volume, Chapter 1).

Access to a domestic garden and well-being

One of the likely consequences of urban densification is that fewer people will have access to a private domestic garden adjacent to their home. There has been relatively little research on how important it is to have access to a domestic garden and how much vegetation it should have for the health benefits to accrue. Most epidemiological research focuses of either public green area or on all vegetation within a certain distance from one's home. Two epidemiological studies looked into the amount of private green space separately (Dennis & James, 2017; Roscoe et al., 2022). Both studies observed beneficial associations with health outcomes. However, both studies used measures of the total surface area of private green space in a neighbourhood, rather than what individuals actually have access to – their own private green space. Brindley et al. (2018) looked at how self-reported health was related to the average domestic garden size per household in urban neighbourhoods, including households without a domestic garden. They concluded that smaller garden sizes were associated with a higher prevalence of poor health. Zhao et al. (2024) also looked at the size of domestic gardens but did so at the household level. They concluded that it was (indirectly) related to subjective well-being.

Garden size is likely to be a good proxy for the (absolute) amount of greenery the garden contains. However, de Vries et al. (2023) looked at the actual amount of greenery in urban gardens. The researchers investigated associations between the amount of greenery in Dutch domestic gardens adjacent to the home and the prevalence of 21 types of disorders, controlling for a wide range of covariates. The amount of garden greenery was assessed based on detailed aerial photographs $(25 \times 25\,\text{cm})$ taken in the summer period. The health data was based on electronic patient records of about 800,000 individuals. Included disorders ranged from cardiac disease to anxiety disorder, and from Attention Deficit Hyperactivity Disorder (ADHD) to infectious disease of the intestinal tract. Adjusted models showed that the amount of garden greenery was beneficially associated with the prevalence of 17 of the 21 disorders, that is, persons with 50 square metres or more of garden greenery showed a lower prevalence than the persons without a domestic garden. For some disorders, already smaller amounts of garden greenery were associated with a lower prevalence. The association was strongest for infectious disease of the intestinal tract, with its prevalence being at least 20% lower when 50 square metres or more of garden greenery was present. Stroke/brain haemorrhage came second (15% lower), followed by heart disease (at least 13% lower) and ADHD (11% lower). Including the total amount of greenery within a wider area around the home (125 metres) in the models did not change these outcomes. The association was less strong for depression, and no association was observed for anxiety disorder. Despite the latter, overall, the aforementioned studies suggest that having access to private green space adjacent to the home is beneficial for one's health.

Exposure, engagement, and experiences in gardens and well-being

On a small scale, Chalmin-Pui, Roe, et al. (2021) evaluated recovery from stress by measuring stress levels before and after adding two containers of ornamental plants to previously bare front gardens in the city of Salford, UK. Outcome measures were physiological (diurnal cortisol concentration) and psychological (self-reported perceived stress and well-being). Over a period of one year, the new plants in front of the home resulted in a 6% drop in residents' perceived stress levels. According to the authors, a 6% decrease is equivalent to the long-term impact of eight weekly mindfulness sessions. As for the physiological results of this intervention study, while 24% of residents had a healthy daily cortisol pattern at the beginning before the intervention, this increased to 53% three months after adding the plants, also suggesting better mental health and recovery from stress in these participants. Effects may be stronger in stressful times: during the Covid-19 pandemic, gardeners considered relaxation, and stress release, one of the most important benefits of gardening, and many of them spent more time gardening (Egerer et al., 2022).

Building on this type of evidence, researchers have also been attempting to qualify how green spaces can be optimised to deliver therapeutic effects, pleasant emotional responses, and stress restoration. In addition to being the practical operationalisation of theoretical pathways, finding the 'active ingredients' for the health benefits of gardens may be even more important in dense urban contexts. Indeed, not all green spaces are alike, and not all are actually fully green in colour. Scientific research has taken place in the form of empirical studies in actual green spaces and under controlled lab conditions, but both focus on the experiences that participants have and the garden features that are present, that are noticed, or that are engaged with. Topics include the role of (perceived) biodiversity (Egerer & Marselle, this volume, Chapter 8; Farris et al., in press), prompting or facilitating engagement (Boyd, 2022), multisensory engagement (Harries et al., in press; Zhang, Dempsey, & Cameron, 2023), and physical, social, or creative activity (Moula et al., 2022; Smyth et al., 2022).

Summarising Harries et al.'s (2023) review applied to private, collective, and public gardens, planting should be diversified to create experiences that will stimulate as many senses as possible across the seasons with different colours, textures, scents, shapes, tastes, and qualities that will attract birds and pollinators, thereby creating opportunities for restoration through 'soft fascination'. These aspects are all likely to have instant impacts on our mood through the stress reduction pathway. Serenity can be fostered even in busy areas by accentuated natural sounds of water and birdsong. Especially, larger public gardens should cater for multiple needs and purposes with distinctive spaces for privacy, social interaction, exploration, and familiarity. This affords residents and users to select a space that fits their needs at that moment in time, and to practice emotional self-regulation (Beckmann, 2023). These practical aspects, taken together and adapted to local climatic and social conditions, can improve the quality of green spaces specifically for their health benefits.

Crowding in public green areas and well-being impacts

With urban densification reducing the amount of public green space per capita, the visitor density in public green areas is likely to increase. It may even increase up to a point where, for some people, the area becomes too busy and visiting it is no longer considered attractive. Indeed, visitors of urban forests preferred experiences with lower densities of visitors, which was perceived as being more conducive to recovery from stress (Arnberger & Eder, 2015; Arnberger et al., 2010). Zhang, Qi, and Zhang (2023) showed crowding in small public green spaces to have a negative effect on mood during a visit, as well as on the intention to revisit the space. At very high densities of overcrowding, anti-social behaviour may result, and conflict may arise between user groups in terms of their needs, values, and expectations (e.g., birdwatching vs football vs family picnic vs teenager hangout vs dog walking; Mori et al., 2023; Oviedo et al., 2022). Negative experiences may result in less future contact with nature. During the Covid-19 pandemic, urban green spaces were among the only places one was allowed to visit for leisure purposes, that is, at least in some countries (in countries with a stricter lockdown, even this was not allowed). As a result, especially where such spaces were scarce, they were often overcrowded, to the point of not being able to keep safe distances from others, and avoided or even closed for that reason (Kleinschroth et al., 2024). This may have exacerbated existing socioeconomic health inequalities (Gao et al., 2023).

Densification also implies an influx of people to the city who are unlikely to have any immediate place attachment to their new residence. Multiple studies have demonstrated the importance of gardens and gardening in adapting to a new home (Strunk & Richardson, 2019), fostering community attachment especially in cases of suburban sprawl (Arnberger & Eder, 2012), keeping in touch with roots by growing familiar plants, including vegetables that may be harder to find commercially (Abramovic et al., 2019). Offering access to green spaces for newcomers to the city is vital for urban social cohesion as a whole, and for the individuals themselves.

Conclusion

Densification tends to lower access to green space, and thereby to negatively affect the health and well-being of citizens. Recovery from stress is likely to be an important pathway. Contact with nature can help cope with stress or, in other words, enhance resilience at the individual level (White et al., 2023). The amount of contact is important and can be increased by easier access to nature. There are indications that the type and characteristics of the green space matter, to begin with it being perceived as safe. However, the evidence with regard to type and characteristics is limited and usually focuses on green areas, that is, areas dominated by vegetation. Incidental contacts with (very nearby) nature such as street trees may be much more frequent than purposeful visits during leisure time. Although such contacts are likely to be less immersive, their high frequency can make them important nevertheless, as evidenced by beneficial associations between green window views and mental well-being.

In this chapter, special attention was paid to domestic gardens adjacent to the home, their size, the amount of greenery present in such gardens, and gardening as a specific type of engagement with nature. Evidence is mounting that having access to a domestic garden positively affects one's health and well-being, especially for larger gardens containing more greenery. The same holds for gardening as a specific form of engagement with nature. An important question is to what extent private and public green spaces are substitutable when it comes to health and well-being. The study by de Vries et al. (2023) suggests that they are not, and that domestic gardens are more important than public green space. To some extent, this is supported by Collins et al. (2023), showing a larger beneficial effect on mental health of having a private garden than of having access to a public green space, regardless of whether the other type is present or not, but only for men. However, other studies suggest that public and private green space are substitutable, at least to some extent (Poortinga et al., 2021).

For each health aspect, the conditions under which public green space can compensate for the absence of private green space merits further research, especially since it is likely that domestic gardens will become less common. More insight into the most relevant mechanisms might help identify the best alternatives for the absence of a domestic garden adjacent to the home. What is it about these gardens that makes them especially important for residents' health and well-being? Bieri et al. (2024) conclude that collective gardens are becoming more popular. But do collective gardens and/or allotment gardens, at the fringe of the city, compensate for the absence of private domestic gardens, and more so than neighbourhood or larger urban parks? Other possibilities to look into are smaller private outdoor spaces, such as (green) balconies, although size is likely to matter (Shentova et al., 2022). Even indoor nature may be considered (Almeida et al., 2023).

Not only the possession of private green space is likely to become less common but also the amount of urban public green space is likely to decrease, at least on a per capita basis. Park management policy options in the pandemic emergency scenario suggested by Geneletti et al. (2022) in Italy and Shoari et al. (2020) in the UK included shift rotations, entry allocation systems, dedicated park times for different age groups or uses, or indeed, entry fees. Anticipating such measures as permanent options for densifying cities may reduce crowding but will surely raise barriers against health benefits for urban citizens. Hence, we would urge that mitigating the negative effects of densification include consideration for providing good access to peri-urban green spaces, including agricultural areas that may be (visually) experienced by foot or bicycle, and prioritising maintaining the available amount of public urban green space per capita.

References

Abramovic, J., Turner, B., & Hope, C. (2019). Entangled recovery: Refugee encounters in community gardens. *Local Environment*, *24*(8), 696–711.

Almeida, I., Lopes, C., Pedroso, R., & Gaspar, R. (2023). The outdoor nature, indoors: Relationship between contact with nature, life satisfaction and affect during a COVID-19 pandemic lockdown. *PsyEcology*, *14*(2), 123–158.

Arnberger, A., Aikoh, T., Eder, R., Shoji, Y., & Mieno, T. (2010). How many people should be in the urban forest? A comparison of trail preferences of Vienna and Sapporo forest visitor segments. *Urban Forestry & Urban Greening*, *9*(3), 215–225.

Arnberger, A., & Eder, R. (2012). The influence of green space on community attachment of urban and suburban residents. *Urban Forestry & Urban Greening*, *11*(1), 41–49.

Arnberger, A., & Eder, R. (2015). Are urban visitors' general preferences for green-spaces similar to their preferences when seeking stress relief? *Urban Forestry & Urban Greening, 14*(4), 872–882.

Balikçi, S., Giezen, M., & Arundel, R. (2022). The paradox of planning the compact and green city: Analyzing land-use change in Amsterdam and Brussels. *Journal of Environmental Planning and Management, 65*(13), 2387–2411.

Baum, A., Garofalo, J. P., & Yali, A. M. (1999). Socioeconomic status and chronic stress: Does stress account for SES effects on health? *Annals of the New York Academy of Sciences, 896*(1), 131–144.

Baxter, D. E., & Pelletier, L. G. (2019). Is nature relatedness a basic human psychological need? A critical examination of the extant literature. *Canadian Psychology/Psychologie Canadienne, 60*(1), 21–34.

Beckmann, J. (2023). Self-regulation of recovery. In M. Kellmann, S. Jakowski, & J. Beckmann (Eds.), *The importance of recovery for physical and mental health: Negotiating the effects of underrecovery* (pp. 53–69). Routledge.

Beute, F., Marselle, M. R., Olszewska-Guizzo, A., Andreucci, M. B., Lammel, A., Davies, Z. G., Glanville, J., Keune, H., O´Brian, L., Remmen, R., Russo, A., & de Vries, S. (2023). How do different types and characteristics of green space impact mental health? A scoping review. *People and Nature, 5*(6), 1839–1876.

Bieri, D., Joshi, N., Wende, W., & Kleinschroth, F. (2024). Increasing demand for urban community gardening before, during and after the COVID-19 pandemic. *Urban Forestry & Urban Greening, 92*, 128206. https://doi.org/10.1016/j.ufug.2024.128206

Bille, R. A., Jensen, K. E., & Buitenwerf, R. (2023). Global patterns in urban green space are strongly linked to human development and population density. *Urban Forestry & Urban Greening, 86*, 127980. https://doi.org/10.1016/j.ufug.2023.127980

Bockarjova, M., Botzen, W. J. W., van Schie, M. H., & Koetse, M. J. (2020). Property price effects of green interventions in cities: A meta-analysis and implications for gentrification. *Environmental Science & Policy, 112*, 293–304.

Boyd, F. (2022). Between the library and lectures: How can nature be integrated into university infrastructure to improve students' mental health. *Frontiers in Psychology, 13*, 865422. https://doi.org/10.3389/fpsyg.2022.865422

Bratman, G. N., Anderson, C. B., Berman, M. G., Cochran, B., de Vries, S., Flanders, J., Folke, C., Frumkin, H., Gross, J. J., Hartig, T., Kahn, P. H., Jr., Kuo, M., Lawler, J. J., Levin, P. S., Lindahl, T., Meyer-Lindenberg, A., Mitchell, R., Ouyang, Z., Roe, J., . . . Daily, G. C. (2019). Nature and mental health: An ecosystem service perspective. *Science Advances, 5*(7), eaax0903. https://doi.org/10.1126/sciadv.aax0903

Brindley, P., Jorgensen, A., & Maheswaran, R. (2018). Domestic gardens and self-reported health: A national population study. *International Journal of Health Geographics, 17*(1), 31. https://doi.org/10.1186/s12942-018-0148-6

Cameron, R. W. F., Brindley, P., Mears, M., McEwan, K., Ferguson, F., Sheffield, D., Jorgensen, A., Riley, J., Goodrick, J., Ballard, L., & Richardson, M. (2020). Where the wild things are! Do urban green spaces with greater avian biodiversity promote more positive emotions in humans? *Urban Ecosystems, 23*(2), 301–317.

Chalmin-Pui, L. S., Griffiths, A., Roe, J., Heaton, T., & Cameron, R. (2021). Why garden? – Attitudes and the perceived health benefits of home gardening. *Cities, 112*, 103118. https://doi.org/10.1016/j.cities.2021.103118

Chalmin-Pui, L. S., Roe, J., Griffiths, A., Smyth, N., Heaton, T., Clayden, A., & Cameron, R. (2021). "It made me feel brighter in myself" – the health and well-being impacts of a residential front garden horticultural intervention. *Landscape and Urban Planning, 205*, 103958. https://doi.org/10.1016/j.landurbplan.2020.103958

Collins, R. M., Smith, D., Ogutu, B. O., Brown, K. A., Eigenbrod, F., & Spake, R. (2023). The relative effects of access to public greenspace and private gardens on mental health. *Landscape and Urban Planning, 240*, 104902. https://doi.org/10.1016/j.landurbplan.2023.104902

Dadvand, P., de Vries, S., Bauer, N., Dayamba, D. S., Feng, X., Morand, S., Payyappallimana, U., Remans, R., Rasolofoson, R., Shackleton, C., Shanley, P., Tyrväinen, L., van den Berg, A., & van den Bosch, M. (2023). The health and wellbeing effects of forests, trees and green space. In C. Konijnendijk, D. Devkota, S. Mansourian, & C. Wildburger (Eds.), *Forest and trees for human health: Pathways, impacts, challenges and response options* (pp. 77–124). IUFRO.

de Vries, S. (2022). Nature, health and well-being: Evidence and examples. In M. Stuiver (Ed.), *The symbiotic city: Voices of nature in urban transformations* (pp. 207–229). Wageningen Academic Publishers.

de Vries, S., Buijs, A. E., & Snep, R. P. (2020). Environmental justice in the Netherlands: Presence and quality of greenspace differ by socioeconomic status of neighbourhoods. *Sustainability, 12*(15), 5889. https://doi.org/10.3390/su12155889

de Vries, S., Kramer, H., Smits, M., Spijker, J., Verheij, R., Dückers, M., Baliatsas, C., & Wiegersma, S. (2023). *Een groene tuin, een gezonde tuin? Onderzoek naar het belang van privégroen bij huis voor de gezondheid van burgers* [A green garden, a healthy garden? Study on the importance of private greenery near home for citizens' health]. Wageningen Environmental Research.

Dennis, M., & James, P. (2017). Evaluating the relative influence on population health of domestic gardens and green space along a rural-urban gradient. *Landscape and Urban Planning, 157*, 343–351.

Dzhambov, A. M., Lercher, P., Browning, M. H. E. M., Stoyanov, D., Petrova, N., Novakov, S., & Dimitrova, D. D. (2021). Does greenery experienced indoors and outdoors provide an escape and support mental health during the COVID-19 quarantine? *Environmental Research, 196*, 110420. https://doi.org/10.1016/j.envres.2020.110420

Egerer, M., Lin, B., Kingsley, J., Marsh, P., Diekmann, L., & Ossola, A. (2022). Gardening can relieve human stress and boost nature connection during the COVID-19 pandemic. *Urban Forestry & Urban Greening, 68*, 127483. https://doi.org/10.1016/j.ufug.2022.127483

Farris, S., Zhang, L., Dempsey, N., McEwan, K., Hoyle, H., & Cameron, R. (in press). 'The Elephant in the Room' – does actual or perceived biodiversity elicit restorative responses in a virtual park? *Cities & Health*, 1–16. https://doi.org/10.1080/23748834.2024.2383825

Gao, S., Zhai, W., & Fu, X. (2023). Green space justice amid COVID-19: Unequal access to public green space across American neighborhoods. *Frontiers in Public Health, 11*, 1055720. https://doi.org/10.3389/fpubh.2023.1055720

Gaston, K. J., & Soga, M. (2020). Extinction of experience: The need to be more specific. *People and Nature, 2*(3), 575–581.

Geneletti, D., Cortinovis, C., & Zardo, L. (2022). Simulating crowding of urban green areas to manage access during lockdowns. *Landscape and Urban Planning, 219*, 104319. https://doi.org/10.1016/j.landurbplan.2021.104319

Gillis, K., & Gatersleben, B. (2015). A review of psychological literature on the health and wellbeing benefits of biophilic design. *Buildings*, *5*(3), 948–963.

Grahn, P., & Stigsdotter, U. K. (2010). The relation between perceived sensory dimensions of urban green space and stress restoration. *Landscape and Urban Planning*, *94*(3–4), 264–275.

Haahtela, T. (2019). A biodiversity hypothesis. *Allergy*, *74*(8), 1445–1456.

Haaland, C., & van den Bosch, C. K. (2015). Challenges and strategies for urban green-space planning in cities undergoing densification: A review. *Urban Forestry & Urban Greening*, *14*(4), 760–771.

Harries, B., Chalmin-Pui, L. S., Gatersleben, B., Griffiths, A., & Ratcliffe, E. (2023). 'Designing a wellbeing garden' a systematic review of design recommendations. *Design for Health*, 7(2), 180–201.

Harries, B., Chalmin-Pui, L. S., Gatersleben, B., Griffiths, A., & Ratcliffe, E. (in press). Identifying features within a garden linked to emotional reactions and perceived restoration. *Cities & Health*, 1–13. https://doi.org/10.1080/23748834.2023.2300235

Hartig, T., Mitchell, R., de Vries, S., & Frumkin, H. (2014). Nature and health. *Annual Review of Public Health*, *35*, 207–228.

Hoffimann, E., Barros, H., & Ribeiro, A. I. (2017). Socioeconomic inequalities in green space quality and accessibility-evidence from a southern European city. *International Journal of Environmental Research and Public Health*, *14*(8), 916. https://doi.org/10.3390/ijerph14080916

Jorgensen, L. J., Ellis, G. D., & Ruddell, E. (2013). Fear perceptions in public parks: Interactions of environmental concealment, the presence of people recreating, and gender. *Environment and Behavior*, *45*(7), 803–820.

Juster, R.-P., McEwen, B. S., & Lupien, S. J. (2010). Allostatic load biomarkers of chronic stress and impact on health and cognition. *Neuroscience & Biobehavioral Reviews*, *35*(1), 2–16.

Kahana, E., Lovegreen, L., Kahana, B., & Kahana, M. (2003). Person, environment, and person-environment fit as influences on residential satisfaction of elders. *Environment and Behavior*, *35*(3), 434–453.

Kaplan, S. (1995). The restorative benefits of nature: Toward an integrative framework. *Journal of Environmental Psychology*, *15*(3), 169–182.

Kellert, S. R., & Wilson, E. O. (Eds.). (1993). *The biophilia hypothesis*. Island Press.

Kleinschroth, F., Savilaakso, S., Kowarik, I., Martinez, P. J., Chang, Y., Jakstis, K., Schneider, J., & Fischer, L. K. (2024). Global disparities in urban green space use during the COVID-19 pandemic from a systematic review. *Nature Cities*, *1*, 136–149.

Korpela, K. M., Hartig, T., Kaiser, F. G., & Fuhrer, U. (2001). Restorative experience and self-regulation in favorite places. *Environment and Behavior*, *33*(4), 572–589.

Korpela, K. M., & Ylén, M. (2007). Perceived health is associated with visiting natural favourite places in the vicinity. *Health & Place*, *13*(1), 138–151.

Kuo, M. (2015). How might contact with nature promote human health? Promising mechanisms and a possible central pathway. *Frontiers in Psychology*, *6*, 1093. https://doi.org/10.3389/fpsyg.2015.01093

Lin, B., Meyers, J., & Barnett, G. (2015). Understanding the potential loss and inequities of green space distribution with urban densification. *Urban Forestry & Urban Greening*, *14*(4), 952–958.

Lin, J., Huang, B., Wang, Q., Chen, M., Lee, H. F., & Kwan, M.-P. (2024). Impacts of street tree abundance, greenery, structure and management on residential house prices in New York City. *Urban Forestry & Urban Greening, 94*, 128288. https://doi.org/10.1016/j.ufug.2024.128288

Lin, Y.-H., Tsai, C.-C., Sullivan, W. C., Chang, P.-J., & Chang, C.-Y. (2014). Does awareness effect the restorative function and perception of street trees? *Frontiers in Psychology, 5*, 906. https://doi.org/10.3389/fpsyg.2014.00906

Loebach, J., Sanches, M., Jaffe, J., & Elton-Marshall, T. (2021). Paving the way for outdoor play: Examining socio-environmental barriers to community-based outdoor play. *International Journal of Environmental Research and Public Health, 18*(7), 3617. https://doi.org/10.3390/ijerph18073617

Markevych, I., Schoierer, J., Hartig, T., Chudnovsky, A., Hystad, P., Dzhambov, A. M., de Vries, S., Triguero-Mas, M., Brauer, M., Nieuwenhuijsen, M. J., Lupp, G., Richardson, E. A., Astell-Burt, T., Dimitrova, D., Feng, X., Sadeh, M., Standl, M., Heinrich, J., & Fuertes, E. (2017). Exploring pathways linking greenspace to health: Theoretical and methodological guidance. *Environmental Research, 158*, 301–317.

Marselle, M. R., Bowler, D. E., Watzema, J., Eichenberg, D., Kirsten, T., & Bonn, A. (2020). Urban street tree biodiversity and antidepressant prescriptions. *Scientific Reports, 10*(1), 22445. https://doi.org/10.1038/s41598-020-79924-5

Marselle, M. R., Hartig, T., Cox, D. T. C., de Bell, S., Knapp, S., Lindley, S., Triguero-Mas, M., Böhning-Gaese, K., Braubach, M., Cook, P. A., de Vries, S., Heintz-Buschart, A., Hofmann, M., Irvine, K. N., Kabisch, N., Kolek, F., Kraemer, R., Markevych, I., Martens, D., . . . Bonn, A. (2021). Pathways linking biodiversity to human health: A conceptual framework. *Environment International, 150*, 106420. https://doi.org/10.1016/j.envint.2021.106420

Martin, L., White, M. P., Hunt, A., Richardson, M., Pahl, S., & Burt, J. (2020). Nature contact, nature connectedness and associations with health, wellbeing and pro-environmental behaviours. *Journal of Environmental Psychology, 68*, 101389. https://doi.org/10.1016/j.jenvp.2020.101389

McDonald, R. I., Aronson, M. F. J., Beatley, T., Beller, E., Bazo, M., Grossinger, R., Jessup, K., Mansur, A. V., Puppim de Oliveira, J. A., Panlasigui, S., Burg, J., Pevzner, N., Shanahan, D., Stoneburner, L., Rudd, A., & Spotswood, E. (2023). Denser and greener cities: Green interventions to achieve both urban density and nature. *People and Nature, 5*(1), 84–102.

Meuwese, D., Dijkstra, K., Maas, J., & Koole, S. L. (2021). Beating the blues by viewing green: Depressive symptoms predict greater restoration from stress and negative affect after viewing a nature video. *Journal of Environmental Psychology, 75*, 101594. https://doi.org/10.1016/j.jenvp.2021.101594

Mori, K., Rock, M., McCormack, G., Liccioli, S., Giunchi, D., Marceau, D., Stefanakis, E., & Massolo, A. (2023). Fecal contamination of urban parks by domestic dogs and tragedy of the commons. *Scientific Reports, 13*(1), 3462. https://doi.org/10.1038/s41598-023-30225-7

Moula, Z., Palmer, K., & Walshe, N. (2022). A systematic review of arts-based interventions delivered to children and young people in nature or outdoor spaces: Impact on nature connectedness, health and wellbeing. *Frontiers in Psychology, 13*, 858781. https://doi.org/10.3389/fpsyg.2022.858781

Neilson, B. N., Craig, C. M., Travis, A. T., & Klein, M. I. (2019). A review of the limitations of attention restoration theory and the importance of its future research for the improvement of well-being in urban living. *Visions for Sustainability, 11*, 59–67.

Nordh, H., & Østby, K. (2013). Pocket parks for people – a study of park design and use. *Urban Forestry & Urban Greening, 12*(1), 12–17.

Osborne, L. P., Cushing, D. F., & Washington, T. L. (2021). Where have all the backyards gone? The decline of usable residential greenspace in Brisbane, Australia. *Australian Planner, 57*(2), 100–113.

Oviedo, M., Drescher, M., & Dean, J. (2022). Urban greenspace access, uses, and values: A case study of user perceptions in metropolitan ravine parks. *Urban Forestry & Urban Greening, 70*, 127522. https://doi.org/10.1016/j.ufug.2022.127522

Padgett, D. A., & Glaser, R. (2003). How stress influences the immune response. *Trends in Immunology, 24*(8), 444–448.

Pasanen, T. P., Neuvonen, M., & Korpela, K. M. (2018). The psychology of recent nature visits: (How) are motives and attentional focus related to post-visit restorative experiences, creativity, and emotional well-being? *Environment and Behavior, 50*(8), 913–944.

Plaut, P., Shach-Pinsly, D., Schreuer, N., & Kizony, R. (2021). The reflection of the fear of falls and risk of falling in walking activity spaces of older adults in various urban environments. *Journal of Transport Geography, 95*, 103152. https://doi.org/10.1016/j.jtrangeo.2021.103152

Poortinga, W., Bird, N., Hallingberg, B., Phillips, R., & Williams, D. (2021). The role of perceived public and private green space in subjective health and wellbeing during and after the first peak of the COVID-19 outbreak. *Landscape and Urban Planning, 211*, 104092. https://doi.org/10.1016/j.landurbplan.2021.104092

Ribeiro, A. I., Fraga, S., Kelly-Irving, M., Delpierre, C., Stringhini, S., Kivimaki, M., Joost, S., Guessous, I., Gandini, M., Vineis, P., & Barros, H. (2019). Neighbourhood socioeconomic deprivation and allostatic load: A multi-cohort study. *Scientific Reports, 9*(1), 8790. https://doi.org/10.1038/s41598-019-45432-4

Rigolon, A., Browning, M., & Jennings, V. (2018). Inequities in the quality of urban park systems: An environmental justice investigation of cities in the United States. *Landscape and Urban Planning, 178*, 156–169.

Rigolon, A., Browning, M. H. E. M., McAnirlin, O., & Yoon, H. V. (2021). Green space and health equity: A systematic review on the potential of green space to reduce health disparities. *International Journal of Environmental Research and Public Health, 18*(5), 2563. https://doi.org/10.3390/ijerph18052563

Roscoe, C., Mackay, C., Gulliver, J., Hodgson, S., Cai, Y., Vineis, P., & Fecht, D. (2022). Associations of private residential gardens versus other greenspace types with cardiovascular and respiratory disease mortality: Observational evidence from UK Biobank. *Environment International, 167*, 107427. https://doi.org/10.1016/j.envint.2022.107427

Shentova, R., de Vries, S., & Verboom, J. (2022). Well-being in the time of corona: Associations of nearby greenery with mental well-being during COVID-19 in The Netherlands. *Sustainability, 14*(16), 10256. https://doi.org/10.3390/su141610256

Shoari, N., Ezzati, M., Baumgartner, J., Malacarne, D., & Fecht, D. (2020). Accessibility and allocation of public parks and gardens in England and Wales: A COVID-19 social distancing perspective. *PLoS One, 15*(10), e0241102. https://doi.org/10.1371/journal.pone.0241102

Smyth, N., Thorn, L., Wood, C., Hall, D., & Lister, C. (2022). Increased wellbeing following engagement in a group nature-based programme: The green gym programme delivered by the conservation volunteers. *Healthcare, 10*(6), 978. https://doi.org/10.3390/healthcare10060978

Soga, M., Evans, M. J., Tsuchiya, K., & Fukano, Y. (2021). A room with a green view: The importance of nearby nature for mental health during the COVID-19 pandemic. *Ecological Applications, 31*(2), e2248. https://doi.org/10.1002/eap.2248

Soga, M., & Gaston, K. J. (2016). Extinction of experience: The loss of human-nature interactions. *Frontiers in Ecology and the Environment*, *14*(2), 94–101.

Soga, M., & Gaston, K. J. (2020). The ecology of human-nature interactions. *Proceedings. Biological Sciences*, *287*(1918), 20191882. https://doi.org/10.1098/rspb.2019.1882

Stoltz, J., & Grahn, P. (2021). Perceived sensory dimensions: Key aesthetic qualities for health-promoting urban green spaces. *Journal of Biomed Research*, *2*(1), 22–29.

Strunk, C., & Richardson, M. (2019). Cultivating belonging: Refugees, urban gardens, and placemaking in the Midwest, U.S.A. *Social & Cultural Geography*, *20*(6), 826–848.

Sun, C., Lin, T., Zhao, Q., Li, X., Ye, H., Zhang, G., Liu, X., & Zhao, Y. (2019). Spatial pattern of urban green spaces in a long-term compact urbanization process – a case study in China. *Ecological Indicators*, *96*(2), 111–119.

Taylor, M. S., Wheeler, B. W., White, M. P., Economou, T., & Osborne, N. J. (2015). Research note: Urban street tree density and antidepressant prescription rates – a cross-sectional study in London, UK. *Landscape and Urban Planning*, *136*, 174–179.

Ulrich, R. S. (1983). Aesthetic and affective response to natural environment. *Human Behavior & Environment: Advances in Theory & Research*, *6*, 85–125.

Wang, R., Feng, Z., & Pearce, J. (2022). Neighbourhood greenspace quantity, quality and socioeconomic inequalities in mental health. *Cities*, *129*, 103815. https://doi.org/10.1016/j.cities.2022.103815

Weimann, H., Rylander, L., van den Bosch, M. A., Albin, M., Skärbäck, E., Grahn, P., & Björk, J. (2017). Perception of safety is a prerequisite for the association between neighbourhood green qualities and physical activity: Results from a cross-sectional study in Sweden. *Health & Place*, *45*, 124–130.

White, M. P., Alcock, I., Grellier, J., Wheeler, B. W., Hartig, T., Warber, S. L., Bone, A., Depledge, M. H., & Fleming, L. E. (2019). Spending at least 120 minutes a week in nature is associated with good health and wellbeing. *Scientific Reports*, *9*(1), 7730. https://doi.org/10.1038/s41598-019-44097-3

White, M. P., Hartig, T., Martin, L., Pahl, S., van den Berg, A. E., Wells, N. M., Costongs, C., Dzhambov, A. M., Elliott, L. R., Godfrey, A., Hartl, A., Konijnendijk, C., Litt, J. S., Lovell, R., Lymeus, F., O'Driscoll, C., Pichler, S., Pouso, C., Razani, N., . . . van den Bosch, M. (2023). Nature-based biopsychosocial resilience: An integrative theoretical framework for research on nature and health. *Environment International*, *181*, 108234. https://doi.org/10.1016/j.envint.2023.108234

Zhang, J., Browning, M. H. E. M., Liu, J., Cheng, Y., Zhao, B., & Dadvand, P. (2023). Is indoor and outdoor greenery associated with fewer depressive symptoms during COVID-19 lockdowns? A mechanistic study in Shanghai, China. *Building and Environment*, *227*(2), 109799. https://doi.org/10.1016/j.buildenv.2022.109799

Zhang, J., Qi, R., & Zhang, H. (2023). Examining the impact of crowding perception on the generation of negative emotions among users of small urban micro public spaces. *Sustainability*, *15*(22), 16104. https://doi.org/10.3390/su152216104

Zhang, L., Dempsey, N., & Cameron, R. (2023). Flowers – sunshine for the soul! How does floral colour influence preference, feelings of relaxation and positive up-lift? *Urban Forestry & Urban Greening*, *79*, 127795. https://doi.org/10.1016/j.ufug.2022.127795

Zhao, Y., van den Berg, P. E. W., Ossokina, I. V., & Arentze, T. A. (2024). How do urban parks, neighborhood open spaces, and private gardens relate to individuals' subjective well-being: Results of a structural equation model. *Sustainable Cities and Society*, *101*, 105094. https://doi.org/10.1016/j.scs.2023.105094

8 A tale of two restorations

Urban biodiversity underpins ecosystem restoration and promotes psychological restoration

Monika Egerer and Melissa Marselle

Introduction

Urban environments present a new frontier in ecosystem restoration and in psychological restoration through nature-based solutions, health interventions, and urban planning strategies that invest in urban greening and green infrastructure. As landscapes where most of the world's population lives and where much land use change is occurring, it is critical that city landscapes are designed considering human health and biodiversity, defined as the variety and variability of life on Earth. Furthermore, as crises and disturbances are increasing from, for example, pandemics and climate change, it is important that city landscapes are designed and planned with a consideration of both ecosystem and psychological resilience. This chapter further elaborates on the interconnection of human recovery and urban resilience, by highlighting opportunities where ecological resilience can foster psychological resilience (Pauleit et al., this volume, Chapter 1).

'Ecosystem resilience' can generally be understood and described as the capacity of a system to cope with disturbances, bounce back from a disturbance, and maintain key system functions and processes (Gunderson & Holling, 2002). For example, in ecology, functions and processes may include natural biological control in agricultural landscapes (Feit et al., 2019) or nutrient cycling in aquatic systems (Pelletier et al., 2020; Swann et al., 2021). In the social-ecological systems literature, the concept of resilience has been described as an interacting process between social and environmental (sub)systems, where nearly all ecosystems and landscapes are the result of the synergistic and antagonistic interactions between human and natural communities (van Oudenhoven et al., 2011). Furthermore, scholars now understand that ecosystems as well as social systems are dynamic, fluctuating, nonlinear systems that may not return to a previous condition(s) even when stressors are removed; thus, systems can have multiple so-called 'stable states', given a certain set of environmental (or social)

Egerer, M., & Marselle, M. (2025). A tale of two restorations: Urban biodiversity underpins ecosystem restoration and promotes psychological restoration. In S. Pauleit, M. Kellmann, & J. Beckmann (Eds.), *Creating Urban and Workplace Environments for Recovery and Well-being* (pp. 151–176). Routledge.

DOI: 10.4324/9781003435471-10

conditions (Oliver et al., 2015). Though a nuanced concept, 'stable states' typically refer to conditions of a system that are resistant to change or disturbance. These states are characterised by equilibrium or stability, where the system tends to return to its original state after experiencing a disturbance. In ecological systems, for example, a 'stable state' might refer to a particular configuration of species composition that persists over time, despite changes in environmental conditions or external disturbances. Thus, biodiversity management approaches must be adaptable and flexible.

'Psychological resilience'[1] is defined as "the process and outcome of successfully adapting to difficult or challenging life experiences" (APA, 2018, w.p.). In the psychological literature, resilience often occurs at the individual (person) level (although it can occur at other scales, for example, family resilience; Walsh, 2021). As a process, psychological resilience involves adversity (e.g., stressful life events) and protective factors in order to facilitate the outcome of positive adaptation. Adversity is defined as difficult, challenging life experiences – such as chronic adversity like poverty or acute adversity like divorce, job loss, death of a family member (Masten & Reed, 2005; Turner & Wheaton, 1997) – that negatively threaten individual functioning or development by increasing the risk of mental ill health (Jordanova et al., 2007; Kessler, 1997). Positive adaptation concerns how well a person is able to maintain good well-being following exposure to adversity (Harrop et al., 2006; Mancini et al., 2010; Wells, 2021). To facilitate resilience, protective factors are required. Protective factors help buffer the negative impacts of adversity, making the ability to positively adapt or 'bounce back' from adversity more likely (Yates et al., 2004). Protective factors occur at the individual, family, and community levels (Marselle et al., 2019). Contact with natural environments is considered a community-level protective factor (Marselle et al., 2019; Masten & Reed, 2005; Masten & Wright, 2009; Wells, 2021; Zautra et al., 2010). This suggests that biodiversity-based interventions to restore ecosystems could also facilitate psychological resilience (White et al., 2023).

In this chapter, we bridge an ecological and psychological perspective of resilience, with urban biodiversity as a fundamental link between the two. In supporting and creating biodiverse environments, urban planning strategies can create win-wins for conservation and human health (Fischer et al., 2017). In regard to human health, the concept of psychological resilience is of focus because this is an increasingly important need for contemporary populations faced with multiple crises and, thus, a demand from urban environments, specifically urban nature. Indeed, restoring ecosystems and their functions can contribute to more healthy and resilient cities (Elmqvist et al., 2015). We specifically focus on how urban biodiversity and biodiverse urban environments can 1) act as habitats for plant and animal biodiversity by providing food and shelter across the urban landscape and restoring ecosystem functioning and 2) promote psychological resilience through the restoration and building of psychological capacities. These two aspects are addressed in the first two sections of the chapter, and the final section of the chapter discusses how to create win-win scenarios for both ecosystems and people through biodiversity.

Biodiversity and ecological resilience and restoration in cities

Biodiversity's components include genetic diversity, species diversity, and ecosystem diversity; thus, interventions should consider the variety of plants that may be (re)introduced, but also the variety of ecosystems of focus (e.g., forests, grasslands, and wetlands). Contact with urban nature, which biodiversity is a part of, is associated with multiple benefits for human health and well-being (Frumkin et al., 2017). However, urban nature is under continuous threat due to more competitive uses of limited land resources and land privatisation (Colding et al., 2020; Lee & Webster, 2006). Forms of urban nature, including single trees, parks, and forests (Andersson et al., 2019; Beatley, 2017), are gaining social-ecological importance for combating climate change and creating health-promoting strategies for current and future cities (Flies et al., 2017). The ecological significance of urban nature is linked to biodiversity via species diversity, structural complexity, and the conservation of rare plant and animal species (Threlfall et al., 2017), while the public health significance of green space has been linked to human health and well-being via reducing harm to environmental stressors (e.g., clean air, reduced noise pollution), restoring our depleted psychological capacities (e.g., stress reduction, attention restoration), and building future capacities to deal with everyday demands (e.g., recreation opportunity, place attachment; Marselle et al., 2021). The health-promoting potential of urban green spaces is not limited to the experience of visual aesthetics but is extended to auditory, olfactory, and haptic stimuli (Franco et al., 2017; Marselle et al., 2021). These multisensory benefits of urban green space are why public health interventions include 'nature prescriptions' to facilitate people's contact with nature for their health (Leavell et al., 2019; Ulmer et al., 2016). For example, spending at least two hours a week in nature is positively associated with reported good health and well-being (White et al., 2019).

Urban environments present new opportunities to restore ecosystems to thereby enhance the resilience and ecological functioning of city landscapes. Biodiversity is specifically linked to ecosystem functioning and stability. Ecosystem restoration in urban environments is relevant in the context of the United Nations (UN) 'Decade on Ecosystem Restoration'. Urban ecosystems are often degraded in both their biotic (i.e., living) and abiotic (i.e., non-living) conditions, including problems such as polluted soils and non-native and invasive plant species (Gulezian & Nyberg, 2010; Klaus & Kiehl, 2021; Pouyat et al., 2010). Furthermore, urban ecosystems often face further degradation through environmental pollution, including from light, sound, and heat. Thus, although urban areas can contain diverse habitats and be 'biodiversity hotspots' with, for example, endemic or endangered species only found within them (Ives et al., 2016; Soanes & Lentini, 2019), the biodiversity of plants and animals in urban areas still generally remains lower than in natural and semi-natural areas, especially when habitat conservation and vegetation availability are low (Aronson et al., 2014).

Ecological restoration is the process of assisting the recovery of degraded, damaged, or destroyed ecosystems in the direction of either a historic reference state with specific abiotic conditions and ecosystem functioning (Society for Ecological Restoration, 2024) or to a system that meets goals for abiotic conditions and ecosystem functioning goals but is essentially 'novel' in its context (Hobbs et al., 2006). In this sense, the novelty of a system depends on an analogue, such as remnant natural habitats or a salt marsh, as well as human influence on the system (Lundholm & Richardson, 2010). In particular, restoration in urban contexts has evolved to broaden ideas around restoration and prior reference states and accept (and sometimes promote) novel ecosystems in cities that can still support biodiversity and promote ecosystem functionality (Ahern, 2016; Hobbs et al., 2014; Teixeira & Fernandes, 2020). Depending on the degree of degradation within urban ecosystems, restoration activities can improve abiotic and biotic conditions to various extents to achieve abiotic conditions and ecosystem functions (Klaus & Kiehl, 2021). Ecological restoration through, for example, 'nature-based solutions' (NBS) that are founded on elevating biodiversity and improving ecosystem functioning can be an important strategy for urban conservation and environmental management (Clement, 2022; Lafortezza et al., 2018). NBS are "actions to protect, sustainably manage and restore natural or modified ecosystems, which address societal challenges (e.g., climate change, food and water security or natural disasters) effectively and adaptively, while simultaneously providing human well-being and biodiversity benefits" (Cohen-Shacham et al., 2016, p. 2). One of the key goals that can be addressed by NBS is the restoration of degraded urban ecosystems to support biodiversity and increase ecosystem resilience and, thereby, the delivery of ecosystem services, that is, the benefits that nature can provide to people (Lafortezza et al., 2018; Millennium Ecosystem Assessment, 2005). For example, the City of Detroit, Michigan, has invested millions of dollars in the restoration of segments of the Detroit River to convert them into a recreational space and a functioning wetland habitat. In removing contaminating sediments and restoring the ecosystem to a wetland of diverse native plants, the restoration efforts of the wetland ecosystem aim to restore functions including water filtration and natural sedimentation, as well as provide habitat for native wildlife, including birds, insects, and amphibians (Matheny, 2020).

In providing such ecosystem functions, the ecological restoration of green spaces (forests, parks, grasslands, gardens, cemeteries, etc.) and blue spaces (streams, lakes, ponds, etc.) can contribute to the development of more resilient urban ecosystems and landscapes (Klaus & Kiehl, 2021). From a theoretical perspective, the ecological characteristics of resilient urban ecosystems are those that incorporate diverse mechanisms for coping with change and disturbance through increased biodiversity within the ecosystem, thereby increasing functional redundancy among species, and diversity in spatial pattern (i.e., landscape heterogeneity; Lafortezza et al., 2018; Pickett et al., 2014). Ecological restoration in cities through NBS that aim to increase biodiversity can improve climate regulation through heat mitigation, increase water storage through soil availability, and reduce pollutants through air filtration through increased vegetation and canopy cover (Elmqvist et al., 2015). As described later, this can be an important overlap with the reducing harm pathway that links biodiversity to human health (Marselle et al., 2021). Thus, supporting and potentially enhancing biodiversity through restoration efforts can contribute to renewal post-disturbance and overall contribute to ecosystem resilience (Elmqvist et al., 2003).

Cities are already making strides through various projects to target biodiversity conservation through NBS and restoration actions. In Munich, Germany, the city has developed and implemented a biodiversity strategy which has supported monitoring initiatives in various ecosystems across the city but also is funding initiatives to promote grassroots conservation initiatives, such as wildflower strips and nature-friendly gardening. These restoration activities can support biodiversity. For example, adding street-side vegetation strips with wildflowers significantly boosted the pollinator abundance (Dietzel et al., 2023). Here, the richness of flowering plants and floral density has been found to have a positive influence on the abundance of honeybees, wild bees, and hoverflies. Increases in pollinators may translate to increases in wild plant pollination, an important ecosystem function and ecosystem service. Globally, the UN Environment Programme aims to support funding initiatives for role model cities interested in starting or scaling up ecosystem restoration efforts, strengthening advocacy, participating in knowledge exchanges, and kickstarting efforts around urban biodiversity. Eight pilot cities highlight innovative policy approaches and initiate implementation of urban ecosystem restoration and nature-based solutions in cities (Generation Restoration Cities, n.d.).

In summary, increasing biodiversity through restoration efforts can improve green space ecosystem functions and, thereby, the resilience of urban ecosystems to perturbations. Yet there are also several important ways in which biodiversity and ecosystem quality produced through restoration activities can mediate the pathways towards human health. In other words, the health and well-being of urban residents benefit from these processes (Wyles et al., 2019).

Biodiversity and psychological resilience and restoration in cities

There is a large body of evidence on the effects of urban nature on mental health and well-being (Beute et al., 2023; van den Berg et al., 2015). But what role might biodiversity of urban nature play in psychological resilience? Is it possible that people who have more contact with biodiversity are more resilient to stressful life events? And if so, what are the mechanisms to explain this? To answer these questions, different areas of psychological research need to be integrated: studies of psychological resilience from developmental and clinical psychology and research on the mental health benefits of natural environments from environmental psychology (Marselle et al., 2019; Wells, 2021; White et al., 2023).

Models of psychological resilience

Models of psychological resilience explain how adversity and protective factors interact to facilitate psychological resilience (Masten, 2014), two of which – the main effect model and the moderator model – are discussed here. In the main effect model of psychological resilience, both adversity and protective factors have a direct impact on mental health, but with opposite impacts – adversity having negative impact, and protective factors having a positive impact, on mental health. Resilience occurs when the positive impacts from the protective factors are greater than the negative impacts of adversity (Masten, 2014; Wells, 2021). For example, frequent group walks in nature were found to have a positive effect on mental health at a greater magnitude than the negative effects of recent stressful life events on mental health, suggesting an 'un-doing effect' (Marselle et al., 2019). During the Covid-19 pandemic, people who had contact with urban nature demonstrated better mental health outcomes than those who had less contact with urban nature (Berdejo-Espinola et al., 2021; Davies & Sanesi, 2022; Sia et al., 2022), suggesting that contact with urban nature benefited mental health over and above the negative impacts to mental health from experiencing a global pandemic. In this way, the main effect model of psychological resilience sounds similar to the idea of balance between stress and recovery in the *Human Recovery Theory* by Kellmann and Kallus (2001) as well as Pauleit et al. (this volume, Chapter 1).

In the moderator model of psychological resilience, there is an interaction between adversity and protective factors whereby the protective factor buffers the negative effect of adversity on mental health, making positive adaptation more likely (Masten, 2014; Wells, 2021). Here, protective factors are statistically analysed as moderators. A moderator is a variable that changes the strength or direction of an association between an independent variable (i.e., adversity) and an outcome variable (i.e., mental health). The strength of the association between adversity and mental health depends on the level of the protective factor, as a moderating variable. For example, Wells and Evans (2003) found the amount of nature around the home buffered the effect of children's stressful life events (e.g., 'getting picked on at school', 'parents arguing') on their psychological distress and self-worth. When there was a high amount of nature near the home, stressful life events had less of an impact on children's distress and self-worth; this buffering effect was greatest for children who experienced the most stressful life events (Wells & Evans, 2003). Regarding biodiversity, Marselle and colleagues (2020) found that living within 100 metres of greater abundance of street trees (but not tree species richness) reduced the risk of being prescribed antidepressants in adults with low socioeconomic status by half.

Nature as a moderator

Figure 8.1 shows biodiverse nature as a moderator. Biodiversity as a community-level protective factor in psychological resilience can be understood as urban design decisions or ecological interventions to increase the amount of biodiverse nature around the home, workplace, or school (Corraliza & Collado, 2011; Leather et al., 1998; Marselle et al., 2020; van den Berg et al., 2010), or as 'nature prescription' to facilitate contact with nature, such as group walks in a national park (Marselle et al., 2019). Here, the relationship between adversity and mental health differs depending on the level of the moderator variable (e.g., more or less street trees around the home; participation vs not participating in nature hikes).

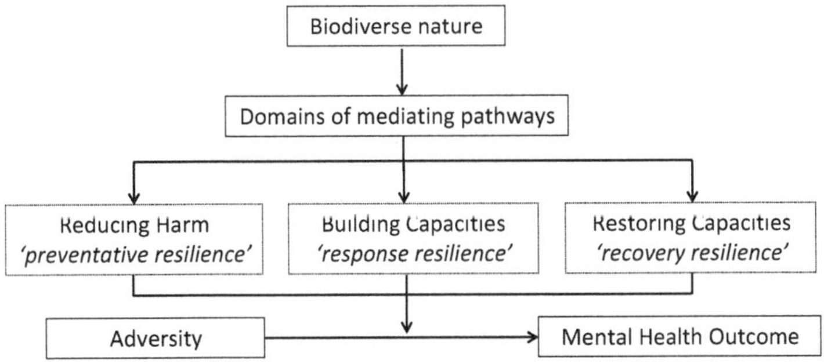

Figure 8.1 A mediated moderation model of resilience in which biodiverse nature indirectly (through a mediating pathway) buffers the negative impact of adversity on mental health to foster psychological resilience. Three domains of mediating pathways are suggested to explain how biodiverse nature moderates (buffers) the negative effect of adversity on a mental health outcome.

Source: Figure based on Marselle et al. (2021), Wells (2021), and White et al. (2023)

Domains of mediating pathways

What are the underlying variables that explain biodiverse nature's role as a protective factor in the moderator model of psychological resilience? Discussion of the underlying variables that explain (or mediate) biodiverse nature's role as a protective factor can be explained by a mediated moderation model of psychological resilience (Figure 8.1). Mediators are explanatory variables that reveal the underlying mechanism or pathway that explains why one variable affects another (Baron & Kenny, 1986).

A conceptual framework identified four domains of mediating pathways by which biodiversity impacts human health in both positive and negative ways (Marselle et al., 2021): 1) *Reducing Harm* (e.g., provision of medicines, decreasing exposure to air and noise pollution), 2) *Restoring Capacities* (e.g., attention restoration, stress reduction), 3) *Building Capacities* (e.g., promoting social cohesion, transcendent experiences), and 4) *Causing Harm* (e.g., dangerous wildlife, zoonotic diseases, allergens). The three domains of mediating pathways that positively impact human health that may explain how/why biodiverse nature has a moderating effect on adversity are detailed in Figure 8.1. Each domain of pathways maps onto the new framework of nature-based biopsychosocial resilience (White et al., 2023). Specifically, we argue that plausible mechanisms from within the *Reducing Harm*, *Building Capacities*, and *Restoring Capacities* domains of pathways may explain nature's ability to foster psychological resilience by reducing exposure to adversity (i.e., preventative resilience), reducing the initial impact or reactivity to adversity (i.e., response resilience), or assisting with recovery following exposure to adversity (i.e., recovery resilience) (White et al., 2023), respectively (Figure 8.1).

Reducing Harm. The *Reducing Harm* domain of pathways highlights the various ways biodiversity reduces harm to human health and well-being by providing to the determinants of health (essential provisioning ecosystem services, like medicines, food, and clean drinking water) and reducing the harm caused by environmental stressors (regulating ecosystem services, like regulation of air and noise pollution or extreme heat). In the context of nature-based biopsychosocial resilience (White et al., 2023), the mediators in the *Reducing Harm* domain contribute to 'preventative resilience' as they could reduce the risk or potency of adversity. An example is the ability of biodiversity to reduce exposure to air and noise pollution (Marselle et al., 2021). As an environmental stressor, air pollution is a well-known cause of negative human health outcomes (Lelieveld et al., 2019; Zivin & Neidell, 2018), particularly for urban dwellers. Tree diversity has a significant impact on the potential to mitigate air pollution in cities (Churkina et al., 2015; Grote et al., 2016). Vegetation with high structural complexity and density has been found to be an effective barrier to ultrafine particles from roads (Hagler et al., 2012).

Building Capacities. The *Building Capacities* domain of pathways refers to the deepening or strengthening of capabilities for meeting everyday demands, rather than the restoration of a depleted resource (Hartig, 2007; Marselle et al., 2021). In the context of nature-based biopsychosocial resilience (White et al., 2023), the mediators in the *Building Capacities* domain contribute to 'response resilience' as they reduce the impact of adversity by strengthening biopsychosocial resources to help individuals better cope.

Transcendent experience is a mediator within the *Building Capacities* domain that may explain why contact with biodiversity could foster psychological resilience (for other potential mediators, see Marselle et al., 2021). Transcendent experiences – such as awe, reflection, or humility – contribute to human health and well-being (Capaldi et al., 2015). In the resilience literature, spirituality and the belief that life has meaning are protective factors moderating the effect of adversity on positive mental health outcomes (Masten, 2014). Biodiverse environments are common settings for spiritual encounters, places to experience meaning and purpose in life, oneness, unity, wonder, and awe (Irvine et al., 2019). Even watching nature documentaries, like Planet Earth, from the comfort of one's own home can foster awe, provide relief following a negative stressful life event, and improve mental well-being (Liu et al., 2023). Self-reflection – thinking about one's life, goals, and priorities (Kaplan & Kaplan, 1989) – is crucial for psychological resilience, as it enables one to 'take stock' of the traumatic event and its impact (Joseph, 2012), which is necessary for identifying, evaluating, and expressing post-adversity change (Joseph, 2012). Self-reflection is a higher-order experience in the *Attention Restoration Theory* (ART) which occurs following attention restoration and depends on the duration of time spent in a high-quality natural environment (Herzog et al., 1997; Kaplan & Kaplan, 1989). Natural environments may foster post-adversity growth by promoting self-reflection (Dallimer et al., 2012; Fuller et al., 2007), spiritual well-being (Irvine et al., 2013; Warber et al., 2015), or the belief that life has meaning (Masten & Wright, 2009). A study of urban parks in the UK found that park visitors reported greater reflection when visiting parks with a greater actual, and perceived, species richness of trees and birds (Dallimer et al., 2012; Fuller et al., 2007).

Restoring capacities. This domain of pathways refers to the recovery of physiological or psychological resources that have been diminished through the demands of dealing with everyday life (Hartig et al., 2017). Without restoration of these resources, a person is unable to cope with new demands (imagine working to meet a new deadline with depleted physiological and psychological resources immediately after meeting the last deadline). Over time, lack of restoration of these resources can lead to mental and physical ill health (von Lindern et al., 2017). In the context of nature-based biopsychosocial resilience (White et al., 2023), the mediators in the *Restoring Capacities* domain contribute to 'recovery resilience' as they help individuals recover from stress or the fatigue of cognitive resources. Environments that facilitate the recovery and restoration of these depleted resources are called restorative environments.

Stress reduction theory

There are two main theories of restorative environments. The first is *Stress Reduction Theory* (SRT; Ulrich, 1983; Ulrich et al., 1991), which considers that natural environments benefit health by helping people recover from stress. Evidence of SRT is reduced physiological arousal, psychological stress, and negative emotions and enhanced positive emotions following exposure to nature (Ulrich et al., 1991). Stress reduction is a well-studied mediator of green space and health (Beute et al., 2023; Markevych et al., 2017) and is a plausible mechanism underlying nature's role as a protective factor for psychological resilience, as adversity is considered a severe acute stressor (Turner & Wheaton, 1997). SRT has been shown to facilitate 'recovery resilience' (White et al., 2023). Ulrich (1984) found that people needed less medication following surgery when recovering in a hospital room with a view of a tree, compared to a hospital room with a view of a brick wall. Viewing urban nature has been shown to help people recover quickly following the experience of an acute stressor, such as viewing a stressful video (Ulrich et al., 1991).

SRT states that environments which contain certain characteristics, or *preferanda*, will be restorative (Ulrich, 1983). Complexity – the number of independently perceived elements in a setting – is one of these *preferanda* (Ulrich, 1983; see Box 8.1). Biodiversity is considered a measure of an environment's complexity (Marselle, 2019). Viewing a meadowlike array of plants led to a greater physiological stress recovery; the stress recovery was greatest when viewing an intermediate level of species richness (32 species) of plants (Lindemann-Matthies & Matthies, 2018). However, Schebella et al. (2019) and Rozario et al. (2024) found no evidence of physiological stress recovery after viewing a

Box 8.1 Stress Reduction Theory

- Natural environments benefit health by facilitating recovery from stress.
- Stress recovery is manifested as reduced physiological arousal, psychological stress, and negative affect and enhanced positive affect.
- *Preferanda*, or the visual characteristics of restorative environments, are:
    - Moderate to high complexity (i.e., number of independently perceived elements in a setting)
    - A focal point in the setting to attract or direct attention; moderate to high level of depth (or openness)
    - A smooth and even ground surface that is conducive for movement
    - A lack of threat
    - Deflected vista (e.g., path bending away)
    - Water
- Biodiversity can be considered as a measure of an environment's complexity.

biodiverse environment, compared to viewing an urban environment; nor was there any significant difference in physiological stress recovery between low, medium, and high biodiverse environments.

Attention restoration theory

Directed attention is another plausible mechanism underlying nature as a protective factor of psychological resilience. Directed attention is an executive cognitive function that enables us to focus and process information and plan and solve problems (Suchy et al., 2017). Problem-solving is an essential protective factor for resilience (Masten, 2014). But the ability to direct attention is a limited cognitive resource that can become fatigued with overuse, impairing our inability to solve problems (Kaplan & Berman, 2017) and deal with adversity (Kaplan, 1995). When this happens, one needs to restore the ability to direct attention. *Attention Restoration Theory* (ART; Kaplan, 1995; Kaplan & Berman, 2017; Kaplan & Kaplan, 1989), the second theory of restorative environments, states that contact with nature can restore the ability to direct attention. Changes in cognitive tests after exposure to a natural environment are used as evidence of attention restoration in ART (for systematic reviews, see Ohly et al., 2016; Stevenson et al., 2018). Attention restoration is a well-studied mediator of green space and health (Markevych et al., 2017; Marselle et al., 2021). ART has been shown to facilitate 'recovery resilience' (White et al., 2023). Women with breast cancer who engaged in nature-based activities three times per week showed significant improvement on directed attention compared to women in the standard-care control group (Cimprich & Ronis, 2003).

According to ART, a person can restore a depleted ability to direct attention when they experience four restorative qualities of an environment (see Box 8.2). While biodiversity was not a concept that was used in the original theoretical writings of the ART, it is hypothesised that biodiverse natural environments may be better environments for restoring directed attention as they may contain fascinating stimuli and afford the experience of being away (Marselle, 2019). Evidence from studies supports this hypothesis. Actual (Scopelliti et al., 2012) and perceived (Marselle et al., 2016) biodiversity have been positively related to being away and fasciation, although contrary evidence has been found (Peschardt & Stigsdotter, 2013). Testing 'recovery resilience' (White et al., 2023), Chiang et al. (2017) found a greater restoration of directed attention following exposure to urban green spaces with high-density vegetation compared to green spaces with medium- and low-density vegetation. Although not testing 'recovery resilience', Rozario et al. (2024) found subjective directed attention increased in forests of varying levels of biodiversity compared to urban environments – but no significant difference between the forests of low, medium, and high tree species richness.

In summary, exposure to biodiverse nature can foster psychological resilience by buffering (moderating) against the negative effects of adversity on

Box 8.2 Attention Restoration Theory

- The ability to direct attention is an executive cognitive function that can become fatigued through overuse.
- The inability to concentrate or focus attention is a sign of directed attention fatigue.
- Restoration from directed attention fatigue requires an individual to experience four restorative qualities in a specific environment: 1) *fascination*, when observation and exploration of the environment attract and hold a person's attention without cognitive effort; 2) *being away* from everyday tasks or demands that draw upon directed attention; 3) *extent*, with the environment perceived as coherently organised and with sufficient scope to sustain exploration; and 4) *compatibility* between the environmental setting and one's purposes and inclinations (Kaplan, 1995; Kaplan & Kaplan, 1989).
- Natural environments tend to afford an experience of these four restorative qualities.

mental health. Biodiversity does this through mediating pathways within three domains of pathways: *Reducing Harm*, *Building Capacities*, and *Restoring Capacities* (Marselle et al., 2021). We posit that the mediators in the *Reducing Harm* domain may explain biodiversity's ability to foster psychological resilience by reducing exposure to adversity (i.e., preventative resilience; White et al., 2023); mediators within the *Building Capacities* domain could explain biodiversity's ability to foster psychological resilience by reducing the reactivity to adversity (i.e., response resilience; White et al., 2023); and mediators within the *Restoring Capacities* domain may explain biodiversity's ability to assist with recovery following exposure to adversity (i.e., recovery resilience; White et al., 2023). Fostering psychological resilience through contact with urban nature and experiences with biodiversity may also foster a sense of and commitment to care for urban nature and biodiversity (Prévot et al., 2018). This may positively feed back to urban restoration activities, such as planting biodiverse gardens and trees along street ways. Such potential 'win-wins' are a topic turned to next.

Creating win-wins for urban planning: Biodiversity as a fundamental link

Creating biodiverse environments can be a win-win for urban planning strategies and NBS that promote conservation and public health (Fischer et al., 2017). Restoring ecosystems and their functions can contribute to healthy ecosystems and healthy human communities, and thereby resilient cities, under social and environmental change (Elmqvist et al., 2015). Few studies have examined the impacts of ecological degradation or restoration on mental health (Kondo et al., 2015; Speldewinde et al., 2009) – although only one focuses on those in need of psychological resilience (South et al., 2018). Ecological restoration of vacant lots in the USA (planting new grass and a small number of trees, removing trash, and performing regular monthly maintenance) in neighbourhoods below the poverty level was associated with a significant decrease in local residents' self-reported feelings of depression, as well as a nonsignificant reduction in overall self-reported poor mental health (South et al., 2018). This public health study suggests that ecological restoration activities in deprived neighbourhoods could foster psychological resilience. But generally, urban regeneration projects fail to assess the mental health benefits – instead focusing on the ecological, economic, recreational, and social benefits (Brückner et al., 2022). Thus, clear relationships and drivers behind win-win outcomes remain unclear and call for future work. Nonetheless, some examples of (eco)systems in cities can provide insight into possible synergies among biodiversity-based ecological resilience and psychological resilience.

Urban gardens are one social-ecological system where increasing biodiversity has impacts for both ecosystem functioning and human health and well-being and support win-win situations in cities. Gardening includes many forms of horticultural activity (cultivating food, herbs, and flower crops for consumption or non-consumption purposes) undertaken in diverse spatial and social contexts, from private properties, including home gardens, to median strips or public spaces, such as schools and parks (McClintock & Simpson, 2018; Milbourne, 2021; Vávra et al., 2018). Gardens can become a nexus of urban greening, human–nature connection, and public health – and can also be refugia for diverse wild-growing plant communities (Cabral et al., 2017; Egerer & Lin, 2022; Lin & Egerer, 2020; Seitz et al., 2022). Conservation gardening, wildlife-friendly gardening, or other forms of horticultural activity can create habitat for native plants and animals as well as create places where people engage intensively with nature, particularly in times of stress, to promote mental health and psychological restoration and resilience (Egerer et al., 2022; Sia et al., 2022; Soga et al., 2017).

The area of cities dedicated to gardening (e.g., allotments, home gardens; de Vries & Chalmin-Pui, this volume, Chapter 7) varies with city context and often exists at a relatively small (residential or communal) scale, but the ecological and social effects of gardens could add up across a city. For example, Europe has approximately three million allotment gardens (Bell et al., 2016). In the UK, approximately 35–47% of green space consists of private home gardens (Loram et al., 2007), and 87% of UK households can access a home garden (Cameron et al., 2012). In Stockholm, Sweden, 2.5% of total green space area is dedicated to allotment gardening, where individual garden parcels are rented and managed by individuals or households (Andersson et al., 2007) and allotments are estimated to involve around 24,000 people and cover 210 hectares of land (discussed in Barthel et al., 2010). The potential for urban gardening to contribute to urban green infrastructure and support food production is also high, though its potential is limited due to land use policy and zoning limitations. For example, in Berlin, Germany, it is estimated that 82% of vegetable demand could be met through the implementation of urban gardening in about 42 square kilometres of area across the city (de Simone et al., 2023).

Much research has shown how urban gardens support biodiversity of plants and animals. For example, studies have found that urban gardens can host a diversity of native and non-native plant species, as well as plant species that are of conservation concern. Work in 18 community gardens in Berlin found 404 taxa representing 255 genera, in which 19 species were of conservation concern and four species were on the Red List in Germany (Seitz et al., 2022). Studies on plant diversity within home domestic gardens in the UK have found high cultivated and spontaneous growing plant species: 1,166 species in 61 gardens in Sheffield (Smith et al., 2013), and 1,051 species in 267 gardens in five cities (Loram et al., 2008).

Biodiversity is related to ecosystem functions such as microclimate regulation, storm water retention, soil nutrient cycling, pollination, and natural pest control (Cabral et al., 2017; Lin et al., 2015). All these ecosystem functions can be linked to ecosystem restoration indicators, such as improved temperature regulation in a parking-lot-turned-urban-garden initiative (Tomatis et al., 2023), or improved soil conditions through active soil remediation/restoration activities using compost for growing fruits and vegetables (Tresch et al., 2019). Reducing impervious surface and increasing vegetation and soil surface within gardens can also improve soil moisture retention and regulation (Lin et al., 2019) and increase storm water capture (Gittleman et al., 2017). Increasing plant diversity can also potentially support more diverse natural enemies (Jha et al., 2023), making garden ecosystems more resilient to pest outbreaks (Arnold et al., 2019).

Engagement in gardening activities can, in turn, promote the health and well-being of gardeners through contact with biodiversity (Lin et al., 2018). Meta-analyses summarise how gardening is a positive 'restorative' activity, and one of the reasons is through interaction with soil and plants, as well as physical activity (Soga et al., 2017). Gardeners often report increased life satisfaction, vigour, psychological well-being, sense of community, and cognitive functioning (Soga et al., 2017). According to White's et al. (2023) framework, we can interpret that gardening may foster psychological resilience by enabling people to draw on these psychological resources in order to reduce exposure to future stressors ('preventive resilience') or reduce the initial impact of adversity ('response resilience') (White et al., 2023). Gardening has also been shown to assist with recovery following exposure to adversity ('recovery resilience'; White et al., 2023). In an experimental study, gardening was found to decrease the stress hormone cortisol and increase positive mood following exposure to an acute stressor, indicating that gardening can promote neuroendocrine and affective restoration from acute stress (van den Berg & Custers, 2011). During crises, these benefits of gardening for psychological resilience can be especially enhanced. For example, during the Covid-19 pandemic, 'crisis gardening' became a 'lifesaver' during lockdowns for many urban residents. In Singapore, surveyed gardeners during the pandemic reported significantly higher mental resilience (of seven resilience factors, including 'emotional regulation', 'relationship/social support', 'confidence', 'positive thinking', 'control', 'flexibility', and 'spirituality') than a control group – and these positive resilience effects were heightened in those that gardened weekly for one to four hours (Sia et al., 2022). This may be through (re)connections to or experiences with nature and biodiversity. Marsh et al. (2021) found that during the Covid-19 pandemic, gardeners reported experiencing heightened senses of joy, beauty, and reassurance, as well as a greater attunement to the natural world and an increased sense of nature connection than they had at other times, where one respondent reported that 'birds felt louder'. These heightened sensory and emotional experiences had therapeutic benefits across diverse demographics and geographic contexts during a psychologically stressful time. People also reported that through this intensive (re)connection to nature around them, they would consider more wildlife-friendly gardening (Kingsley et al., 2022).

Thus, as a common way in which people have direct contact with nature, 'doses' of urban gardening can be a mainstreamed public health intervention to potentially foster psychological resilience, which may be especially beneficial during times of crisis (Kingsley et al., 2022; Lin et al., 2021). Nature prescriptions, where a healthcare provider provides a written prescription for a person to spend time in nature (Kondo et al., 2020), might be one such public health intervention. Activities for a nature prescription might include gardening (Howarth et al., 2020), walking groups (Lahart et al., 2019), or nature conservation (Lovell et al.,

2015). Indeed, horticultural therapy is an increasingly popular yet not necessarily new nature-based form of mental health treatment that can aid in mental health recovery of patients (Cipriani et al., 2017; Gonzalez et al., 2010). Regarding psychological resilience, female victims of domestic violence reported that gardening helped reduce feelings of stress, negative affect, and depression and enhanced feelings of relaxation and empowerment (Stuart, 2005). A dose–response relationship was also found where women who spent six hours or more per week gardening reported experiencing more therapeutic and positive feelings than women who spent three hours or less per week gardening (Stuart, 2005). Taken together, this suggests that urban gardening could be a nature prescription to those experiencing adversity to help foster psychological resilience.

This could have spillover effects on the biodiversity and functioning of gardens if people spend more time in gardens and feel a sense of duty to increase biodiversity within the gardens (Prévot et al., 2018; Robinson & Breed, 2019). Such a positive and synergistic relationship between garden ecosystems and human health could be especially beneficial given the land area that gardening occupies in urban landscapes, as discussed earlier. In Berlin, for example, there are initiatives and projects to involve citizen scientists in the propagation and cultivation of threatened plant species in gardens (Fišer et al., 2021), accompanied by conservation authorities and botanical gardens (Godefroid et al., 2011; Lauterbach et al., 2019). Here, the idea is that gardens are where restoration of ecosystem functioning through species conservation where people live and recreate may be most feasible or achievable. Gardens across a city supporting a wide range of plant species, in which people experience biodiversity and where both human needs and nature's biological diversity align. Such gardening can present a system for win-wins in urban restoration and psychological resilience.

Yet it remains unclear how exactly biodiversity in urban gardens impacts psychological well-being (Marselle et al., 2021; Rozario et al., 2024). The feedback loops between biodiversity and ecological restoration, for example, via wildlife-friendly gardening and psychological restoration are also largely unclear and nonlinear (Garfinkel et al., 2024). Research in urban gardens in Israel found that individual characteristics, such as affinity to nature, influence the relationship between psychological well-being and biodiversity present within the garden (Shwartz et al., 2023). Thus, there is no 'one-size-fits-all' when it comes to making recommendations around biodiversity-based interventions in gardens (Shwartz et al., 2023) or how to 'turbo-boost' a recovery process through biodiversity-related nature experiences. It may largely depend on the person themselves and their characteristics. These are some ways in which ecosystem restoration and psychological resilience based on biodiversity can align to create win-wins for people and nature.

Conclusion

Researchers working in urban environments are often confronted with the questions: What is the most liveable city, or sustainable city, or biodiverse city, or healthy city? What are innovative concepts in urban planning that bridge urban greening, ecosystem restoration, and human health? What will the ideal future cities look like? These are all good questions, and one way to think about this is through a restoration-and-resilience lens. In ecology, resilient ecosystems are characterised by their biodiversity and the functions of this biodiversity in relation to ecosystem processes. Thus, creating or sustaining resilience requires sustaining or restoring biodiversity. In public health and environmental psychology, psychological resilience is related to restoring and rebuilding pathways that can be influenced by biodiversity exposure and biodiversity-based nature interactions.

There are diverse ways in which to think about restoration and resilience and how to promote both. This chapter shares examples of where parallels in ecosystem restoration and psychological restoration may occur, with resilience as a goal. Biodiversity can be a key link between ecological and psychological resilience – city environments can be managed to support biodiverse urban ecosystems that create opportunities for psychological restoration and human health. Whether it is biodiverse gardens and parks, streams and waterways, or green mobility corridors for both animals and people movement, these are ways to create city environments for both people and nature (Heiland et al., 2019).

In conclusion, planning future cities is a tale of two restorations and of dual resilience, underpinned by biodiversity. Biodiversity creates functioning and resilient ecosystems, and biodiversity can foster human health for psychological resilience.

Note

1 Despite coming from different psychological disciplines, there are similarities between the theories of psychological resilience and human recovery (see Pauleit et al., this volume, Chapter 1). Both focus on the process by which individuals recover from stressors, and both discuss stress buffers. Protective factors in psychological resilience theory are similar to the personal resources and strategies to cope with stress identified in the theory of human recovery (Pauleit et al., this volume, Chapter 1). However, differences exist. Adversity differs from the everyday demands (e.g., noise pollution, work stress, traffic congestion; see Pauleit et al., this volume, Chapter 1) discussed in the theory of human recovery by severity of the stressor, and its health impacts. While the human recovery theory posits a balance between stress and recovery – that an increasing stress must co-occur with an increase in recovery to prevent negative health effects from stress (Kellmann & Kallus, 2001; Pauleit et al., this volume, Chapter 1) and cultivate resilience (Beckmann & Kellmann, 2024) – it is unclear what increased recovery is needed to facilitate a recovery resilience from acute or chronic adverse life experiences.

References

Ahern, J. (2016). Novel urban ecosystems: Concepts, definitions and a strategy to support urban sustainability and resilience. *Landscape Architecture Frontiers*, *4*, 10–21.

Andersson, E., Barthel, S., & Ahrné, K. (2007). Measuring social – ecological dynamics behind the generation of ecosystem services. *Ecological Applications*, *17*(5), 1267–1278.

Andersson, E., Langemeyer, J., Borgström, S., McPhearson, T., Haase, D., Kronenberg, J., Barton, D. N., Davis, M., Naumann, S., Röschel, L., & Baró, F. (2019). Enabling green and blue infrastructure to improve contributions to human well-being and equity in urban systems. *BioScience*, *69*, 566–574.

APA. (2018). *APA dictionary of psychology: Resilience.* American Psychological Association. Retrieved May 14, 2024 from https://dictionary.apa.org/resilience

Arnold, J. E., Egerer, M., & Daane, K. M. (2019). Local and landscape effects to biological controls in urban agriculture – a review. *Insects, 10*(7), 215. https://doi.org/10.3390/insects10070215

Aronson, M. F., La Sorte, F. A., Nilon, C. H., Katti, M., Goddard, M. A., Lepczyk, C. A., Warren, P. S., Williams, N. S. G., Cilliers, S., Clarkson, B., Dobbs, C., Dolan, R., Hedblom, M., Klotz, S., Kooijmans, J. L., Kühn, I., MacGregor-Fors, I., McDonnell, M., Mörtberg, U., . . . Winter, M. (2014). A global analysis of the impacts of urbanization on bird and plant diversity reveals key anthropogenic drivers. *Proceedings of the Royal Society B: Biological Sciences, 281*(1780), 20133330. https://doi.org/10.1098/rspb.2013.3330

Baron, R. M., & Kenny, D. A. (1986). The moderator-mediator variable distinction in social psychological research: Conceptual, strategic, and statistical considerations. *Journal of Personality and Social Psychology, 51*(6), 1173–1182.

Barthel, S., Folke, C., & Colding, J. (2010). Social–ecological memory in urban gardens – retaining the capacity for management of ecosystem services. *Global Environmental Change, 20*(2), 255–265.

Beatley, T. (2017). *Handbook of biophilic city planning and design.* Island Press-Center for Resource Economics.

Beckmann, J., & Kellmann, M. (2024). Fostering recovery and well-being in a healthy lifestyle: A concluding summary. In M. Kellmann & J. Beckmann (Eds.), *Fostering recovery and well-being in a healthy lifestyle: Psychological, somatic, and organizational prevention approaches* (pp. 218–222). Routledge.

Bell, S., Fox-Kämper, R., Keshavarz, N., Benson, M., Caputo, S., Noori, S., & Voigt, A. (Eds.). (2016). *Urban allotment gardens in Europe.* Routledge.

Berdejo-Espinola, V., Suárez-Castro, A. F., Amano, T., Fielding, K. S., Oh, R. R. Y., & Fuller, R. A. (2021). Urban green space use during a time of stress: A case study during the COVID-19 pandemic in Brisbane, Australia. *People and Nature, 3*(3), 597–609.

Beute, F., Marselle, M. R., Olszewska-Guizzo, A., Andreucci, M. B., Lammel, A., Davies, Z. G., Glanville, J., Keune, H., O'Brien, L., Remmen, R., Russo, A., & de Vries, S. (2023). How do different types and characteristics of green space impact mental health? A scoping review. *People and Nature, 5*, 1839–1876.

Brückner, A., Falkenberg, T., Heinzel, C., & Kistemann, T. (2022). The regeneration of urban blue spaces: A public health intervention? Reviewing the evidence. *Frontiers in Public Health, 9*, 782101. https://doi.org/10.3389/fpubh.2021.782101

Cabral, I., Keim, J., Engelmann, R., Kraemer, R., Siebert, J., & Bonn, A. (2017). Ecosystem services of allotment and community gardens: A Leipzig, Germany case study. *Urban Forestry & Urban Greening, 23*, 44–53.

Cameron, R. W., Blanuša, T., Taylor, J. E., Salisbury, A., Halstead, A. J., Henricot, B., & Thompson, K. (2012). The domestic garden – its contribution to urban green infrastructure. *Urban Forestry & Urban Greening, 11*(2), 129–137.

Capaldi, C. A., Passmore, H.-A., Nisbet, E. K., Zelenski, J. M., & Dopko, R. L. (2015). Flourishing in nature: A review of the benefits of connecting with nature and its application as a wellbeing intervention. *International Journal of Wellbeing, 5*(4), 1–16. https://doi.org/10.5502/ijw.v5i4.449

Chiang, Y. C., Li, D., & Jane, H. A. (2017). Wild or tended nature? The effects of landscape location and vegetation density on physiological and psychological responses. *Landscape and Urban Planning, 167*, 72–83.

Churkina, G., Grote, R., Butler, T. M., & Lawrence, M. (2015). Natural selection? Picking the right trees for urban greening. *Environmental Science and Policy, 47*, 12–17.

Cimprich, B., & Ronis, D. (2003). An environmental intervention to restore attention in women with newly diagnosed breast cancer. *Cancer Nursing, 26*, 284–292.

Cipriani, J., Benz, A., Holmgren, A., Kinter, D., McGarry, J., & Rufino, G. (2017). A systematic review of the effects of horticultural therapy on persons with mental health conditions. *Occupational Therapy in Mental Health, 33*(1), 47–69.

Clement, S. (2022). Nature-based solutions for urban biodiversity. In E. Croci & B. Lucchitta (Eds.), *Nature-based solutions for more sustainable cities – a framework approach for planning and evaluation* (pp. 33–45). Emerald Publishing Limited.

Cohen-Shacham, E., Walters, G., Janzen, C., & Maginnis, S. (Eds.). (2016). *Nature-based solutions to address global societal challenges.* IUCN. Retrieved May 31, 2024 from http://dx.doi.org/10.2305/IUCN.CH.2016.13.en

Colding, J., Gren, Å., & Barthel, S. (2020). The incremental demise of urban green spaces. *Land, 9*(5), 162. https://doi.org/10.3390/land9050162

Corraliza, J. A., & Collado, S. (2011). La naturaleza cercana como moderadora del estrés infantil [Close nature as a moderator of childhood stress]. *Psicothema, 23*(2), 221–226.

Dallimer, M., Irvine, K. N., Skinner, A. M. J., Davies, Z. G., Rouquette, J. R., Maltby, L. L., Warren, P. H., Armsworth, P. R., & Gaston, K. J. (2012). Biodiversity and the feel-good factor: Understanding associations between self-reported human well-being and species richness. *BioScience, 62*, 47–55.

Davies, C., & Sanesi, G. (2022). COVID-19 and the importance of urban green spaces. *Urban Forestry & Urban Greening, 74*, 127654. https://doi.org/10.1016/j.ufug.2022.127654

de Simone, M., Pradhan, P., Kropp, J. P., & Rybski, D. (2023). A large share of Berlin's vegetable consumption can be produced within the city. *Sustainable Cities and Society, 91*, 104362. https://doi.org/10.1016/j.scs.2022.104362

Dietzel, S., Rojas-Botero, S., Kollmann, J., & Fischer, C. (2023). Enhanced urban roadside vegetation increases pollinator abundance whereas landscape characteristics drive pollination. *Ecological Indicators, 147*, 109980. https://doi.org/10.1016/j.ecolind.2023.109980

Egerer, M., & Lin, B. (2022). Balancing urban agriculture with sustaining ecosystem services. *CABI Reviews, 17*(003). https://doi.org/10.1079/cabireviews202217003

Egerer, M., Lin, B., Kingsley, J., Marsh, P., Diekmann, L., & Ossola, A. (2022). Gardening can relieve human stress and boost nature connection during the COVID-19 pandemic. *Urban Forestry & Urban Greening, 68*, 127483. https://doi.org/10.1016/j.ufug.2022.127483

Elmqvist, T., Folke, C., Nyström, M., Peterson, G., Bengtsson, J., Walker, B., & Norberg, J. (2003). Response diversity, ecosystem change, and resilience. *Frontiers in Ecology and the Environment, 1*(9), 488–494.

Elmqvist, T., Setälä, H., Handel, S. N., van der Ploeg, S., Aronson, J., Blignaut, J. N., Gómez-Baggethun, E., Nowak, D. J., Kronenberg, J., & de Groot, R. (2015). Benefits of restoring ecosystem services in urban areas. *Current Opinion in Environmental Sustainability, 14*, 101–108.

Feit, B., Blüthgen, N., Traugott, M., & Jonsson, M. (2019). Resilience of ecosystem processes: A new approach shows that functional redundancy of biological control services is reduced by landscape simplification. *Ecology Letters, 22*(10), 1568–1577.

Fischer, J., Meacham, M., & Queiroz, C. (2017). A plea for multifunctional landscapes. *Frontiers in Ecology and the Environment, 15*(2), 59–59.

Fišer, Ž., Aronne, G., Aavik, T., Akin, M., Alizoti, P., Aravanopoulos, F., Bacchetta, G., Balant, M., Ballian, D., Barazani, O., Bellia, A. F., Bernhardt, N., Kharrat, M. B. D., Douglas, A. B., Burkart, M., Calic, D., Carapeto, A., Carlson, T., Castro, S., . . . Zippel, E. (2021). ConservePlants: An integrated approach to conservation of threatened plants for the 21st Century. *Research Ideas and Outcomes*, 7, e62810. https://doi.org/10.3897/rio.7.e62810

Flies, E. J., Skelly, C., Negi, S. S., Prabhakaran, P., Liu, Q., Liu, K., Goldizen, F. C., Lease, C., & Weinstein, P. (2017). Biodiverse green spaces: A prescription for global urban health. *Frontiers in Ecology and the Environment*, *15*(9), 510–516.

Franco, L. S., Shanahan, D. F., & Fuller, R. A. (2017). A review of the benefits of nature experiences: More than meets the eye. *International Journal of Environmental Research and Public Health*, *14*(8), 864. https://doi.org/10.3390/ijerph14080864

Frumkin, H., Bratman, G. N., Breslow, S. J., Cochran, B., Kahn Jr, P. H., Lawler, J. J., Levin, P. S., Tandon, P. S., Varanasi, U., Wolf, K. L., & Wood, S. A. (2017). Nature contact and human health: A research agenda. *Environmental Health Perspectives*, *125*(7), 075001. https://doi.org/10.1289/EHP1663

Fuller, R. A., Irvine, K. N., Devine-Wright, P., Warren, P. H., & Gaston, K. J. (2007). Psychological benefits of greenspace increase with biodiversity. *Biology Letters*, *3*, 390–394.

Garfinkel, M., Belaire, A., Whelan, C., & Minor, E. (2024). Wildlife gardening initiates a feedback loop to reverse the "extinction of experience". *Biological Conservation*, *289*, 110400. https://doi.org/10.1016/j.biocon.2023.110400

Generation Restoration Cities. (n.d.). *Generation restoration cities*. Retrieved May 13, 2024 from https://www.decadeonrestoration.org/call-proposals-pilot-cities-urban-ecosystem-restoration

Gittleman, M., Farmer, C. J., Kremer, P., & McPhearson, T. (2017). Estimating stormwater runoff for community gardens in New York City. *Urban Ecosystems*, *20*, 129–139.

Godefroid, S., Piazza, C., Rossi, G., Buord, S., Stevens, A.-D., Aguraiuja, R., Cowell, C., Weekley, C. W., Vogg, G., Iriondo, J. M., Johnson, I., Dixom, B., Gordon, D., Magnanon, S., Valentin, B., Bjureke, K., Koopman, R., Vicens, M., Virevaire, M., & Vanderborght, T. (2011). How successful are plant species reintroductions? *Biological Conservation*, *144*(2), 672–682.

Gonzalez, M. T., Hartig, T., Patil, G. G., Martinsen, E. W., & Kirkevold, M. (2010). Therapeutic horticulture in clinical depression: A prospective study of active components. *Journal of Advanced Nursing*, *66*(9), 2002–2013.

Grote, R., Samson, R., Alonso, R., Amorim, J. H., Cariñanos, P., Churkina, G., Fares, S., Thiec, D. L., Niinemets, Ü., Mikkelsen, T. N., Paoletti, E., Tiwary, A., & Calfapietra, C. (2016). Functional traits of urban trees: Air pollution mitigation potential. *Frontiers in Ecology and the Environment*, *14*(10), 543–550.

Gulezian, P. Z., & Nyberg, D. W. (2010). Distribution of invasive plants in a spatially structured urban landscape. *Landscape and Urban Planning*, *95*, 161–168.

Gunderson, L. H., & Holling, C. S. (2002). *Panarchy: Understanding transformations in human and natural systems*. Island Press.

Hagler, G. S. W., Lin, M. Y., Khlystov, A., Baldauf, R. W., Isakov, V., Faircloth, J., & Jackson, L. E. (2012). Field investigation of roadside vegetative and structural barrier impact on near-road ultrafine particle concentrations under a variety of wind conditions. *Science of the Total Environment*, *419*, 7–15.

Harrop, E., Addis, S., Elliott, E., & Williams, G. (2006). *Resilience, coping and salutogenic approaches to maintaining and generating health: A review*. Cardiff University. Retrieved

May 13, 2024 from https://www.nice.org.uk/guidance/ph6/evidence/behaviour-change-review-3-resilience-coping-and-salutogenic-approaches-to-maintainingand-generating-health-pdf-369664527

Hartig, T. (2007). Three steps to understanding restorative environments as health resources. In T. Hartig & P. Travlou (Eds.), *Open space: People space* (pp. 183–200). Taylor & Francis.

Hartig, T. (2017). Restorative environments. In *Reference Module in Neuroscience and Biobehavioral Psychology*. Elsevier. https://doi.org/10.1016/B978-0-12-809324-5.05699-6

Heiland, S., Weidenweber, J., & Ward Thompson, C. (2019). Linking landscape planning and health. In M. Marselle, J. Stadler, H. Korn, K. N. Irvine, & A. Bonn (Eds.), *Biodiversity and health in the face of climate change* (pp. 425–448). Springer.

Herzog, T. R., Black, A. M., Fountaine, K. A., & Knotts, D. J. (1997). Reflection and attentional recovery as distinctive benefits of restorative environments. *Journal of Environmental Psychology*, *17*(2), 165–170.

Hobbs, R. J., Arico, S., Aronson, J., Baron, J. S., Bridgewater, P., Cramer, V. A., Epstein, P. R., Ewel, J. J., Klink, C. A., Lugo, A. E., Norton, D., Ojima, D., Richardson, D. M., Sanderson, E. W., Valladares, F., Vila, M., Zamora, R., & Zobel, M. (2006). Novel ecosystems: Theoretical and management aspects of the new ecological world order. *Global Ecology and Biogeography*, *15*(1), 1–7.

Hobbs, R. J., Higgs, E., Hall, C. M., Bridgewater, P., Chapin III, F. S., Ellis, E. C., Ewel, J. J., Hallett, L. M., Harris, J., Hulvey, K. B., Jackson, S. T., Kennedy, P. L., Kueffer, C., Lach, L., Lantz, T. C., Lugo, A. E., Mascaro, J., Murphy, S. D., Nelson, C. R., . . . Yung, L. (2014). Managing the whole landscape: Historical, hybrid, and novel ecosystems. *Frontiers in Ecology and the Environment*, *12*(10), 557–564.

Howarth, M., Brettle, A., Hardman, M., & Maden, M. (2020). What is the evidence for the impact of gardens and gardening on health and well-being: A scoping review and evidence-based logic model to guide healthcare strategy decision making on the use of gardening approaches as a social prescription. *BMJ Open*, *10*(7), e036923. https://doi.org/10.1136/bmjopen-2020-036923

Irvine, K. N., Hoesly, D., Bell-Williams, R., & Warber, S. L. (2019). Biodiversity and spiritual well-being. In M. R. Marselle, J. Stadler, H. Korn, K. N. Irvine, & A. Bonn (Eds.), *Biodiversity and health in the face of climate change* (pp. 213–247). Springer.

Irvine, K. N., Warber, S. L., Devine-Wright, P., & Gaston, K. J. (2013). Understanding urban green space as a health resource: A qualitative comparison of visit motivation and derived effects among park users in Sheffield, UK. *International Journal of Environmental Research and Public Health*, *10*(1), 417–442.

Ives, C. D., Lentini, P. E., Threlfall, C. G., Ikin, K., Shanahan, D. F., Garrard, G. E., Bekessy, S. A., Fuller, R. A., Mumaw, L., Rayner, L., Rowe, R., Valentine, L. E., & Kendal, D. (2016). Cities are hotspots for threatened species. *Global Ecology and Biogeography*, *25*, 117–126.

Jha, S., Egerer, M., Bichier, P., Cohen, H., Liere, H., Lin, B., Lucatero, A., & Philpott, S. M. (2023). Multiple ecosystem service synergies and landscape mediation of biodiversity within urban agroecosystems. *Ecology Letters*, *26*(3), 369–383.

Jordanova, V., Stewart, R., Goldberg, D., Bebbington, P. E., Brugha, T., Singleton, N., Lindesay, J. E., Jenkins, R., Prince, M., & Meltzer, H. (2007). Age variation in life events and their relationship with common mental disorders in a national survey population. *Social Psychiatry and Psychiatric Epidemiology*, *42*, 611–616.

Joseph, S. (2012). What doesn't kill us . . . *The Psychologist*, *25*(11), 816–819. Retrieved September 19, 2024 from https://www.bps.org.uk/psychologist/what-doesnt-kill-us

Kaplan, R., & Kaplan, S. (1989). *The experience of nature: A psychological perspective.* Cambridge University Press.

Kaplan, S. (1995). The restorative benefits of nature: Toward an integrative framework. *Journal of Environmental Psychology, 15*(3), 169–182.

Kaplan, S., & Berman, M. G. (2017). Directed attention as a common resource for executive functioning and self-regulation. *Perspectives on Psychological Science, 5*(1), 43–57.

Kellmann, M., & Kallus, K. W. (2001). *The Recovery-Stress Questionnaire for Athletes; manual.* Human Kinetics.

Kessler, R. (1997). The effects of stressful life events on depression. *Annual Review of Psychololgy, 48*, 191–214.

Kingsley, J., Diekmann, L., Egerer, M. H., Lin, B. B., Ossola, A., & Marsh, P. (2022). Experiences of gardening during the early stages of the COVID-19 pandemic. *Health & Place, 76*, 102854. https://doi.org/10.1016/j.healthplace.2022.102854

Klaus, V. H., & Kiehl, K. (2021). A conceptual framework for urban ecological restoration and rehabilitation. *Basic and Applied Ecology, 52*, 82–94.

Kondo, M. C., Low, S. C., Henning, J., & Branas, C. C. (2015). The impact of green stormwater infrastructure installation on surrounding health and safety. *American Journal of Public Health, 105*(3), 114–121.

Kondo, M. C., Oyekanmi, K. O., Gibosn, A., South, E. C., Bocarro, J., & Hipp, A. (2020). Nature prescriptions for health: A review of evidence and research opportunities. *International Journal of Environmental Research and Public Health, 17*(12), 4213. https://doi.org/10.3390/ijerph17124213

Lafortezza, R., Chen, J., Van Den Bosch, C. K., & Randrup, T. B. (2018). Nature-based solutions for resilient landscapes and cities. *Environmental Research, 165*, 431–441.

Lahart, I., Darcy, P., Gidlow, C., & Calogiuri, G. (2019). The effects of green exercise on physical and mental wellbeing: A systematic review. *International Journal of Environmental Research and Public Health, 16*(8), 1352. https://doi.org/10.3390/ijerph16081352

Lauterbach, D., Burkart, M., Dreilich, A., Loewenstein, P., Stevens, A.-D., & Zippel, E. (2019). Beiträge der Botanischen Gärten Potsdam und Berlin zum Botanischen Artenschutz in Brandenburg [Contributions of the Potsdam and Berlin Botanic Gardens to botanical species conservation in Brandenburg]. *Naturschutz und Landschaftspflege in Brandenburg, 28*(1), 4–23.

Leather, P., Pyrgas, M., Beale, D., & Lawrence, C. (1998). Windows in the workplace: Sunlight, view, and occupational stress. *Environment and Behavior, 30*, 739–762.

Leavell, M. A., Leiferman, J. A., Gascon, M., Braddick, F., Gonzalez, J. C., & Litt, J. S. (2019). Nature-based social prescribing in urban settings to improve social connectedness and mental well-being: A review. *Current Environmental Health Reports, 6*, 297–308.

Lee, S., & Webster, C. (2006). Enclosure of the urban commons. *GeoJournal, 66*, 27–42.

Lelieveld, J., Klingmüller, K., Pozzer, A., Pöschl, U., Fnais, M., Daiber, A., & Münzel, T. (2019). Cardiovascular disease burden from ambient air pollution in Europe reassessed using novel hazard ratio functions. *European Heart Journal, 40*, 1590–1596.

Lin, B. B., & Egerer, M. H. (2020). Global social and environmental change drives the management and delivery of ecosystem services from urban gardens: A case study from Central Coast, California. *Global Environmental Change, 60*, 102006. https://doi.org/10.1016/j.gloenvcha.2019.102006

Lin, B. B., Egerer, M. H., Kingsley, J., Marsh, P., Diekmann, L., & Ossola, A. (2021). COVID-19 gardening could herald a greener, healthier future. *Frontiers in Ecology and the Environment, 19*(9), 491–493.

Lin, B. B., Egerer, M. H., Liere, H., Jha, S., & Philpott, S. M. (2019). Soil management is key to maintaining soil moisture in urban gardens facing changing climatic conditions. *Scientific Reports*, *8*(1), 17565. https://doi.org/10.1038/s41598-018-35731-7

Lin, B. B., Egerer, M. H., & Ossola, A. (2018). Urban gardens as a space to engender biophilia: Evidence and ways forward. *Frontiers in Built Environment*, *4*, 79. https://doi.org/10.3389/fbuil.2018.00079

Lin, B. B., Philpott, S. M., & Jha, S. (2015). The future of urban agriculture and biodiversity-ecosystem services: Challenges and next steps. *Basic and Applied Ecology*, *16*(3), 189–201.

Lindemann-Matthies, P., & Matthies, D. (2018). The influence of plant species richness on stress recovery of humans. *Web Ecology*, *18*(2), 121–128.

Liu, J., Huo, Y., Wang, J., Bai, Y., Zhao, M., & Di, M. (2023). Awe of nature and well-being: Roles of nature connectedness and powerlessness. *Personality and Individual Differences*, *201*, 111946. https://doi.org/10.1016/j.paid.2022.111946

Loram, A., Thompson, K., Warren, P. H., & Gaston, K. J. (2008). Urban domestic gardens (XII): The richness and composition of the flora in five UK cities. *Journal of Vegetation Science*, *19*(3), 321–330.

Loram, A., Tratalos, J., Warren, P. H., & Gaston, K. J. (2007). Urban domestic gardens (X): The extent & structure of the resource in five major cities. *Landscape Ecology*, *22*, 601–615.

Lovell, R., Husk, K., Cooper, C., Stahl-Timmins, W., & Garside, R. (2015). Understanding how environmental enhancement and conservation activities may benefit health and wellbeing: A systematic review. *BMC Public Health*, *15*, 864. https://doi.org/10.1186/s12889-015-2214-3

Lundholm, J. T., & Richardson, P. J. (2010). Habitat analogues for reconciliation ecology in urban and industrial environments. *Journal of Applied Ecology*, *47*(5), 966–975.

Mancini, A. D., & Bonanno, G. A. (2010). Resilience to potential trauma: Toward a lifespan approach. In J. W. Reich, A. J. Zautra, & J. S. Hall (Eds.), *Handbook of adult resilience* (pp. 258–282). The Guilford Press.

Markevych, I., Schoierer, J., Hartig, T., Chudnovsky, A., Hystad, P., Dzhambov, A. M., de Vries, S., Triguero-Mas, M., Brauer, M., Nieuwenhuijsen, M. J., Lupp, G., Richardson, E. A., Astell-Burt, T., Dimitrova, D., Feng, X., Sadeh, M., Standl, M., Heinrich, J., & Fuertes, E. (2017). Exploring pathways linking greenspace to health: Theoretical and methodological guidance. *Environmental Research*, *158*, 301–317.

Marselle, M. R., Irvine, K. N., Lorenzo-Arribas, A., & Warber, S. L. (2016). Does perceived restorativeness mediate the effects of perceived biodiversity and perceived naturalness on emotional well-being following group walks in nature? *Journal of Environmental Psychology*, *46*, 217–232.

Marselle, M. R. (2019). Theoretical foundations of biodiversity and mental well-being relationships. In M. R. Marselle, J. Stadler, H. Korn, K. N. Irvine, & A. Bonn (Eds.), *Biodiversity and health in the face of climate change* (pp. 133–158). Springer.

Marselle, M. R., Bowler, D. E., Watzema, J., Eichenberg, D., Kirsten, T., & Bonn, A. (2020). Urban street tree biodiversity and anti-depressant prescriptions. *Scientific Reports*, *10*, 22445. https://doi.org/10.1038/s41598-020-79924-5

Marselle, M. R., Hartig, T., Cox, D. T. C., de Bell, S., Knapp, S., Lindley, S., Triguero-Mas, M., Böhning-Gaese, K., Braubach, M., Cook, P. A., de Vries, S., Heintz-Buschart, A., Hofmann, M., Irvine, K. N., Kabisch, N., Kolek, F., Kraemer, R., Markevych, I., Martens, D., . . . Bonn, A. (2021). Pathways linking biodiversity to human health: A conceptual framework. *Environment International*, *150*, 106420. https://doi.org/10.1016/j.envint.2021.106420

Marselle, M. R., Warber, S. L., & Irvine, K. N. (2019). Growing resilience through interaction with nature: Can group walks in nature buffer the effects of stressful life events on mental health? *International Journal of Environmental Research and Public Health, 16*(6), 986. https://doi.org/10.3390/ijerph16060986

Marsh, P., Diekmann, L. O., Egerer, M., Lin, B., Ossola, A., & Kingsley, J. (2021). Where birds felt louder: The garden as a refuge during COVID-19. *Wellbeing, Space and Society, 2*, 100055. https://doi.org/10.1016/j.wss.2021.100055

Masten, A. S. (2014). *Ordinary magic: Resilience in development*. Guilford Press.

Masten, A. S., & Reed, M. J. (2005). Resilience in development. In C. R. Snyder & S. J. Lopez (Eds.), *Handbook of positive psychology* (pp. 74–88). Oxford University Press.

Masten, A. S., & Wright, M. O. (2009). Resilience over the lifespan: Developmental perspectives on resistance, recovery, and transformation. In J. W. Reich, A. J. Zautra, & S. Hall (Eds.), *Handbook of adult resilience* (pp. 213–237). Guilford Press.

Matheny, K. (2020, August 27). *RiverWalk extension project will allow riverfront strolls from Windsor tunnel to Belle Isle*. Detroit Free Press. Retrieved May 31, 2024 from https://eu.freep.com/story/news/local/michigan/wayne/2020/08/27/detroit-cleanup-riverwalk-extension/5646371002/

McClintock, N., & Simpson, M. (2018). Stacking functions: Identifying motivational frames guiding urban agriculture organizations and businesses in the United States and Canada. *Agriculture and Human Values, 35*, 19–39.

Milbourne, P. (2021). Growing public spaces in the city: Community gardening and the making of new urban environments of publicness. *Urban Studies, 58*(14), 2901–2919.

Millennium Ecosystem Assessment (MEA). (2005). *Ecosystems and human well-being: Synthesis*. Island Press.

Ohly, H., White, M. P., Wheeler, B. W., Bethel, A., Ukoumunne, O. C., Nikolaou, V., & Garside, R. (2016). Attention restoration theory: A systematic review of the attention restoration potential of exposure to natural environments. *Journal of Toxicology and Environmental Health, Part B, 19*(7), 305–343.

Oliver, T. H., Heard, M. S., Isaac, N. J. B., Roy, D. B., Procter, D., Eigenbrod, F., Freckleton, R., Hector, A., Orme, C. D. L., Petchey, O. L., Proença, V., Raffaelli, D., Suttle, K. B., Mace, G. M., Martín-López, B., Woodcock, B. A., & Bullock, J. M. (2015). Biodiversity and resilience of ecosystem functions. *Trends in Ecology & Evolution, 30*, 673–684.

Pelletier, M. C., Ebersole, J., Mulvaney, K., Rashleigh, B., Gutierrez, M. N., Chintala, M., Kuhn, A., Molina, M., Bagley, M., & Lane, C. (2020). Resilience of aquatic systems: Review and management implications. *Aquatic Sciences, 82*, 44. https://doi.org/10.1007/s00027-020-00717-z

Peschardt, K. K., & Stigsdotter, U. K. (2013). Associations between park characteristics and perceived restorativeness of small public urban green spaces. *Landscape and Urban Planning, 112*(1), 26–39.

Pickett, S. T., McGrath, B., Cadenasso, M. L., & Felson, A. J. (2014). Ecological resilience and resilient cities. *Building Research & Information, 42*(2), 143–157.

Pouyat, R. V., Yesilonis, I. D., Groffman, P. M., Szlavecz, K., & Schwarz, K. (2010). Chemical, physical and biological characteristics of urban soils. *Urban Ecosystem Ecology, 55*, 119–152.

Prévot, A.-C., Cheval, H., Raymond, R., & Cosquer, A. (2018). Routine experiences of nature in cities can increase personal commitment toward biodiversity conservation. *Biological Conservation, 226*, 1–8. https://doi.org/10.1016/j.biocon.2018.07.008

Robinson, J. M., & Breed, M. F. (2019). Green prescriptions and their co-benefits: Integrative strategies for public and environmental health. *Challenges, 10*(1), 9. https://doi.org/10.3390/challe10010009

Rozario, K., Oh, R. R. Y., Marselle, M., Schröger, E., Gillerot, L., Ponette, Q., Godbold, D., Haluza, D., Kilpi, K., Müller, D., Roeber, U., Verheyen, K., Muys, B., Müller, S., Shaw, T., & Bonn, A. (2024). The more the merrier? Perceived forest biodiversity promotes short-term mental health and well-being – a multicentre study. *People and Nature, 6*(1), 180–201.

Schebella, M. F., Weber, D., Schultz, L., & Weinstein, P. (2019). The wellbeing benefits associated with perceived and measured biodiversity in Australian urban green spaces. *Sustainability, 11*(3), 802. https://doi.org/10.3390/su11030802

Scopelliti, M., Carrus, G., Cini, F., Mastandrea, S., Ferrini, F., Lafortezza, R., Agrimi, M., Salbitano, F., Sanesi, G., & Semenzato, P. (2012). Biodiversity, perceived restorativeness and benefits of nature: A study on the psychological processes and outcomes of on-site experiences in urban and peri-urban green areas in Italy. In S. Kabisch, A. Kunath, P. Schweizer-Ries, & A. Steinführer (Eds.), *Vulnerability, risks and complexity. Impacts of global change on human habitats* (pp. 255–270). Hogrefe.

Seitz, B., Buchholz, S., Kowarik, I., Herrmann, J., Neuerburg, L., Wendler, J., Winker, L., & Egerer, M. (2022). Land sharing between cultivated and wild plants: Urban gardens as hotspots for plant diversity in cities. *Urban Ecosystems, 25*(3), 927–939.

Shwartz, A., Tzunz, M., Gafter, L., & Colléony, A. (2023). One size does not fit all: The complex relationship between biodiversity and psychological well-being. *Urban Forestry & Urban Greening, 86*, 128008. https://doi.org/10.1016/j.ufug.2023.128008

Sia, A., Tan, P. Y., Wong, J. C. M., Araib, S., Ang, W. F., & Er, K. B. H. (2022). The impact of gardening on mental resilience in times of stress: A case study during the COVID-19 pandemic in Singapore. *Urban Forestry & Urban Greening, 68*, 127448. https://doi.org/10.1016/j.ufug.2021.127448

Smith, V. M., Greene, R. B., & Silbernagel, J. (2013). The social and spatial dynamics of community food production: A landscape approach to policy and program development. *Landscape Ecology, 28*, 1415–1426.

Soanes, K., & Lentini, P. E. (2019). When cities are the last chance for saving species. *Frontiers in Ecology and the Environment, 17*, 225–231.

Society for Ecological Restoration. (2024, May 30). *What is ecological restoration?* Society for Ecological Restoration. Retrieved May 30, 2024 from https://ser-rrc.org/what-is-ecological-restoration/

Soga, M., Gaston, K. J., & Yamaura, Y. (2017). Gardening is beneficial for health: A meta-analysis. *Preventive Medicine Reports, 5*, 92–99.

South, E. C., Hohl, B. C., Kondo, M. C., MacDonald, J. M., & Branas, C. C. (2018). Effect of greening vacant land on mental health of community-dwelling adults: A cluster randomized trial. *The Journal of the American Medical Association Network Open, 1*(3), e180298. https://doi.org/10.1001/jamanetworkopen.2018.0298

Speldewinde, P. C., Cook, A., Davies, P., & Weinstein, P. (2009). A relationship between environmental degradation and mental health in rural Western Australia. *Health & Place, 15*, 880–887.

Stevenson, M. P., Schilhab, T., & Bentsen, P. (2018). Attention restoration theory II: A systematic review to clarify attention processes affected by exposure to natural environments. *Journal of Toxicology and Environmental Health, Part B, 21*(4), 227–268.

Stuart, S. M. (2005). Lifting spirits: Creating gardens in California domestic violence shelters. In P. F. Barlett (Ed.), *Urban place: Reconnecting with the natural world* (pp. 61–88). MIT Press.

Suchy, Y., Ziemnik, R. E., & Niermeyer, M. A. (2017). Assessment of executive functions in clinical settings. In E. Goldberg (Ed.), *Executive functions in health and disease* (pp. 551–569). Academic Press.

Swann, G. E. A., Panizzo, V. N., Piccolroaz, S., Pashley, V., Horstwood, M. S. A., Roberts, S., Vologina, E., Piotrowska, N., Sturm, M., Zhdanov, A., Granin, N., Norman, C., McGowan, S., & Mackay, A. (2021). Changing nutrient cycling in Lake Baikal, the world's oldest lake. *Proceedings of the National Academy of Sciences, 117*(44), 27211–27217.

Teixeira, C. P., & Fernandes, C. O. (2020). Novel ecosystems: A review of the concept in non-urban and urban contexts. *Landscape Ecology, 35*(1), 23–39.

Threlfall, C. G., Mata, L., Mackie, J. A., Hahs, A. K., Stork, N. E., Williams, N. S. G., & Livesley, S. J. (2017). Increasing biodiversity in urban green spaces through simple vegetation interventions. *Journal of Applied Ecology, 54*, 1874–1883.

Tomatis, F., Diez, F. J., Wilhelm, M. S., & Navas-Gracia, L. M. (2023). Prediction of daily ambient temperature and its hourly estimation using artificial neural networks in urban allotment gardens and an urban park in Valladolid, Castilla y León, Spain. *Agronomy, 14*(1), 60. https://doi.org/10.3390/agronomy14010060

Tresch, S., Frey, D., Le Bayon, R.-C., Mäder, P., Stehle, B., Fliessbach, A., & Moretti, M. (2019). Direct and indirect effects of urban gardening on aboveground and belowground diversity influencing soil multifunctionality. *Scientific Reports, 9*(1), 9769. https://doi.org/10.1038/s41598-019-46024-y

Turner, R. J., & Wheaton, B. (1997). Checklist measurement of stressful life events. In S. Cohen, R. C. Kessler, & L. Underwood Gordon (Eds.), *Measuring stress: A guide for health and social scientists* (pp. 29–58). Oxford University Press.

Ulmer, J. M., Wolf, K. L., Backman, D. R., Tretheway, R. L., Blain, C. J., O'Neil-Dunne, J. P., & Frank, L. D. (2016). Multiple health benefits of urban tree canopy: the mounting evidence for a green prescription. *Health Place, 42*, 54–62.

Ulrich, R. S. (1983). Aesthetic and affective response to natural environment. In I. Altman & J. F. Wohlwill (Eds.), *Human behavior and the natural environment* (pp. 85–125). Plenum Press.

Ulrich, R. S. (1984). View through a window may influence recovery from surgery. *Science, 224*(4647), 420–421.

Ulrich, R. S., Simons, R. F., Losito, B. D., Fiorito, E., Miles, M. A., & Zelson, M. (1991). Stress recovery during exposure to natural and urban environments. *Journal of Environmental Psychology, 11*(3), 201–230.

van den Berg, A. E., & Custers, M. H. G. (2011). Gardening promotes neuroendocrine and affective restoration from stress. *Journal of Health Psychology, 16*(1), 3–11.

van den Berg, A. E., Maas, J., Verheij, R. A., & Groenewegen, P. P. (2010). Green space as a buffer between stressful life events and health. *Social Science & Medicine, 70*(8), 1203–1210.

van den Berg, M., Wendel-Vos, W., van Poppel, M., Kemper, H., van Mechelen, W., & Maas, J. (2015). Health benefits of green spaces in the living environment: A systematic review of epidemiological studies. *Urban Forestry & Urban Greening, 14*(4), 806–816.

van Oudenhoven, F. J. W., Mijatovic, D., & Eyzaguirre, P. B. (2011). Social-ecological indicators of resilience in agrarian and natural landscapes. *Management of Environmental Quality, 22*, 154–173.

Vávra, J., Megyesi, B., Duží, B., Craig, T., Klufová, R., Lapka, M., & Cudlínová, E. (2018). Food self-provisioning in Europe: An exploration of sociodemographic factors in five regions. *Rural Sociology, 83*(2), 431–461.

von Lindern, E., Lymeus, F., & Hartig, T. (2017). The restorative environment: A complementary concept for salutogenesis studies. In M. B. Mittelmark, S. Sagy, M. Eriksson, G. F. Bauer, J. Pelikan, B. Lindström, & G. A. Espnes (Eds.), *The handbook of salutogenesis* (pp. 181–195). Springer.

Walsh, F. (2021). Family resilience: A dynamic systemic framework. In M. Ungar (Ed.), *Multisystemic resilience: Adaptation and transformation in contexts of change* (pp. 255–270). Oxford Academic.

Warber, S. L., DeHudy, A. A., Bialko, M. F., Marselle, M. R., & Irvine, K. N. (2015). Addressing "Nature-Deficit Disorder": A mixed methods pilot study of young adults attending a wilderness camp. *Evidence-Based Complementary and Alternative Medicine*, 651827. https://doi.org/10.1155/2015/651827

Wells, N. M. (2021). The natural environment as a resilience factor: Nature's role as a buffer of the effects of risk and adversity. In A. R. Schutte, J. C. Torquati, & J. R. Stevens (Eds.), *Nature and psychology: Biological, cognitive, development and social pathways to well-being* (pp. 195–233). Springer.

Wells, N. M., & Evans, G. W. (2003). Nearby nature: A buffer of life stress among rural children. *Environment and Behavior, 35*(3), 311–330.

White, M. P., Alcock, I., Grellier, J., Wheeler, B. W., Hartig, T., Warber, S. L., Bone, A., Depledge, M. H., & Fleming, L. E. (2019). Spending at least 120 minutes a week in nature is associated with good health and wellbeing. *Scientific Reports, 9*(1), 7730. https://doi.org/10.1038/s41598-019-44097-3

White, M. P., Hartig, T., Martin, L., Pahl, S., van den Berg, A. E., Wells, N. M., Costongs, C., Dzhambov, A. M., Elliott, L. R., Godfrey, A., Hartl, A., Konijnendijk, C., Litt, J. S., Lovell, R., Lymeus, F., O'Driscoll, C., Pichler, C., Pouso, S., Razani, N., . . . van den Bosch, M. (2023). Nature-based biopsychosocial resilience: An integrative theoretical framework for research on nature and health. *Environment International, 181*, 108234. https://doi.org/10.1016/j.envint.2023.108234

Wyles, K. J., White, M. P., Hattam, C., Pahl, S., King, H., & Austen, M. (2019). Are some natural environments more psychologically beneficial than others? The importance of type and quality on connectedness to nature and psychological restoration. *Environment and Behavior, 51*(2), 111–143.

Yates, T. M., & Masten, A. S. (2004). Fostering the future: Resilience theory and the practice of positive psychology. In P. A. Linley & S. Joseph (Eds.), *Positive psychology in practice* (pp. 521–539). Wiley & Sons.

Zautra, A. J., Hall, J. S., & Murray, K. E. (2010). Resilience: A new definition of health for people and communities. In J. R. Reich, A. J. Zautra, & J. S. Hall (Eds.), *Handbook of adult resilience* (pp. 3–30). Guilford Press.

Zivin, J. G., & Neidell, M. (2018). Air pollution's hidden impacts. *Science, 359*, 39–40.

Part III

Urban planning and management for recovery

9 Impacts of heat on human well-being

Creating restorative indoor and outdoor thermal environments in a changing climate

Amelie Bauer, Hannah Lehmann, Teresa Zölch, and Stephan Pauleit

Introduction

Climate change leads not only to an increase of mean annual temperatures but also to more frequent and intense heatwaves. This constitutes a major health risk, as excessive heat triggers a series of physiological processes that can lead to heat-related health problems or even death (Arsad et al., 2022; Lüthi et al., 2023). In addition to heat stroke, heat exhaustion, and dehydration, heat-related morbidity includes chronic kidney diseases (Kenny et al., 2018), exacerbation of cardiovascular diseases (de Blois et al., 2015; Wang et al., 2018), and respiratory diseases, diabetes, and impaired digestion (Mora et al., 2017). Deterioration of mental health and cognitive impairment (Razmjou, 1996; Stearns et al., 2015; van Loenhout et al., 2016) and reduced well-being are also associated with heat stress (Ioannou et al., 2017; Legault et al., 2017; van Hoof et al., 2017; van Loenhout et al., 2016), although knowledge about the relationship between heat and mental health is still limited (Liu et al., 2021). While there is some evidence that there is an increase in suicide rates during heatwaves and that existing mental health conditions can worsen and increase vulnerability to heat-related illnesses, little is known about the mechanisms and the links of the impact on mental well-being (Ebi et al., 2021; Lõhmus, 2018; Thompson et al., 2018).

How strongly heat affects a person depends on a combination of exposure (severity and duration of heat), sensitivity, as well as the available resources for adaptation and recovery (see Figure 9.1). These factors vary geographically, but also between population groups and individuals, and are often influenced by existing inequalities, such as income. Physiologically, infants, young children, the elderly, and the chronically ill are particularly vulnerable to heat due to

Bauer, A., Lehmann, H., Zölch, T., & Pauleit, S. (2025). Impacts of heat on human well-being: Creating restorative indoor and outdoor thermal environments in a changing climate. In S. Pauleit, M. Kellmann, & J. Beckmann (Eds.), *Creating Urban and Workplace Environments for Recovery and Well-being* (pp. 179–198). Routledge.

DOI: 10.4324/9781003435471-12

their limited capacity for thermoregulation (Kenny et al., 2020). Due to their heightened exposure, heat also poses a serious health risk to people who work outdoors (Kjellstrom et al., 2009). Heat in the workplace means higher physical exertion and faster dehydration and can lead to a reduced ability to concentrate, increasing the risk of workplace accidents (Fatima et al., 2021; Kenny et al., 2020). Employees in agriculture, construction, manufacturing, and the service sector are most at risk.

Geographically, regions with hotter climates will be more strongly affected by increasing temperatures, and heat is especially risky to health in combination with high humidity (IPCC, 2023). Research gaps exist exactly for those regions where, in the future, the most extreme heatwaves are expected (Campbell et al., 2018). Yet regions with historically more temperate climates are also affected by heat and its consequences, especially as these societies are often ill-prepared for heat. For Europe, it has been estimated that repeated heatwaves led to the premature death of over 70,000 people in 2003 and over 60,000 in 2022 (Ballester et al., 2023). In temperate Germany, more than 6,000 additional heat-related deaths were recorded each year between 2006 and 2018 (Umweltbundesamt, 2019), with clear increases in hospital admissions and deaths during heat events (an der Heiden et al., 2019, 2020; Gabriel & Endlicher, 2011; Steul et al., 2018).

Urban areas will be more affected by negative impacts of increasing temperatures than rural areas – not only because most people live and work in cities, but also because cities can be considerably warmer than surrounding rural areas, a phenomenon called the urban heat island (UHI) effect (Oke, 1973). The UHI is particularly strong in densely built areas, such as city centres, due to the high amount of built and sealed surfaces that absorb incoming solar radiation, which is reradiated as sensible heat. Correspondingly, there is a lack of green infrastructure[1] that may provide cooling via shading and evapotranspiration of water (Oke et al., 2017).

Heat exposure as well as possibilities for adaptation and recovery also vary between population groups and can be connected to existing inequalities. For example, poorer households are often situated in areas with lower levels of green space provision, accessibility, and quality (Schüle et al., 2019; Wolch et al., 2014).

Human recovery is directly impacted by rising temperatures. Higher temperatures will imply more people are stressed by heat. Heat also interferes with recovery from other stressors, affecting passive recovery, such as night-time sleep, as well as active recovery, such as physical activity. Physical activity becomes more strenuous or even dangerous in high temperatures, although it is needed to mitigate civilisation diseases caused by sedentary behaviour (Kellmann & Beckmann, 2024). At the same time, increasing obesity levels exacerbate heat stress, as obese people overheat more quickly (Zhou et al., 2023).

Air conditioning as a technical solution for adaptation to heat is expected to increase in many world regions, despite its high energy consumption (Li, Yang, et al., 2012) and excess heat production, which intensifies the UHI in cities (Hsieh et al., 2007). This presents a conflict between climate change adaptation and mitigation. In some climates or for certain populations, air conditioning may be unavoidable in the future to protect against health risks or mortality. However, for many contexts, air conditioning is currently the sole solution, where other measures might be equally helpful. Air conditioning has even been introduced to regions previously well-adapted to heat, often as a harbinger of 'modernity' – for example, concrete buildings with glass facades that can only be kept comfortable with air conditioning, replacing traditional vernacular architecture much better suited to hotter climates (Lundgren & Kjellstrom, 2013; Wilhite, 2009). Future efforts should therefore focus on adaptation measures that aid human recovery from heat stress with no adverse or even beneficial environmental effects. Ideally, adaptation measures should contribute towards climate change mitigation.

Both the roles of indoor and outdoor environments for prevention of and recovery from human heat stress need to be considered. In industrialised societies, humans spend between 80 and 90% of their day in buildings (Rupp et al., 2015) – mostly at home and, for working adults, at the workplace. Exposure to work environments is mostly not a matter of choice, and people are limited in their adaptive opportunities. Thus, residential and office buildings will be a special focus of this chapter. However, the outdoor environment also influences indoor temperatures by heating up building mass and can hinder effective indoor recovery (e.g., when sleep quality is impaired in an overheated bedroom). With proper design, outdoor temperatures can be reduced, mitigating the UHI effect, while offering restorative environments, such as cool, shaded, and greened spaces. Both environments can complement each other for recovery (e.g., indoor 'cooling areas' for outdoor workers, or a cool park to recover from an overheated apartment or office).

To cope with the negative effects of increasing heat, societies have to adapt on different levels, such as city planning, building and landscape design, as well as organisation and daily routines. This chapter will draw from literature on health, occupational medicine, thermal comfort, and heat stress, as well as place-based results from prior studies situated in Germany, to give recommendations for adapting indoor and outdoor environments at different levels of action: individual as well as infrastructural (building technology, social organisation) and urban planning. The last section will discuss policy implications.

Heat stress, thermal comfort, and recovery

The human body functions best at a core temperature of approximately 36.8°C +/- 0.5°C (Hanna & Tait, 2015). If there is a deviation from this optimum temperature range, the body initiates thermoregulatory processes (e.g., sweating, dilation of the skin vessels) in order to regulate the core temperature. In addition to thermoregulation as the body's short-term physiological response to heat, acclimatisation can serve as a long-term resource to regulate the body's core temperature and thus adapt to heat. Gradual and continuous acclimatisation to heat exposure improves thermoregulatory capacity and increases heat tolerance to a certain threshold (Kirby & Convertino, 1986; Pallubinsky et al., 2017).

The range of heat tolerance can be further increased through behavioural and technical adaptation measures (Hanna & Tait, 2015). However, if external influences or physical activity lead to an increase in core temperature that exceeds the body's ability to release heat, *heat stress* occurs (Hanna & Tait, 2015).

Thermal comfort describes the 'condition of mind that expresses satisfaction with the thermal environment and is assessed by subjective evaluation' (American Society of Heating, 2013). The most popular index is based on calculations for indoor environments at given clothing and activity levels and 'average' physiology (Fanger, 1970). Fanger's concept posits that 'comfort' is obtained when individuals perceive the thermal environment as 'neutral', or slightly warm/ slightly cool. Discomfort is reached when individuals describe the environment as warm/hot or cool/cold, or when the human body has to initiate thermoregulatory processes (sweat/shiver).

Building codes define temperature thresholds in order to avoid or reduce the experience of thermal discomfort or heat stress indoors. For instance, German building code DIN EN 16798–1 specifies the maximum indoor operative temperatures (a combination of radiant and ambient temperature) for mechanically ventilated buildings during the cooling period between 25.5°C and 28°C (depending on the building category, for example, office or factory building). Also, German Technical Rules for Workplaces (BAuA, 2010) prescribe that from air temperatures of 26°C and above, heat protection measures 'should' be taken, while above 30°C, 'effective measures must be taken' (with a separate protocol for especially vulnerable groups, for example, teenagers, elderly, or pregnant workers). Such standards do not exist for outdoor environments, however.

Outdoor thermal comfort depends not only on the sensation of the human body but also on the fluctuation of the relevant meteorological parameters. Therefore, defined reference individuals are used to assess outdoor thermal comfort, and differences in outdoor thermal comfort indices relate to the dynamics of the weather patterns (Höppe, 2002; Staiger et al., 1997; Verein Deutscher Ingenieure, 2022). A broad range of such indices have been proposed to quantify thermal comfort (Staiger et al., 2019). Some of the most widely used indices are the Universal Thermal Comfort Index (Jendritzky et al., 2012), the Perceived Temperature (Staiger et al., 2012), the Physiologically Equivalent Temperature (PET; Höppe, 1999) and Wet Bulb Globe Temperature (Yaglou & Minard, 1957).

Reference temperatures for thermal (dis)comfort are based on models of 'average human' reaction to heat and then generalised to a wider population. For example, the PET is based on the so-called 'Climate Michael' (in German: 'Klima-Michel'), a 35-year-old healthy male. How a given thermal stimulus actually affects health and well-being of an individual depends on a range of different factors (Figure 9.1).

Because of these interrelating factors, each individual has a different level of stress capacity, depending on their personal vulnerability (physiological/psychological), as well as their exposure to heat (magnitude, duration, and context of the exposure to heat stress). For recovery, individuals have different resources at their disposal. Besides individual constitution and behaviour, the design and

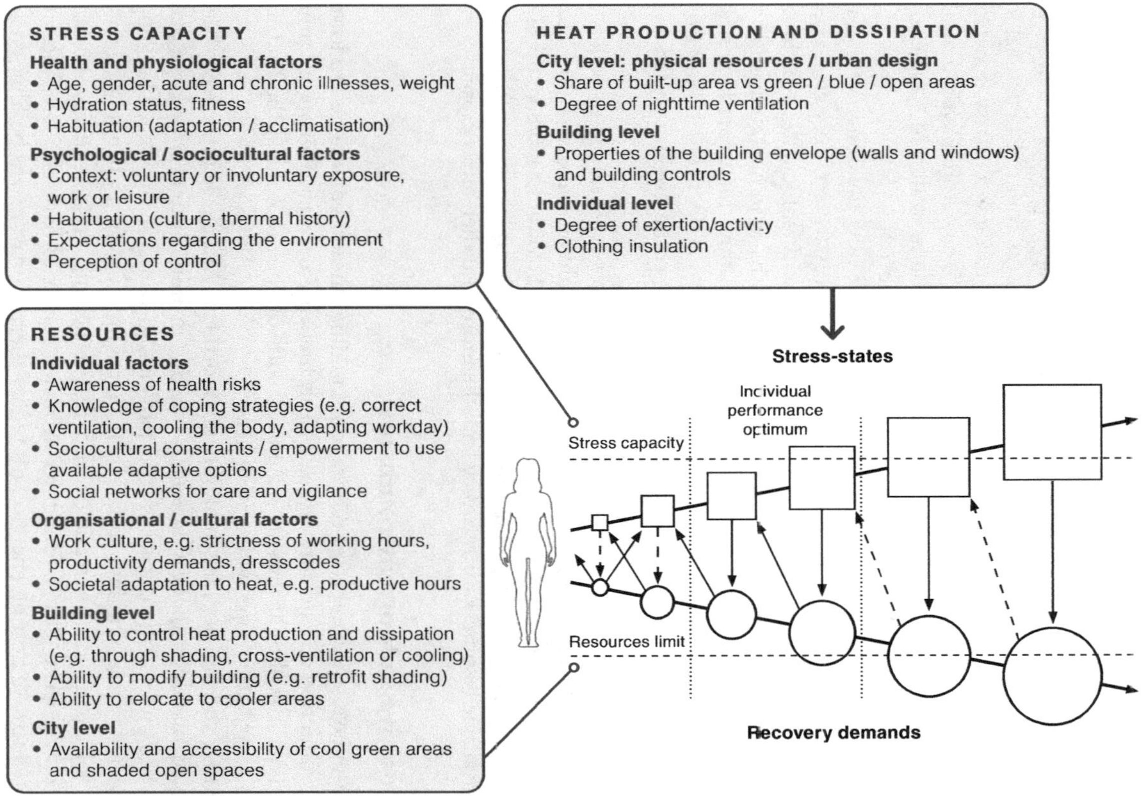

Figure 9.1 Factors influencing thermal comfort, heat stress, and recovery.

management of indoor and outdoor environments play a crucial role in reducing heat stress and enhancing recovery from it.

Lastly, there is an important distinction between thermal discomfort and heat stress. According to the earlier definition, thermal discomfort occurs when individuals perceive an environment to be warm/hot or initiate the thermoregulatory process of sweating. With thermal comfort in mind, environments are therefore currently designed to be 'thermally neutral'. However, recent research indicates that diseases related to metabolic syndrome appear linked to constantly comfortable environments and that – at least for healthy persons – temporary exposure to 'uncomfortable' hot and cold environments could be beneficial for metabolic health, possibly through 'exercising' the cardiovascular system (van Marken Lichtenbelt et al., 2017). While heat stress is therefore physiologically detrimental, the notion of thermal comfort should be re-evaluated – especially when high amounts of energy are consumed to achieve it.

The following sections of this chapter will explore how the design of indoor and outdoor environments can increase the resources for recovery from heat stress, for example, by providing neighbourhoods with sufficient green infrastructure. However, recovery and *prevention* often go hand in hand: measures to keep residential buildings cool will prevent residents from incurring heat stress and its adverse health effects but will also allow them to effectively recover from the heat stress they may have encountered in other contexts throughout their day, for example, at work or while jogging outside.

Thus, similar to the *Scissors Model* of human recovery (developed by Kallus & Kellmann, 2000, and presented in Pauleit et al., this volume, Chapter 1), the goals for designing restorative thermal environments are to 1) lower heat where possible so that people do not surpass the limit of their stress capacity, and to 2) increase their available resources for recovery and, therefore, also their stress capacity.

Restorative indoor environments

To avoid heat stress and assist restoration, buildings should be designed to lower heat production and quickly dissipate heat, reducing occupants' exposure time. Also, buildings should provide occupants with options to control the thermal situation or better cope with arising heat.

During the last decades, buildings in Northern/Middle Europe have been designed mainly with heating energy savings in mind, often with large glass facades to increase the uptake of solar radiation in winter. Many office buildings also include large window surfaces for better lighting. In a changing climate, these solar gains can increasingly lead to overheating in the summer months (Lomas & Porritt, 2017). Buildings in many countries have also been heavily insulated to save heating energy. This higher thermal mass means buildings react slowly to outdoor thermal conditions – taking longer to heat up, but also to cool down again after a heat event (Verbeke & Audenaert, 2018).

Aside from these characteristics of the building envelope, indoor environments are largely influenced by the available building controls, such as shading, cooling, and ventilation devices. Increasing the availability and accessibility of such control options can empower individuals to better manage the conditions of the thermal environment according to their needs. It can also increase their stress capacity: an important psychological factor for the perception of thermal sensations is the amount of control people feel they have over their environment. When building occupants feel that they can exert control over their thermal environment, they are more 'forgiving' of the building, more satisfied with the thermal environment (Humphreys & Nicol, 1998), and even have higher thermal comfort (Langevin et al., 2012). This would also help residents manage their stress experience, as individual temperature preferences show large variations. However, not only the availability is important but also whether people are empowered and understand how to use the available controls. For example, many office workers do not understand available building controls or cannot agree on a setting with their coworkers. When control options are available and usable, they can serve as an effective resource for the prevention of and recovery from heat stress.

While these technical-infrastructural properties have a large influence on heat exposure and recovery capacities, there can also be organisational practices and individual strategies in indoor environments that reduce heat/exposure and assist recovery from heat stress. For example, many work environments prescribe certain dress codes which could be adapted to hotter temperatures. Working hours or workloads could also be distributed according to heat, with physically or mentally more demanding tasks during cooler hours and easier tasks – or even larger recovery breaks – scheduled during the hottest hours.

However, not all these measures are currently widespread or well-accepted. Table 9.1 shows an overview from a recent survey in Munich, Southern Germany, which reported the availability and perceived helpfulness of heat protection measures during a three-day heatwave.[2]

By far, the most helpful measures were using a cooler room and adapting the workday. However, unlike workday modifications, cooler rooms were not widely available. Both the adaptation of clothing levels and of eating/drinking habits (e.g., lighter meals, more water intake) were deemed as highly helpful. Apparently, these practices are already well known and widely used in the study group. Lesser-known or not as socially acceptable measures (mentioned by study participants in additional comments), such as cool foot baths or face mist, might be 'good practices' that can be implemented more widely. Shading windows to avoid solar heat gains was perceived as helpful by about half of the respondents who took the measure. However, 12% of the total 210 office workers did not have exterior shading at their disposal. Windows, opened for ventilation during cooler hours and closed during hotter hours, were rated as helpful by about half of the respondents who had taken these actions, with the more effective cross-ventilation rated especially helpful. Additional ventilation with personal desk fans (aimed at body or face) was deemed helpful by 67% of the respondents who had them at their disposal.

The thermal qualities of the indoor environment at home can also be considered a resource (or an additional stressor). Since homes increasingly double as workspaces, their design becomes even more important. Generally, it appears

Table 9.1 Heat protection measures taken by office workers ($N = 165$) on the hottest day of a heatwave, with outdoor temperatures up to 33.6°C.

Measure (sorted by perceived helpfulness)	*Number of respondents who took the measure*	*Measure helped against heat*	*Measure did not help against heat*
Use a cooler room	18	83.3%	16.7%
Adapt workday	60	78.3%	21.7%
Adapt eating/ drinking habits	99	68.7%	31.3%
Adapt clothing	123	66.7%	33.3%
Use fan	57	66.7%	33.3%
Cross-ventilate	97	61.9%	38.1%
Shade windows/ darken rooms	115	53.0%	47.0%
Keep windows closed	92	51.1%	48.9%
Open windows	98	44.9%	55.1%

that people are more comfortable in their living spaces, even when working from home, which might be related to easier-to-understand controls (Karjalainen, 2009) and higher autonomy, for example, to adapt clothing, transfer location, or even change the work schedule to reduce heat stress and suit recovery as needed. From this perspective, working from home during heatwaves should be encouraged where possible, especially when the home is cooler or more comfortable than the work environment. Homes are also the environment where most people recover from the workday. Night-time recovery during sleep is especially important for health and is impaired by high temperatures (Beckmann et al., 2021). For instance, during the three-day heatwave, 44% of the surveyed Munich office workers reported that their sleep quality was '(rather) not impaired' by heat, 20% 'partially', and 37% '(rather) impaired'. Moreover, 29% of the interviewees could 'not' or 'rather not' recover from the day's heat stress at night, while 33% were able to only 'partially', and 38% to 'rather' or 'fully', recover.

Adapting work locations, schedules, or dress codes, however, is not available for everyone and mostly limited to 'white-collar' jobs. A study of nurses and nursing assistants working in personal protective equipment showed a much narrower spectrum for heat adaptation. Only 9% of employees were able to take more and/or longer breaks to recover, make changes to their care planning, or carry out strenuous work at cooler times of the day. Shorter working days were only possible for 6% of employees in outpatient care, and almost all respondents (97%) stated that no additional nursing staff were available to support the regular nursing staff (Jegodka et al., 2021). Similarly, in Munich day-care centres, only 1.1% of pedagogical staff surveyed $(N = 176)$ stated that they were able to adjust their working hours during a heatwave (Lehmann et al., 2023). This highlights how organisational practices – that might be equally or even more important for recovery than technical building properties – are constrained by labour demands and inflexible schedules or workflows.

While the factors discussed until now apply to buildings and people in general, designing restorative indoor environments should also pay attention to the specific characteristics of their inhabitants. The climate-responsive design for occupants with higher vulnerability to heat should be prioritised, for example, in care homes.

In many instances, heat exposure and possibilities for indoor restoration are influenced by socioeconomic factors and existing environmental injustices. For example, poorer households are often situated in areas with lower levels of green space provision, accessibility, and quality (Schüle et al., 2019; Wolch et al., 2014). Consequently, heat stress is higher in such areas (Jenerette et al., 2011), and this situation is often exacerbated by the proximity to noisy roads, which makes it more difficult to ventilate during night-time, increasing heat in apartments.

Restorative outdoor environments

Outdoor environments should be designed to reduce heat – determined by temperature, radiation, humidity, and wind speed – so that urban residents experience less heat stress and can better recover. At city scale, temperatures correspond directly with the city's physical makeup and are highest in areas of high building density and surface sealing. It is well established that the heat storage capacity of artificial materials leads to the phenomenon of the urban heat island effect (Oke, 1973), whereas green infrastructure provides the ecosystem services of shading and evapotranspiration (Bowler et al., 2010; Pauleit et al., 2020). Therefore, areas with a high share of green infrastructure spaces show the lowest temperatures. In a systematic review, vegetation cover turned out to be the second strongest influence on the UHI effect of surface temperatures, only surpassed by the cover of built and other impervious surfaces (Deilami et al., 2018). While the UHI effect may be offset within large urban parks or woodlands, however, the capacity to cool adjacent built areas is mostly limited (Lin et al., 2015; Upmanis et al., 1998). Therefore, it has been suggested that a network of green infrastructure such as gardens and street trees should permeate built areas to increase especially shading effects (de Vries & Suyin Chalmin-Pui, this volume, Chapter 7; Ettinger et al., 2024; Li, Zhou, et al., 2012; van den Bosch & Jarvis, this volume, Chapter 6).

Green areas are also subjectively perceived as cooler. For instance, research in the city of Munich, Southern Germany, showed that the highest heat exposure is perceived in streets (30% of 731 respondents experienced high or very high heat stress), whereas lowest exposure was expressed for parks and green spaces (60% of respondents experienced no or low heat stress; Bauer et al., 2021). Hence, priority should be given to the protection and enhancement of existing green infrastructures within a city's boundaries.

Besides the overall green share, at city scale, it is also important to protect ventilation corridors that connect the surroundings with inner-city districts and provide them with cold air (Barlag & Kuttler, 1990/91). Maps of urban climate functions support urban planners in detecting such important structures (Bründl, 1988). These maps are synthetic products displaying all climatological aspects relevant in the urban context, for example, the map for Munich (Landeshauptstadt München, 2014). Especially with urban green infrastructure as strategically developed networks of green and blue spaces at city and neighbourhood scales, the aims of a high green share and of ventilation corridors can be achieved to lower heat and to counter climate change impacts (Pauleit et al., 2020).

The implementation of green infrastructure measures is also an important approach to reduce heat at local level and support human recovery by providing cooler green spaces in easy reach. Recovery is enhanced in such 'oases' not only by allowing the body to cool down but, at the same time, also by having beneficial impacts on mental well-being, as described in several other chapters of this book. At the local level, a sufficient green cover of a neighbourhood should be achieved for a cooling effect, where sufficient relates to approximately 25% of green cover in densely built inner areas, according to Pauleit et al. (2023), while other research, such as Rahman et al. (2022), showed that heat stress is reduced by 50% when green cover reaches 30–40%. Moreover, different types of green infrastructure provide a different quality of regulating ecosystem services due to their shading and evapotranspiring features. Research clearly shows that trees are by far the most effective measure to reduce heat stress (Klemm, 2018; Rahman et al., 2019; Zölch et al., 2016) and should be prioritised in urban planning. To achieve the best cooling effects, nevertheless, the implementation needs to take local conditions into account and place green infrastructure measures strategically and adapted to the area of interest (Erlwein et al., 2021; Zölch et al., 2019). This can, for example, mean that trees are planted in heat hotspots and, at the same time, are clustered outside of ventilation corridors to not prevent local air exchange (Middel et al., 2015).

Green infrastructure types of larger size, such as parks and green spaces, not only improve the urban microclimate but are also important resources for citizens' recovery. With rising urban heat, the number of visitors will increase, and 'cooling' characteristics, such as woodlands and opportunities for swimming, are expected to become more important (Welling et al., 2021). Thus, urban planning should not only prioritise protecting green infrastructure but also adapt their functions for human heat recovery. One important aspect is accessibility: in Munich, larger green spaces at the urban edges ('green belt') were generally visited mostly by bike (38%), but elderly citizens had a higher share of car use (34%), and for lower-income citizens, public transport was more important (36%). Most people visited the 'green belt' spaces closest to their home (Welling et al., 2021). Accessibility is even more important for people with limited mobility, who cannot easily reach larger green areas at the city's edge. For these citizens, green infrastructure types of smaller sizes near the home – for example, so-called 'pocket parks', but also inner courtyards with trees and green facades – are an important recovery resource.

Finally, it should be noted that outdoor workers are especially exposed and cannot move freely to adapt to urban heat. For them, actively implementing shading [e.g., shaded break station, (re)park cars in shade, awnings], adapting daily routines to heat (start earlier, adapt break times, follow the sun's course), and increasing opportunities for hydration and cooling through water (keep water accessible, hourly water breaks to drink, and cool forearms, torso, and face with water) can be strategies to decrease heat stress (Lehmann & Gutknecht, 2023). These measures could be transferred to other population groups with high exposure times outdoors and limited mobility. For best effect, such strategies should be developed in a participatory manner, so they are suited to the specific context and (work) culture.

Conclusion and policy implications

In regions with historically more moderate climates, both building stocks and societies are still not well adapted to coping with excessive heat. Therefore, it is important to design indoor as well as outdoor environments that reduce heat and offer effective restoration from heat exposure.

Currently, urbanisation often leads to an increase of building density. This process endangers urban green spaces and, thus, the regulating ecosystem services (ventilation, evapotranspiration, night-time cooling) important for urban cooling and, simultaneously, residents' ability to recover from heat stress. Urban planning should therefore prioritise the protection and creation of urban green spaces and ventilation corridors and keep them free from encroachment. Results from studies briefly presented in this chapter show that even in dense inner-city neighbourhoods of central European cities, an increase of the share of green infrastructure from 10% to 20–30% would be feasible (Zölch et al., 2016). Well-greened open spaces and building greening, such as green roofs and facades, can reduce indoor heat gains. Having easy access to green spaces which serve as cool islands during heat weaves is even more important. However, it requires a dramatic transformation of streets and other open spaces. The change from streets for cars to streets for pedestrians, bicycles, and public transport is key in this context. It will require a major effort of interdisciplinary approaches where urban planners, landscape architects, and urban ecologists closely collaborate with engineers to retrofit above- and belowground infrastructures. Moreover, intense citizen participation is needed to duly recognise their needs and values in the planning process. The aim should be to develop strategic networks of green infrastructure that enhance the microclimate and simultaneously promote physical activity in liveable and biodiverse cities. A city-wide approach informed by climatic assessments, such as maps of urban climate functions, could identify 'hotspots' with high temperatures and low green supply, which should then be prioritised to ensure at least a minimum level of green space provision. Such an assessment should also be intertwined with sociodemographic risk factors at smaller scales, for example, mapping of care facility locations to identify especially vulnerable populations in 'high-risk' areas. Green spaces should also be (re)designed with their recovery function in mind, providing areas with different thermal sensations (e.g., shaded as well as sun-exposed, cooling water features) from which individuals can choose according to their individual needs (Klemm, 2018). For this, design guidelines should be based on people's thermal and spatial perception (Coutts et al., 2014; Lang et al., 2020; Lenzholzer et al., 2018).

Urban outdoor spaces designed for recovery and according to the needs of locals could reintroduce more malleable boundaries between indoor and outdoor spaces that have historically helped climate adaptation. For example, when residents can sit in front of their buildings during summer evenings, this provides both cooling and vigilance for vulnerable neighbours (Brown & Walker, 2010; Wilhite, 2009), not only addressing climate adaptation needs but, simultaneously, allowing for more social interaction, which could also reduce the risk of loneliness that has become a major mental health threat in modern cities (Solmi et al., 2020).

At the building level, the need for air conditioning is expected to increase along with higher temperatures, although it is undesirable from a climate protection standpoint because of its high energy consumption. Therefore, passive measures to assist heat prevention and recovery – retrofitting exterior shading and implementing night-time ventilation – should be prioritised. Less reliance on mechanical cooling would also increase urban resilience by reducing electricity demands and lowering the likelihood of blackouts. However, passive measures are often hindered by conflicting aims with existing regulations. For example, in the Munich office worker survey, the retrofit of exterior shading was prohibited by an architect as the building's copyright owner, as well as by heritage protection laws or security guidelines. These and other existing policies and building standards urgently need to be checked and revised for their compatibility with climate adaptation goals. Smaller-scale measures, such as individual desk fans, could be a low-effort measure to make indoor environments more comfortable in increasing heat (Vesely & Zeiler, 2014) and can be implemented relatively easily and at low cost.

However, the 'designing of environments' should refer not only to physical properties but also to the social practices that take place in these environments. Important recovery resources can be found at the organisational level. At home, many people feel more satisfied with the thermal comfort, as well as better able to control their environment, than in the office (Langevin et al., 2012). Thus, offering remote work more broadly might decrease stress for many. For example, worker protection laws could specify that during heatwaves or from specific indoor temperatures on, workers are automatically free to choose their work location. Next to presence at offices, dress codes form another sociocultural practice that could be adapted. For example, the CoolBiz campaign in Japan aimed at increasing the acceptability and use of cooler business clothing for men (short sleeves instead of a full suit and tie) so that indoor temperatures could rise from 22 to 28°C, reducing the energy used for air conditioning (Granier et al., 2018). Such initiatives make effective recovery practices more available, that is, both more socially acceptable and more widely known. Often, effective strategies for heat reduction and recovery are still not 'learnt' culturally – for example, many of the surveyed office workers still opened windows during the hottest times of day. Such cultural change should be supported by raising awareness and providing information on good practices. The latter could also be gained by learning from cultures with traditionally higher temperatures that already have developed 'recovery practices', such as the traditional Spanish siesta (Nieto, 2015).

As apparent throughout this chapter, both heat exposure and as well as available resources for recovery are often unequally distributed. Outdoor workers and nursing staff who work in personal protective equipment are more exposed to heat and have fewer resources (such as adapting schedules or working from home) at their disposal than 'white-collar' office workers. Lower socioeconomic status is also associated with lower green space provision and lower-quality housing (Ellena et al., 2020). Urban climate adaptation is therefore also an equity issue.

Generally, the balance between prevention of and recovery from heat stress on the one hand, and climate change mitigation on the other, needs to be considered on a wider scale. Widespread mechanical cooling through air conditioning would compromise climate protection goals (Bettgenhäuser et al., 2011) but might, in some cases, be necessary when passive cooling becomes increasingly ineffective (e.g., night-time ventilation brings no cooling when outdoor and indoor temperature are the same during heatwaves). A wider societal discourse on the definition of demands and needs is therefore necessary. For example, healthy office workers could tolerate certain amounts of discomfort, or even heat stress, when exposure is only temporary at the end of the workday (Koth et al., 2022, 2024) and adequate recovery is possible afterwards. On the other hand, an intensive care unit with vulnerable patients and workers in full protective equipment has much higher internal heat gains, and individuals have both reduced stress capacity and fewer resources for recovery at their disposal. Therefore, a sufficiency perspective should be considered: Who really *needs* energy-intensive cooling, and who can 'make do with less' because of higher stress capacity and adequate recovery resources? Also, simply accepting a decline in productivity or work hours during hot periods might be the most climate-adapted and healthy measure. Splitting up an 8-hour workday into the cooler morning and evening hours would help productivity and reduce heat stress or energy consumption at work (Hooyberghs et al., 2017), but it might also mean missing out on active recovery opportunities, such as sports, which are not possible or even unhealthy during the hot hours.

Vulnerable population groups should be prioritised in urban planning as well as general climate adaptation policies. To this end, cities could undertake vulnerability assessments that identify 'high-risk' population groups or locations, for example, homeless people, care homes, or child day-care centres located in areas with little green infrastructure.

In both indoor and outdoor environments – as well as their interrelationships – the different climate-adaptive design measures highlighted in this chapter could help prevent heat stress events and often simultaneously assist recovery as well as increase stress capacity. When opportunities for recovery are available in some contexts, urban dwellers could replenish resources and re-establish a recovery-stress balance and, in this way, develop a 'stress buffer', as described by Kallus and Kellmann (2000), making them more resilient to (heat) stress in other contexts. Measures such as urban greening and passive cooling have multiple co-benefits for climate adaptation, mitigation, individual recovery, and many other functions. These 'no regret' measures should therefore be prioritised in policies and urban planning and ensure that all city dwellers possess at least some recovery options independent of their occupation and socioeconomic status. At the same time, recovery demands and opportunities often differ according to individual, organisational, cultural, and socioeconomic conditions. Especially the measures with high energy consumption should be guided by an assessment of the stress capacity levels and available resources for different population groups and be considered also on a society-wide scale.

Notes

1 *Green infrastructure* is defined as strategically developed networks of multifunctional green and blue spaces at city and neighbourhood scales and covers different types, such as green spaces, parks, trees, green roofs, and facades (Pauleit et al., 2020).

2 2023 mixed-methods field study conducted in Munich, Southern Germany, featuring 210 office workers from 20 companies with different workplace characteristics. Between 20.-23.6.2023 participants filled in an online survey on their thermal comfort, heat stress and control satisfaction on the respective workday. The 22nd June was the hottest day with mean outdoor air temperature (24 h, measured at 2m) of 24.4°C, relative humidity of 64.3%, maximum outdoor temperature 33.6°C, and mean indoor temperature of offices 27.22°C. The research was funded by the Bavarian State Ministry of the Environment and Consumer Protection as well as the Bavarian State Ministry of Health, Care and Prevention through the project 'Leistungsfähigkeit im Klimawandel sichern' ('Ensuring performance in the face of climate change') within the scope of the compound project "Climate Change and Health II".

References

American Society of Heating. (2013). *ANSI/AHRAE standard 55 – thermal environmental conditions for human occupancy*. Retrieved March 20, 2024 from https://ierga.com/hr/wp-content/uploads/sites/2/2017/10/ASHRAE-55-2013.pdf

an der Heiden, M., Buchholz, U., & Uphoff, H. (2020). Schätzung der Zahl hitzebedingter Sterbefälle infolge der Hitzewelle 2018 [Estimate of the number of heat-related deaths as a result of the 2018 heatwave]. *UMID, 29*(1), 77–90.

an der Heiden, M., Muthers, S., Niemann, H., Buchholz, U., Grabenhenrich, L., & Matzarakis, A. (2019). Schätzung hitzebedingter Todesfälle in Deutschland zwischen 2001 und 2015 [Estimate of heat-related deaths in Germany between 2001 and 2015]. *Bundesgesundheitsblatt – Gesundheitsforschung – Gesundheitsschutz, 62*, 571–579.

Arsad, F. S., Hod, R., Ahmad, N., Ismail, R., Mohamed, N., Baharom, M., Osman, Y., Radi, M. F. M., & Tangang, F. (2022). The impact of heatwaves on mortality and morbidity and the associated vulnerability factors: A systematic review. *International Journal of Environmental Research and Public Health, 19*(23), 16356. https://doi.org/10.3390/ijerph192316356

Ballester, J., Quijal-Zamorano, M., Méndez Turrubiates, R. F., Pegenaute, F., Herrmann, F. R., Robine, J. M., Basagaña, X., Tonne, C., Antó, J. M., & Achebak, H. (2023). Heat-related mortality in Europe during the summer of 2022. *Nature Medicine, 29*, 1857–1866.

Barlag, A.-B., & Kuttler, W. (1990/91). The significance of country breezes for urban planning. *Energy and Buildings, 15*(3–4), 291–297.

Bauer, A., Mittermüller, J., Rupp, J., & Wutz, S. (2021). *Grün in der wachsenden Stadt. Perspektiven und Aktivierung der Stadtgesellschaft* [Green in the growing city. Perspectives and activation of urban society]. Technical University Munich. Retrieved March 20, 2024 from https://www.lss.ls.tum.de/fileadmin/w00bds/lapl/Bilder/Projekte/GrueneStadt/Broschure_3.pdf

Beckmann, S. K., Hiete, M., & Beck, C. (2021). Threshold temperatures for subjective heat stress in urban apartments – analysing nocturnal bedroom temperatures during a heat wave in Germany. *Climate Risk Management, 32*, 100286. https://doi.org/10.1016/j.crm.2021.100286

Bettgenhäuser, K., Boermans, T., Offermann, M., Krechting, A., & Becker, D. (2011). *Klimaschutz durch Reduzierung des Energiebedarfs für Gebäudekühlung* [Climate protection by reducing the energy requirement for cooling buildings]. Umweltbundesamt. Retrieved March 20, 2024 from https://www.umweltbundesamt.de/sites/default/files/medien/461/publikationen/3979.pdf

Bowler, D. E., Buyung-Ali, L., Knight, T. M., & Pullin, A. S. (2010). Urban greening to cool towns and cities: A systematic review of the empirical evidence. *Landscape and Urban Planning, 97*(3), 147–155.

Brown, S., & Walker, G. (2010). Understanding heat wave vulnerability in nursing and residential homes. In E. Shove, H. Chappells, & L. Lutzenhiser (Eds.), *Comfort in a lower carbon society* (pp. 59–68). Routledge.

Bründl, W. (1988). Climate function maps and urban planning. *Energy and Buildings, 11*(1–3), 123–127.

Bundesanstalt für Arbeitsschutz und Arbeitsmedizin (BAuA). (2010). *Technische Regeln für Arbeitsstätten – Raumtemperatur (ASR A3.5)* [Technical rules for workplaces – room temperature (ASR A3.5)]. Retrieved March 20, 2024 from https://www.baua.de/DE/Angebote/Regelwerk/ASR/pdf/ASR-A3-5.pdf?__blob=publicationFile&v=5

Campbell, S., Remenyi, T. A., White, C. J., & Johnston, F. H. (2018). Heatwave and health impact research: A global review. *Health & Place, 53*, 210–218.

Coutts, A., Loughnan, M., Tapper, N., White, E., Thom, J., Broadbent, A., & Harris, R. (2014). *Impacts of water sensitive urban design solutions on human thermal comfort. Green cities and microclimate.* CRC for Water Sensitive Cities. Retrieved March 20, 2024 from https://watersensitivecities.org.au/wp-content/uploads/2016/07/TMR_B3-1_WSUD_thermal_comfort_no2.pdf

de Blois, J., Kjellstrom, T., Agewall, S., Ezekowitz, J. A., Armstrong, P. W., & Atar, D. (2015). The effects of climate change on cardiac health. *Cardiology, 131*(4), 209–217.

Deilami, K., Kamruzzaman, Md., & Liu, Y. (2018). Urban heat island effect: A systematic review of spatio-temporal factors, data, methods, and mitigation measures. *International Journal of Applied Earth Observation and Geoinformation, 67*, 30–42.

Ebi, K. L., Capon, A., Berry, P., Broderick, C., de Dear, R., Havenith, G., Honda, Y., Kovats, R. S., Ma, W., Malik, A., Morris, N. B., Nybo, L., Seneviratne, S. I., Vanos, J., & Jay, O. (2021). Hot weather and heat extremes: Health risks. *The Lancet, 398*(10301), 698–708.

Ellena, M., Breil, M., & Soriani, S. (2020). The heat-health nexus in the urban context: A systematic literature review exploring the socio-economic vulnerabilities and built environment characteristics. *Urban Climate, 34*, 100676. https://doi.org/10.1016/j.uclim.2020.100676

Erlwein, S., Zölch, T., & Pauleit, S. (2021). Regulating the microclimate with urban green in densifying cities: Joint assessment on two scales. *Building and Environment, 205*, 108233. https://doi.org/10.1016/j.buildenv.2021.108233

Ettinger, A. K., Bratman, G. N., Carey, M., Hebert, R., Hill, O., Kett, H., Levin, P., Murphy-Williams, M., & Wyse, L. (2024). Street trees provide an opportunity to mitigate urban heat and reduce risk of high heat exposure. *Scientific Reports, 14*, 3266. https://doi.org/10.1038/s41598-024-51921-y

Fanger, P. O. (1970). *Thermal comfort: Analysis and applications in environmental engineering*. Danish Technical Press.

Fatima, S. H., Rothmore, P., Giles, L. C., Varghese, B. M., & Bi, P. (2021). Extreme heat and occupational injuries in different climate zones: A systematic review and meta-analysis of epidemiological evidence. *Environment International, 148*, 106384. https://doi.org/10.1016/j.envint.2021.106384

Gabriel, K. M., & Endlicher, W. R. (2011). Urban and rural mortality rates during heat waves in Berlin and Brandenburg, Germany. *Environmental Pollution, 159*, 2044–2050.

Granier, B., Shove, E., & Poskanzer, D. (2018). *"Cool Biz" in Japan: Transnational circulation of practices and policies* [Conference paper]. ACEEE Summer Study on Energy Efficiency in Buildings, Pacific Grove, CA, United States.

Hanna, E. G., & Tait, P. W. (2015). Limitations to thermoregulation and acclimatization challenge human adaptation to global warming. *International Journal of Environmental Research and Public Health, 12*, 8034–8074.

Höppe, P. (1999). The physiological equivalent temperature – a universal index for the biometeorological assessment of the thermal environment. *International Journal of Biometeorology, 43*, 71–75.

Höppe, P. (2002). Different aspects of assessing indoor and outdoor thermal comfort. *Energy and Buildings, 34*(6), 661–665.

Hooyberghs, H., Verbeke, S., Lauwaet, D., Costa, H., Floater, G., & De Ridder, K. (2017). Influence of climate change on summer cooling costs and heat stress in urban office buildings. *Climatic Change, 144*(4), 721–735.

Hsieh, C. M., Aramaki, T., & Hanaki, K. (2007). The feedback of heat rejection to air conditioning load during the nighttime in subtropical climate. *Energy and Buildings, 39*(11), 1175–1182.

Humphreys, M., & Nicol, F. (1998). Understanding the adaptive approach to thermal comfort. *ASHRAE Transactions, 104*(1B), 991–1004.

Ioannou, L. G., Tsoutsoubi, L., Samoutis, G., Bogataj, L. K., Kenny, G. P., Nybo, L., Kjellstrom, T., & Flouris, A. D. (2017). Time-motion analysis as a novel approach for evaluating the impact of environmental heat exposure on labor loss in agriculture workers. *Temperature, 4*(3), 330–340.

IPCC. (2023). *Climate change 2023: Synthesis report*. IPCC. Retrieved March 20, 2024 from https://doi.org/10.59327/IPCC/AR6–9789291691647

Jegodka, Y., Lagally, L., Mertes, H., Deering, K., Schoierer, J., Buchberger, B., & Bose-O'Reilly, S. (2021). Hot days and Covid-19: Online survey of nurses and nursing assistants to assess occupational heat stress in Germany during summer 2020. *The Journal of Climate Change and Health, 3*, 100031. https://doi.org/10.1016/j.joclim.2021.100031

Jendritzky, G., de Dear, R., & Havenith, G. (2012). UTCI – why another thermal index? *International Journal of Biometeorology, 56*(3), 421–428.

Jenerette, G. D., Harlan, S. L., Stefanov, W. L., & Martin, C. A. (2011). Ecosystem services and urban heat riskscape moderation: Water, green spaces, and social inequality in Phoenix, USA. *Ecological Applications, 21*(7), 2637–2651.

Kallus, K. W., & Kellmann, M. (2000). Burnout in athletes and coaches. In Y. L. Hanin (Ed.), *Emotions in sport* (pp. 209–230). Human Kinetics.

Karjalainen, S. (2009). Thermal comfort and use of thermostats in Finnish homes and offices. *Building and Environment, 44*(6), 1237–1245.

Kellmann, M., & Beckmann, J. (Eds.). (2024). *Fostering recovery and well-being in a healthy lifestyle: Psychological, somatic, and organizational prevention approaches*. Routledge.

Kenny, G. P., Notley, S. R., Flouris, A. D., & Grundstein, A. (2020). Climate change and heat exposure: Impact on health in occupational and general populations. In W. Adams & J. Jardine (Eds.), *Exertional heat illness* (pp. 225–261). Springer.

Kenny, G. P., Wilson, T. E., Flouris, A. D., & Fujii, N. (2018). Heat exhaustion. *Handbook of Clinical Neurology, 157*, 505–529.

Kirby, C. R., & Convertino, V. A. (1986). Plasma aldosterone and sweat sodium concentrations after exercise and heat acclimation. *American Journal of Physiology, 161*, 967–970.

Kjellstrom, T., Holmer, I., & Lemke, B. (2009). Workplace heat stress, health and productivity – an increasing challenge for low and middle-income countries during climate change. *Global Health Action, 2*(1). https://doi.org/10.3402/gha.v2i0.2047

Klemm, W. (2018). *Clever and cool: Generating design guidelines for climate responsive urban green infrastructure* [Doctoral dissertation]. Wageningen University. https://doi.org/10.18174/453958

Koth, S. C., Kobas, B., Bausch, K., & Auer, T. (2022). Mitigating climate change through healthy discomfort. *IOP Conference Series: Earth and Environmental Science, 1078*(1), 012034. http://dx.doi.org/10.1088/1755-1315/1078/1/012034

Koth, S. C., Kobas, B., Reitmayer, A., Hepf, C., & Auer, T. (2024). Dynamic cooling – a concept of time-sensitive thermal regulation to cut cooling energy demand in office buildings. *Energy and Buildings, 322*, 114734. https://doi.org/10.1016/j.enbuild.2024.114734

Landeshauptstadt München. (2014). *Stadtklimaanalyse Landeshauptstadt München* [Urban climate analysis City of Munich]. Retrieved March 20, 2024 from https://stadt.muenchen.de/dam/jcr:1d8eeb94-d4fd-4933-b48f-00b58ef1c63b/Bericht_Stadtklimaanalyse_LHM.pdf

Lang, W., Pauleit, S., Brasche, J., Hausladen, G., Maderspacher, J., Schelle, R., & Zölch, T. (2020). *Guidelines for climate-oriented communities in Bavaria*. Centre for Urban Ecology and Climate Adaptation. Retrieved March 20, 2024 from https://www.zsk.tum.de/fileadmin/w00bqp/www/PDFs/Guideline_English_final-komprimiert.pdf

Langevin, J., Wen, J., & Gurian, P. L. (2012). Relating occupant perceived control and thermal comfort: Statistical analysis on the ASHRAE RP-884 database. *HVAC&R Research, 18*(1–2), 179–194.

Legault, G., Clement, A., Kenny, G. P., Hardcastle, S., & Keller, N. (2017). Cognitive consequences of sleep deprivation, shiftwork, and heat exposure for underground miners. *Applied Ergonomics, 58*, 144–150.

Lehmann, H., Bose-O'Reilly, S., Schoierer, J., & Garschagen, M. (2023). Climate change-related health hazards in daycare centers in Munich, Germany: Risk perception and adaptation measures. *Regional Environmental Change, 23*, 147. https://doi.org/10.1007/s10113-023-02136-w

Lehmann, H., & Gutknecht, T. (2023). *Klimawandel und Gesundheit in der Holzbaubranche*. [Climate change and health in the timber construction industry]. BIFA. Retrieved March 20, 2024 from https://www.bifa.de/fileadmin/_migrated/pics/Projekte/Broschuere__Klimawandel_und_Gesundheit.pdf

Lenzholzer, S., Klemm, W., & Vasilikou, C. (2018). Qualitative methods to explore thermo-spatial perception in outdoor urban spaces. *Urban Climate, 23*, 231–249.

Li, D. H. W., Yang, L., & Lam, J. C. (2012). Impact of climate change on energy use in the built environment in different climate zones – a review. *Energy, 42*(1), 103–112.

Li, X. M., Zhou, W. Q., Ouyang, Z. Y., Xu, W. H., & Zheng, H. (2012). Spatial pattern of green space affects land surface temperature: Evidence from the heavily urbanized Beijing metropolitan area, China. *Landscape Ecology, 27*, 887–898.

Lin, W., Ting, Y., Chang, X., Wu, W., & Zhang, Y. (2015). Calculating cooling extents of green parks using remote sensing: Method and test. *Landscape and Urban Planning, 134*, 66–75.

Liu, J., Varghese, B. M., Hansen, A., Xiang, J., Zhang, Y., Dear, K., Gourley, M., Driscoll, T., Morgan, G., Capon, A., & Bi, P. (2021). Is there an association between hot weather and poor mental health outcomes? A systematic review and meta-analysis. *Environment International, 153*, 106533. https://doi.org/10.1016/j.envint.2021.106533

Lõhmus, M. (2018). Possible biological mechanisms linking mental health and heat – a contemplative review. *International Journal of Environmental Research and Public Health, 15*(7), 1515. https://doi.org/10.3390/ijerph15071515

Lomas, K. J., & Porritt, S. M. (2017). Overheating in buildings: Lessons from research. *Building Research & Information, 45*(1–2), 1–18.

Lundgren, K., & Kjellstrom, T. (2013). Sustainability challenges from climate change and air conditioning use in urban areas. *Sustainability, 5*(7), 3116–3128.

Lüthi, S., Fairless, C., Fischer, E. M., Scovronick, N., Armstrong, B., Coelho, M. D. S. Z. S., Guo, Y. L., Guo, Y., Honda, Y., Huber, V., Kyselý, J., Lavigne, E., Royé, D., Ryti, N., Silva, S., Urban, A., Gasparrini, A., Bresch, D. N., & Vicedo-Cabrera, A. M. (2023). Rapid increase in the risk of heat-related mortality. *Nature Communications, 14*(1), 4894. https://doi.org/10.1038/s41467-023-40599-x

Middel, A., Häb, K., Brazel, A. J., Martin, C. A., & Guhathakurta, S. (2015). Impact of urban form and design on mid-afternoon microclimate in phoenix local climate zones. *Landscape and Urban Planning, 122*, 16–28.

Mora, C., Counsell, C. W., Bielecki, C. R., & Louis, L. V. (2017). Twenty-seven ways a heat wave can kill you: Deadly heat in the era of climate change. *Circulation: Cardiovascular Quality and Outcomes, 10*(11), e004233. https://doi.org/10.1161/circoutcomes.117.004233

Nieto, F. J. (2015). Siesta by decree or sound policy to promote sleep health? Lessons from a municipal proclamation in a rural Spanish town. *Sleep Health, 1*(4), 227–228.

Oke, T. R. (1973). City size and the urban heat island. *Atmospheric Environment*, 7(8), 769–779.

Oke, T. R., Mills, G., Christen, A., & Voogt, J. A. (2017). *Urban climates*. Cambridge University Press.

Pallubinsky, H., Schellen, L., Kingma, B. R. M., Dautzenberg, B., van Baak, M. A., & van Marken Lichtenbelt, W. D. (2017). Thermophysiological adaptations to passive mild heat acclimation. *Temperature, 4*(2), 176–186.

Pauleit, S., Erlwein, S., Linke, S., Rahman, M., Zölch, T., & Rötzer, T. (2023). Grün-blaue Infrastruktur für die Klimawandelanpassung der Stadt [Green-blue infrastructure for the city's climate change adaptation]. *Promet, 106*, 79–88. https://doi.org/10.5676/DWD_pub/promet_106_08

Pauleit, S., Fryd, O., Backhaus, A., & Jensen, M. B. (2020). Green infrastructures to face climate change in an urbanizing world. In V. Loftness (Ed.), *Sustainable built environments* (pp. 207–234). Springer.

Rahman, M., Franceschi, E., Pattnaik, N., Moser-Reischl, A., Hartmann, C., Paeth, H., Pretzsch, H., Rötzer, T., & Pauleit, S. (2022). Spatial and temporal changes of outdoor thermal stress: Influence of urban land cover types. *Scientific Reports, 12*, 671. https://doi.org/10.1038/s41598-021-04669-8

Rahman, M. A., Moser, A., Rötzer, T., & Pauleit, S. (2019). Comparing the transpirational and shading effects of two contrasting urban tree species. *Urban Ecosystems, 22*(4), 683–697.

Razmjou, S. (1996). Mental workload in heat: Toward a framework for analyses of stress states. *Aviation, Space, and Environmental Medicine, 67*(6), 530–538.

Rupp, R. F., Vásquez, N. G., & Lamberts, R. (2015). A review of human thermal comfort in the built environment. *Energy and Buildings, 105*, 178–205.

Schüle, S. A., Hilz, L. K., Dreger, S., & Bolte, G. (2019). Social inequalities in environmental resources of green and blue spaces: A review of evidence in the WHO European region. *International Journal of Environmental Research and Public Health, 16*(7), 1216. https://doi.org/10.3390/ijerph16071216

Solmi, M., Veronese, N., Galvano, D., Favaro, A., Ostinelli, E. G., Noventa, V., Favaretto, E., Tudor, F., Finessi, M., Shin, J. I., Smith, L., Koyanagi, A., Cester, A., Bolzetta, F., Cotroneo, A., Maggi, S., Demurtas, J., De Leo, D., & Trabucchi, M. (2020). Factors associated with loneliness: An umbrella review of observational studies. *Journal of Affective Disorders, 271*, 131–138.

Staiger, H., Bucher, K., & Jendritzky, G. (1997). Gefühlte Temperatur. Die physiologisch gerechte Bewertung von Wärmebelastung und Kältestress beim Aufenthalt im Freien in der Maßzahl Grad Celsius [Perceived temperature. The physiologically fair assessment of heat stress and cold stress when outdoors in degrees Celsius]. *Annalen der Meteorologie, Deutscher Wetterdienst, 33*, 100–107.

Staiger, H., Laschewski, G., & Grätz, A. (2012). The perceived temperature – a versatile index for the assessment of the human thermal environment. Part A: Scientific basics. *International Journal of Biometeorology, 56*, 165–176.

Staiger, H., Laschewski, G., & Matzarakis, A. (2019). Selection of appropriate thermal indices for applications in human biometeorological studies. *Atmosphere, 10*(1), 18. https://doi.org/10.3390/atmos10010018

Stearns, R. L., O'Connor, F. G., Casa, D. J., & Kenny, G. P. (2015). Exertional heat stroke. In D. J. Casa & R. L. Stearns (Eds.), *Emergency management for sport and physical activity* (pp. 61–79). Jones and Bartlett Learning.

Steul, K., Schade, M., & Heudorf, U. (2018). Mortality during heatwaves 2003–2015 in Frankfurt-Main – the 2003 heatwave and its implications. *International Journal of Hygiene and Environmental Health, 221*, 81–86.

Thompson, R., Hornigold, R., Page, L., & Waite, T. (2018). Associations between high ambient temperatures and heat waves with mental health outcomes: A systematic review. *Public Health, 161*, 171–191.

Umweltbundesamt. (2019). *Monitoringbericht 2019 zur Deutschen Anpassungsstrategie an den Klimawandel* [2019 Monitoring report on the German strategy for adaptation to climate change]. Retrieved March 20, 2024 from https://www.umweltbundesamt.de/sites/default/files/medien/1410/publikationen/das_monitoringbericht_2019_barrierefrei.pdf

Upmanis, H., Eliasson, I., & Lindqvist, S. (1998). The influence of green areas on nocturnal temperatures in a high latitude city (Goteborg, Sweden). *International Journal of Climatology, 18*, 681–700.

van Hoof, J., Schellen, L., Soebarto, V., Wong, J. K. W., & Kazak, J. K. (2017). Ten questions concerning thermal comfort and ageing. *Building and Environment, 120*, 123–133.

van Marken Lichtenbelt, W., Hanssen, M., Pallubinsky, H., Kingma, B., & Schellen, L. (2017). Healthy excursions outside the thermal comfort zone. *Building Research & Information, 45*(7), 819–827.

van Loenhout, J. A., le Grand, A., Duijm, F., Greven, F., Vinak, N. M., Hoek, G., & Zuurbier, M. (2016). The effect of high indoor temperatures on self-perceived health of elderly persons. *Environmental Research, 146*, 27–34.

Verbeke, S., & Audenaert, A. (2018). Thermal inertia in buildings: A review of impacts across climate and building use. *Renewable and Sustainable Energy Reviews, 82*, 2300–2318.

Verein Deutscher Ingenieure. (VDI). (2022). *Guideline on environmental meteorology – methods for human-biometeorological evaluation of the thermal component of the climate* (VDI 3787, Part 2). Retrieved March 20, 2024 from https://www.vdi.de/richtlinien/details/vdi-3787-blatt-2-environmental-meteorology-methods-for-human-biometeorological-evaluation-of-the-thermal-component-of-the-climate

Vesely, M., & Zeiler, W. (2014). Personalized conditioning and its impact on thermal comfort and energy performance – a review. *Renewable Sustainability Energy Review, 34*, 401–408.

Wang, Y., An, S., Xing, M., Wan, Y., & Liu, Q. (2018). Global warming and heart disease prevention. *European Journal of Preventive Cardiology, 25*(12), 1342. https://doi.org/10.1177/2047487318774846

Welling, M., Hirsch, I., Linke, S., Zölch, T., Bauer, A., & Mittermüller, J. (2021). *Potenziale des Münchner Grüngürtels für die klimaresiliente Stadtentwicklung* [The potential of Munich's green belt for climate-resilient urban development]. Technische Universität München, Lehrstuhl für Strategie und Management der Landschaftsentwicklung. Retrieved March 20, 2024 from https://www.lss.ls.tum.de/fileadmin/w00bds/lapl/Bilder/Projekte/GrueneStadt/FS_Gruenguertel_Leseversion.pdf

Wilhite, H. (2009). The conditioning of comfort. *Building Research & Information, 37*(1), 84–88.

Wolch, J. R., Byrne, J., & Newell, J. P. (2014). Urban green space, public health, and environmental justice: The challenge of making cities 'just green enough'. *Landscape and Urban Planning, 125*, 234–244.

Yaglou, C. P., & Minard, D. (1957). Control of heat casualties at military training centers. *Archives of Industrial Health, 16*, 302–316.

Zölch, T., Maderspacher, J., Wamsler, C., & Pauleit, S. (2016). Using green infrastructure for urban climate-proofing: An evaluation of heat mitigation measures at the micro-scale. *Urban Forestry & Urban Greening, 20*, 305–316.

Zölch, T., Rahman, M., Pfleiderer, E., Wagner, G., & Pauleit, S. (2019). Designing public squares with green infrastructure to optimize human thermal comfort. *Building and Environment, 149*, 640–654.

Zhou, H., Xie, D., & Xiao, P. (2023). Research on thermal comfort of obese and overweight people during indoor running exercise. *Building and Environment, 242*, 110574. https://doi.org/10.1016/j.buildenv.2023.110574

10 Urban safety as a prerequisite for reduced stress and recovery opportunities in the city of tomorrow

Reflections beyond gender-neutral planning practices

Vania Ceccato

Introduction

Growing up in Brazil, I know that going about our daily activities, such as going to school or work, is never worry-free. Women carefully plan their daily routine, including choosing the right bus at the right time. If the bus is late in the evening, women may consider crossing the neighbourhood park and rushing home in alert mode, choosing to walk in the more illuminated spots of the streets. What has been described is not only typical of Brazilians, or women in Brazil, but is, to a greater or smaller extent, also a general problem for women all around the world (Ceccato & Loukaitou-Sideris, 2020). Although men are statistically more likely to be victims of certain types of violent crimes in public spaces, studies consistently show that women report higher levels of fear of crime (Morgan & Smith, 2012). This phenomenon is observed across different cultures and urban settings worldwide and is influenced by a complex interplay of social, cultural, and environmental factors. In countries in the Global South, the situation is more severe, as women are often transit captives, lacking alternative modes of transportation apart from public transport (Ceccato, 2017). This is a global public health problem, because exposure to unsafe or threatening environments can cause chronic stress, anxiety, and fear (Chu et al., 2004; Matheson et al., 2020; Sivak et al., 2021). Evidence shows that poorly perceived safety impacts stress levels and the ability of individuals to recover from daily urban stressors.

This chapter aims to emphasise the pressing necessity of ensuring safety for all individuals in public spaces. In recent years, it has been recognised that simply

Ceccato, V. (2025). Urban safety as a prerequisite for reduced stress and recovery opportunities in the city of tomorrow: Reflections beyond gender-neutral planning practices. In S. Pauleit, M. Kellmann, & J. Beckmann (Eds.), *Creating Urban and Workplace Environments for Recovery and Well-being* (pp. 199–214). Routledge.

DOI: 10.4324/9781003435471-13

reducing stress factors is not sufficient for health and well-being (Kellmann et al., 2023). Instead, the aim is to achieve a balance between stress and recovery. In many cases, the main problem is underrecovery (Kellmann et al., 2023). It is essential that the home and living environment is a place of retreat that offers the opportunity for recovery and thus avoids underrecovery and enables stress to be balanced out through recovery. Urban living spaces must be designed with this in mind. A very important aspect is safety, especially for women and older adults. It is argued that achieving safety in the cities of tomorrow requires moving beyond gender-neutral planning practices to acknowledge and address the varied experiences and needs of all city users for housing, mobility, and recovery. Recognising the diverse experiences of individuals is important when it comes to addressing urban safety. I adopt the concepts of recovery and urban recovery as outlined by Kallus (1995) and Kellmann (2002) as of central importance for my analysis. While recovery is a highly individual process, contingent upon personal evaluations of stress, *resilience* or *urban recovery* involves establishing institutional, political, and infrastructural frameworks that ensure satisfactory living standards and bolstering the resilience of urban systems. Recovery and resilience have emerged as a key concept for future urban development in times of crisis and great uncertainty.

The concept of recovery involves recognising the integral role safe, inclusive, and resilient cities play in the recovery process for individuals and communities affected by crime and victimisation, linking directly to the Sustainable Development Goals, in particular, SDG 11, much of which is reflected in the policy and programmatic work of UN-Habitat and partners, such as UNODC (2020) and UN Women (2017).

This chapter explores potential scenarios for the cities of the future. These scenarios highlight the role of interconnected system thinking (Meadows, 2008) in enhancing urban safety. Three scenarios are presented in order to demonstrate how future cities can prioritise safety by implementing innovative design, informed policies, and community engagement strategies. Scenario 1 explores design techniques that go beyond traditional, gender-neutral planning to cater for diverse urban experiences. Scenario 2 shows how strategic policymaking can prioritise inclusivity and safety for all city users. Finally, scenario 3 focuses on community engagement strategies, emphasising the importance of collective action in creating safer urban environments. By considering these interconnected approaches, future cities can become havens of safety, inclusivity, and resilience. Additionally, I offer examples showcasing existing initiatives from around the globe based on these principles described in scenarios.

Background

The impact of poorly perceived safety on urban life

Drawing on first-hand accounts from women on the effects of sexual harassment in public spaces, Vera-Gray (2018) illustrates the amount of 'safety work' women do every day in order to feel safe. Despite the fact that prior studies of crime safety and physical activity present conflicting results (da Silva et al., 2016; Rees-Punia et al., 2018), there is evidence of the impact of violent crime on the readiness of individuals to walk rather than take public transport (Janke et al., 2016) and on the demand for healthcare (Janke et al., 2016). Fear and perceptions of insecurity in urban areas can lead to precautionary measures, which can include less physical activity, such as walking or cycling, and limited access to social and recreational activities. These contribute to sedentary lifestyles, accumulate stress, reduce recovery, and increase health risks associated with them.

There is no doubt about the effect of the environment on our health and well-being. In an early study in this area, Chu et al. (2004) show evidence of the impact of the urban environment on mental well-being, calling for an integrated view of the relationship between the environment and mental well-being. More recently, Sivak et al. (2021) conducted a systematic review of the effects of poor-quality green spaces' (e.g., vacant lots) impact on human health (e.g., stress) and health risks (e.g., crime). They found that the 'greening' of vacant lots primarily showed consistent improvements in health, feelings of depression, self-reported stress, physical activity, the use of outdoor areas for relaxation and socialisation, and heart rates. Thus, it seems that addressing fear of crime begins with understanding its causes and implementing environmental strategies to both reduce the actual risk of crime and alleviate the fear itself.

The effect of the environment on health is not only direct. The fear of victimisation can segregate communities, restrict the use of public spaces, and erode the sense of belonging among residents, undermining the social well-being of residents (Roberts, 2009; Spinks, 2001). Urban safety also has significant economic implications. Areas perceived to be safe attract more residents, businesses, and tourists, stimulating local economies and fostering economic development. On the other hand, high crime rates can depress property values, deter investment, and increase public spending on law enforcement and healthcare services (Caudill et al., 2015; Ceccato & Wilhelmsson, 2020; Wilhelmsson et al., 2022).

Disparities in urban safety: An intersectional perspective

Urban safety is a multifaceted concept that encompasses protecting individuals and communities from physical harm, crime, and psychological distress within urban environments. The relationship between urban safety and public health is critical and complex. Unsafe urban environments can lead to direct physical harm through violence or accidents, but the implications for public health extend further. However, stress and fear are gender-related. Recent research shows gender differences in anxiety and stress responses: women showed higher anxiety levels compared to men, influenced by factors such as increased caregiving responsibilities and greater exposure to domestic stressors, including domestic violence (Graves et al., 2021; Hou et al., 2020).

The concept of intersectionality is essential here to discuss how these diverse factors combine to shape a woman's fear and vulnerability to crime (Crenshaw,

1994). Women, children, the elderly, and LGBTQI+ community members can encounter specific safety issues and feelings of vulnerability within urban environments. These precautions are just part of an array of symptoms that arise ranging from stress, anxiety, and trouble sleeping to paralysis. It is essential to acknowledge the relationship between recovery from stress and the environment humans inhabit and use it for recovery. Yates and Ceccato (2020), when studying Stockholm, found that the most fearful women share a number of similarities: they have often previously been victimised and were often born abroad. Whilst older women are commonly recognised as more fearful than younger individuals, our attention should turn to equally considering the fearful, young, single mother, whose fears are often lesser known and deemed less worthy of intervention. Findings also show that the most fearful women were most likely to restrict their use of public space by avoiding certain places.

Due to an increased vulnerability to sexual harassment, women's freedom of movement tends to be more restricted compared to men's, mirroring and perpetuating existing gender-based inequalities to access to public spaces (Massey, 2013). Victims often alter their travel habits, such as changing their travel times, modes, or routes, travelling with others, avoiding certain times or staying at home, positioning themselves strategically within a vehicle, or staying close to perceived safe individuals, typically other women. These actions can help some regain a sense of security, though others may still experience heightened vigilance, anxiety, and trauma-related stress (d'Arbois de Jubainville & Vanier, 2017; Yates & Ceccato, 2020).

The interplay between mobility and immobility shapes the power structures and dynamics inherent in gender relations, while gender itself influences mobility and transportation, leading to distinct travel patterns and behaviours (Loukaitou-Sideris, 2016). In their study of 18 cities in all, Ceccato and Loukaitou-Sideris (2020) found that varying percentages of male students also indicated experiences of sexual harassment in transit settings, particularly verbal harassment, but women dominate these statistics in all countries (Figure 10.1a). In this same study, the authors showed that the percentage of female students 'always' or 'often' feeling safe after dark on the bus and at the bus stop, or walking to the bus stop, varied highly. While about half of the respondents felt safe in Stockholm and in Mexico City, in Bogotá and Milan, the share was lower than one-fifth of the respondents. A similar result was found for individuals taking precautions against crime when using public transportation, such as avoiding places, routes, buses, or dressing in a particular way. While in Lagos, Nigeria, all respondents among women took precautionary measures, less than half did so in Guangzhou, China (Figure 10.1b).

People may feel unsafe for various reasons. Research from around the world, despite some mixed results, has consistently shown that having been a victim in the past significantly influences how safe people feel (Hale, 1996). Additionally, seeing someone else, especially a friend or family member, become a victim can also impact an individual's sense of safety [Skogan (1992) provides a comprehensive review]. Various personal factors can affect both the likelihood of being

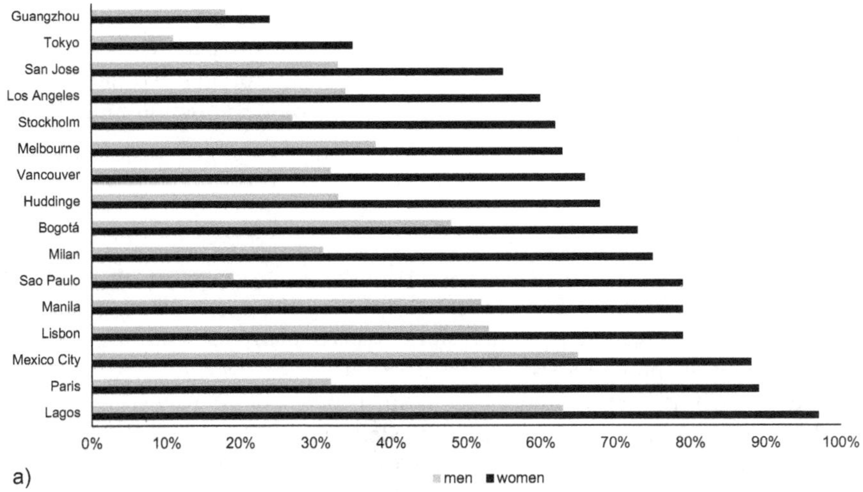

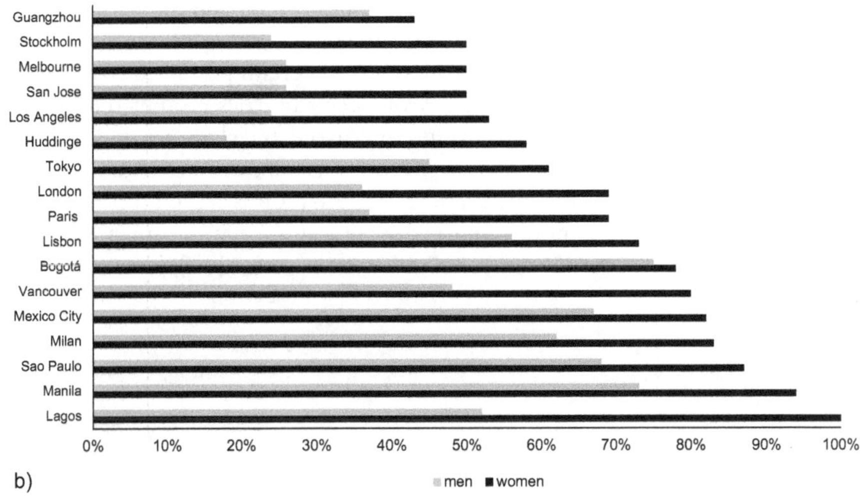

Figure 10.1 a) Percentage of respondents experiencing harassment in the train system. b) Percentage of respondents who felt it necessary to take precautions against crime when using public transportation, such as avoiding places, routes, buses, and dressing in a particular way.

Source: Ceccato and Loukaitou-Sideris (2020, pp. 190–191).

victimised and feelings of safety. Studies indicate that certain groups, including women, older adults, young people living in disadvantaged urban areas, ethnic minorities, members of the LGBTQI+ community, individuals with disabilities, and those facing economic challenges, often experience a greater fear of crime

(Ceccato & Nalla, 2020). Safety concerns may escalate during rush hours due to crimes such as pickpocketing, which are more easily perpetrated in crowded settings, or during off-peak times, when fewer people around may lead to more serious offences. I turn now to temporal aspects of victimisation and fear of crime in cities.

Temporality of crime and fear

People often feel less secure after dark, attributing to a rise in violent incidents at transport hubs during evenings, when there is minimal survivability and fewer bystanders. This heightened fear after sunset is particularly acute among women, influenced by the prevalent risk of sexual assault.

Crimes such as rape outdoors by unknown perpetrators may happen close to where women live. In Stockholm, Sweden, women were raped in familiar places, close to home, on average around 1.6 kilometres from their front door. More than half of cases happen within one kilometre from the victims' residence (Figure 10.2). Almost 50% of all outdoor rapes occur during the summer in the city centre, most often at weekends, between 11:00 p.m. and 3:00 a.m., when bars, restaurants, and other entertainment venues are open.

Fear of sexual violence leads to the adoption of certain precautionary behaviours on the part of transit passengers. Avoidance strategies prompt transit passengers to travel only at particular times and avoid travel routes and settings deemed as particularly risky, or even to avoid using transit routes completely. In Mexico City and São Paulo, where crime victimisation is high, both male and female students reported more often taking precautionary measures than did those living in other cities (Ceccato & Loukaitou-Sideris, 2022).

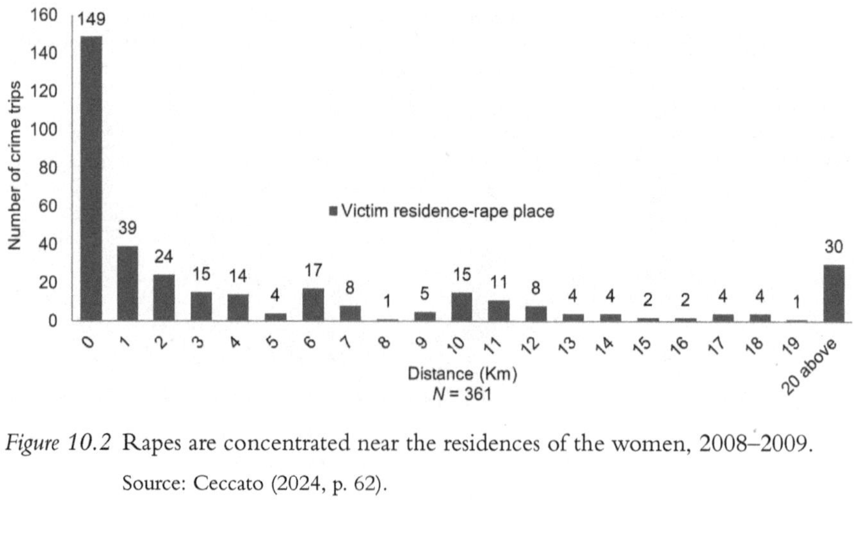

Figure 10.2 Rapes are concentrated near the residences of the women, 2008–2009.

Source: Ceccato (2024, p. 62).

Gender-neutral planning: Beyond women's concerns

Traditional planning often prioritises efficiency and neglecting throughout the varied needs and experiences of its diverse users, particularly in terms of safety and comfort (Greed, 2016). I have so far argued in this chapter that while gender-neutral planning aims for equality, it often overlooks the unique needs, experiences, and safety needs and concerns of different genders, particularly those of women, older, or non-binary, and transgender individuals. Cultural background, socioeconomic status, age, and race affect safety concerns, with age being a critical risk factor for sexual victimisation (Berkowitz, 2020). A common goal for recovery is to promote health and well-being, and for that, gender-specific considerations in urban planning are needed to achieve equitable urban spaces.

The design of public conveniences often follows a gender-neutral model that fails to cater to the needs of all users adequately (Bovens & Marcoci, 2023). The lack of consideration for non-binary and transgender individuals – who may not feel safe or comfortable using strictly gendered facilities – highlights a significant gap in the inclusivity and safety of urban infrastructure. The incorporation of gender-inclusive conveniences with individual stalls and common washing areas could mitigate these issues, providing a safer and more accommodating environment for all users. These changes should not be limited to modification of the physical environment and involve the training of the staff to be sensitive to the needs of all visitors, in this particular case, LGBTQI+ individuals. This could include recognising the importance of privacy, addressing individuals by their correct pronouns, and understanding the challenges faced by transgender and non-binary people. Another example is to provide family-friendly rooms in both men's and women's facilities, as well as in gender-neutral areas, to support caregivers of all genders.

Recovery and urban recovery and urban safety

A common goal of recovery is to promote health and well-being. *Recovery* varies based on the nature and length of stress experienced. Moreover, recovery is intricately linked to the context of the situation and manifests itself in various forms, including passive, active, and pro-active approaches. It is important to recognise that recovery and stress are independent yet interrelated concepts (Pauleit et al., this volume, Chapter 1). A basic level of recovery is necessary for individuals to cope with and manage stress as it arises. This relationship suggests that understanding and implementing recovery strategies are key to maintaining overall well-being, irrespective of the stress levels one might encounter.

Recovery, in the context of health and well-being, can be closely linked to safety, both in physical and psychological terms (Kellmann, 2002). When individuals feel safe in their environment, their stress levels are likely to decrease, fostering conditions conducive to recovery from various stressors, such as being more active outside, physical activity such as jogging, meeting friends, sitting

Table 10.1 Recovery: Individual and city-level characteristics.

Human recovery	*Urban recovery and resilience*
• Is not merely regeneration or healing but an inter- and intraindividual multilevel (e.g., psychological, physiological, social) process in time for the re-establishment of personal resources and their full functional capacity. • Involves gaining or recapturing meaning and purpose in life, and self-determination, resulting in personal empowerment and resilience. • Urban structures should be created that provide suitable conditions for this and thus contribute to solving the demands and challenges of modern societies.	• Urban areas need to fundamentally change in terms of their physical makeup, their functionality, and the ways in which they are organised and governed, to meet the challenges outlined before. • Recovery and resilience have emerged as key concepts for future urban development in times of crisis and great uncertainty. • *Evolutionary resilience* means the capacity of a system to fundamentally change existing structures in order to respond successfully to future challenges.

Source: Adapted from Pauleit et al. (this volume, Chapter 1).

in the sun. In essence, the perception of safety can provide a foundation upon which various recovery processes can be built, enabling individuals to effectively restore their health and well-being after experiencing stress. In this chapter, I differentiate between the individual characteristic of recovery from that of the city level, urban recovery, and resilience, as described in Table 10.1.

Currently, Allan and Bryant (2011, p. 34) warn that "the disciplines of recovery planning and urban design appear to be strangely disconnected" in cases of recovery from major crises, such as earthquakes, and may be sometimes contradictory. The long-run resilience of cities to many forms of physical destruction has been well-documented (Glaeser, 2021) despite the fact that it has been dominated by earthquakes, flooding, volcanic eruption, landslides, hurricanes, and wildfires (Cimellaro, 2016), but less so to mundane daily events that affect individuals unequally, such as crime and sexual harassment. Focusing on the impact of conflicts as collective violence, protests, and organised armed riots, Elfversson and Höglund (2023) found several occasions when city growth increased the risk of violence, for example, when city growth results in the redrawing of borders, clearance of areas for gentrification, and land tenure change, or when immigrants end up living segregated along identity lines, generating conflicts. They suggest that urban planning and the built environment are crucial in determining a city's resilience and ability to recover from the challenges posed by rapid growth; in particular, cities characterised by segregation and social inequality face increased vulnerability and struggle more to cope with the pressures of swift expansion. The social fabric is also important. Elfversson and Höglund (2023) found that the ability of communities to adapt in the face of urban growth challenges varied significantly, with important implications for resilience to violence.

These findings show the interconnectedness of the physical and social environments for urban recovery. In the next section, three scenarios highlight the role of this interconnectedness in enhancing urban safety and urban recovery.

Looking ahead: Future city scenarios

Scenario 1 explores innovative design techniques that go beyond traditional, gender-neutral planning to cater to diverse urban experiences. Scenario 2 examines how strategic policymaking can prioritise inclusivity and safety for all city dwellers. Lastly, scenario 3 focuses on community engagement strategies, emphasising the importance of collective action in creating safer urban environments. I argue here that urban design can create spaces that promote a sense of security and well-being, incorporating elements such as green spaces, adequate lighting, and pedestrian-friendly pathways. These design choices not only enhance the perceived safety of an area but also provide residents with opportunities to recover from the stress of urban living, improving their overall mental health and quality of life, and to build up recovery buffers.

By considering these interconnected approaches, future cities can come close to achieving sustainable development goals by promoting good experiences in dealing with issues of safety and inclusivity. Also important are the Sustainable Development Goals: Goal 5, gender equality (users of the city, of different kinds, public transportation in particular), and Goal 17, which consider the role of partnerships in achieving the goals by implementing cooperation between transport operators, municipal planners, safety experts, policies, and the private sector. By considering the recovery principles, researchers can contribute to Goal 10, reduced inequalities (improving life chances), and Goal 3, good health and well-being. In other words, a pleasant and safe environment leads to higher levels of walkability in an area and a city and, consequently, to better health.

Scenario 1: Gender-informed design

Creating inclusive community spaces that encourage social cohesion and a collective sense of security. These spaces are designed with input from diverse community members to ensure they meet the varied needs and preferences of all residents. Knowing there are safe, well-lit, and well-monitored routes and areas within the city encourages greater mobility and participation in urban life, contributing to physical and mental recovery. Utilising the principles of Crime Prevention Through Environmental Design (CPTED; Crowe & Fennelly, 2013; van Soomeren, 2013), gender-informed design can significantly contribute to creating safer, more inclusive urban spaces that promote social cohesion and a collective sense of security. CPTED is a multidisciplinary approach to deterring criminal behaviour through environmental design. CPTED strategies aim to reduce vulnerability to crime and increase safety by influencing decisions made by offenders preceding criminal acts. The core principles of CPTED include natural surveillance, natural access control, territorial reinforcement, and maintenance (Colquhoun, 2004). These principles have been used to promote behaviours in people that discourage crime and increase community safety, essentially by making spaces less attractive for potential offenders and more comfortable and secure for city users (Cozens & Love, 2015).

Urban spaces can be reimagined with safety at their core, utilising principles of situational crime prevention to tailor and address the unique vulnerabilities of especially women, the elderly, as well as transgender and gender-nonconforming individuals (Ceccato, 2011). This includes implementing extensive, well-distributed lighting in public spaces, along pathways, and around public transport stations to enhance visibility and deter crime. Since many women feel unsafe on their way to and from public transportation, it is essential to design safe routes, namely, multiple 'safe routes', through the city with good visibility, emergency call points, and avoiding deserted spots. These routes are well-publicised and integrated into city maps and GPS applications, offering safe passage at any hour; enhanced visibility and surveillance reduce opportunities for crime, thereby lowering stress and fear among individuals.

One example of evolutionary resilience, meaning, the capacity of a system to fundamentally change existing structures to respond successfully to future challenges, has been illustrated recently in cities in Brazil. To enhance women's safety at deserted bus stops, particularly at night, bus shelter ads turn into video call stations from 8:00 p.m. to 5:00 a.m., connecting passengers with a call centre to keep them company until their bus arrives. By day, the screens will show ads as usual. This innovation is called *guarded bus stops*.[1] The impact of this type of innovation is visible, and a new phase of expansion is underway, with 100 locations across São Paulo, Rio de Janeiro, and other smaller cities.

Scenario 2: Intersectionality of transit safety and gender-sensitive urban policies

Initiating and enforcing policies that address and safeguard against the gender-specific aspects of urban safety are crucial, but it is equally crucial also to consider the intersectionality of safety. Factors such as cultural background, socioeconomic status, age, and race affect these safety concerns, with age being a critical risk factor for sexual victimisation. The concept of intersectionality (Crenshaw, 1994) is essential in understanding how these diverse factors combine to shape an individual's fear, stress, and vulnerability to crime. Implementing campaigns not only offers protection to vulnerable populations but also cultivates a culture of respect and safety, which is fundamental for an individual's recovery. Here the focus is on particular on individual's on the move, in transit across the city.

Adopting gender-focused transport policies such as late-night buses and safe, budget-friendly taxis for women and vulnerable groups enhances safety (Baruah & Biskupski-Mujanovic, 2021) and is an essential element for recovery from stress. Moreover, this is fundamental when it comes to strengthening legal systems for fast, fair justice for crimes mainly targeting women and gender-nonconforming people. These efforts ought to be supported by educational campaigns aimed at increasing public understanding and awareness of these critical issues.

Having women in visible roles within transportation can boost the security of female passengers, signalling a commitment to everyone's safety and comfort (Loukaitou-Sideris, 2020). These women can inspire greater gender diversity in the transportation sector, fostering innovation and inclusivity and, not least, promoting individual recovery. Finally, their involvement in decision-making ensures that policies and measures will have a positive effect on those most impacted by safety concerns, leading to more effective solutions, such as safer transit routes and targeted safety campaigns. Ultimately, just as is the case with gender diversity, having LGBTQI+ representation in transportation planning and operations can drive innovation and lead to the development of more comprehensive safety measures, benefiting not only LGBTQI+ individuals but also all users of public transit.

Urban areas need to fundamentally change in terms of their physical makeup, functionality, and the ways in which they are organised and governed to meet the challenges outlined earlier (Pauleit et al., this volume, Chapter 1). For example, Transport for London, New York City Subway, and San Francisco Municipal Transportation Agency have been pro-active in promoting diversity and inclusion, including efforts aimed at the LGBTQI+ community (Sant, 2022). Stockholm's public transportation authority, Storstockholms Lokaltrafik, operates with a commitment to diversity and inclusivity, but programmes targeting LGBTQI+ inclusivity in transportation planning and operations might not be readily available (Ceccato et al., 2019). Cities such as Warsaw and Kraków have hosted Pride parades and events that signal a growing visibility and advocacy for LGBTQI+ rights. In Poland, there is no widespread, publicly known initiative specifically aimed at promoting LGBTQI+ inclusivity within the Polish public transport system (Golebiewski, 2015). Thus, by adopting a gender-sensitive approach to urban transport planning, these cities not only make public transport safer for women but also improve the overall quality and accessibility of the service for all users. This approach demonstrates a commitment to addressing the causes of inequality and vulnerability in urban spaces and can be key for daily life stresses, promoting means of recovery.

Scenario 3: Empowering communities

Empowering community involvement is crucial for enhancing urban safety. Active engagement helps instil a sense of ownership and responsibility towards public spaces, which boosts social bonds and resilience. Educating communities and encouraging cooperation can lead to more inclusive and respectful societal norms, alleviating stress and supporting recovery from urban challenges. Effective strategies include creating liaison units for gender and minority issues to foster trustful policing, initiating programmes on gender sensitivity and bystander intervention to shift public attitudes, and performing community-led safety audits. These audits, paying special attention to the needs of women, the elderly, and LGBTQI+ individuals, help pinpoint and rectify local safety concerns, making urban environments safer and more inclusive for everyone.

One ongoing example is from Nairobi, Kenya, part of a gender-sensitive programme. Nairobi has seen the implementation of gender-sensitive urban planning initiatives. This involves engaging community members, especially women, in the planning and development of urban spaces to ensure they meet the safety needs of all residents (Mwendwa, 2020). In South America, in Bogotá, community watch programmes have been developed in various neighbourhoods to enhance safety (Rubio et al., 2022).

Worldwide resources provided to empower women and vulnerable individuals to manage their safety and recovery processes can make a significant difference. This includes access to mental health services, legal assistance, and educational programmes that equip them with the knowledge and tools to navigate their environments safely (WHO, 2020). UN Women has focused extensively on issues related to gender equality and the empowerment of women. Their programmes often include components related to safety, legal rights, and access to services (UN Women, 2017). These examples underscore the importance of a multifaceted approach to supporting the safety and recovery of women and vulnerable populations, highlighting ongoing strategies and the need for continued commitment and resources.

Conclusion

Have you ever thought about how much work goes into avoiding certain places – an effort that often remains invisible both to the individuals who practise it and to society at large (Vera-Gray, 2018)? Therefore, people in charge need to plan and build environments that have the potential to be examples of safety, of inclusivity, and thus provide opportunities for recovery. Urban environments should be created that provide suitable conditions for this and thus contribute to solving the demands and challenges of modern societies (Pauleit et al., this volume, Chapter 1). Achieving this vision requires a concerted effort to address unequal victimisation through thoughtful design, progressive policies, and community empowerment. By prioritising the safety and well-being of all citizens, especially those traditionally marginalised, cities run higher chances to become spaces where fear and stress are not part of everyday life and can boost recovery for the individual. The need for recovery, as discussed in this chapter, emphasises the importance of creating cities that are safe, inclusive, and resilient, which is crucial for the healing of individuals and communities impacted by crime and victimisation. This principle is closely aligned with the 2030 Sustainable Development Goals and should be an integral part of the planning of cities of tomorrow.

In practice, it is highly urged to urban planners, policymakers, and communities to adopt a more nuanced approach to urban planning that acknowledges and addresses the diverse needs of all its inhabitants, moving beyond gender-neutral to truly inclusive and equitable urban spaces which promote both individual recovery and full urban resilience. This evolving landscape requires urban planners, policymakers, and community leaders to embrace a more inclusive approach to urban safety, one that acknowledges and addresses the unique experiences and needs of all city residents. Although achieving this ideal remains a distant goal, this chapter presents examples that demonstrate that it can be done.

Note

1 https://eletromidia.com.br/case/guarded-bus-stop/

References

Allan, P., & Bryant, M. (2011). Resilience as a framework for urbanism and recovery. *Journal of Landscape Architecture*, *6*(2), 34–45.

Baruah, B., & Biskupski-Mujanovic, S. (2021). Gender analysis of policymaking in construction and transportation. In G. L. Magnusdottir & A. Kronsell (Eds.), *Gender, intersectionality and climate institutions in industrialised states* (pp. 143–163). Routledge.

Berkowitz, R. (2020). Students' physical victimization in schools: The role of gender, grade level, socioeconomic background and ethnocultural affiliation. *Children and Youth Services Review*, *114*, 105048. https://doi.org/10.1016/j.childyouth.2020.105048

Bovens, L., & Marcoci, A. (2023). The gender-neutral bathroom: A new frame and some nudges. *Behavioural Public Policy*, 7(1), 1–24.

Caudill, S. B., Affuso, E., & Yang, M. (2015). Registered sex offenders and house prices: An hedonic analysis. *Urban Studies*, *52*(13), 2425–2440.

Ceccato, V. (2011). The urban fabric of crime and fear. In V. Ceccato (Ed.), *The urban fabric of crime and fear* (pp. 1–33). Springer.

Ceccato, V. (2017). Women's victimisation and safety in transit environments. *Crime Prevention and Community Safety*, *19*(3–4), 163–167.

Ceccato, V. (2024). *Säkra städer: Aktivt arbete mot brottskoncentration* [Safe cities: Active work against concentration of crime]. Studentlitteratur.

Ceccato, V., & Loukaitou-Sideris, A. (Eds.). (2020). *Transit crime and sexual violence in cities: International evidence and prevention*. Routledge.

Ceccato, V., & Loukaitou-Sideris, A. (2022). Fear of sexual harassment and its impact on safety perceptions in transit environments: A global perspective. *Violence Against Women*, *28*(1), 26–48.

Ceccato, V., & Nalla, M. K. (Eds.). (2020). *Crime and fear in public places: Towards safe, inclusive and sustainable cities*. Taylor & Francis.

Ceccato, V., Näsman, P., Sundling, C., & Langefors, L. (2019). *Trygghet i kollektivtrafiken i Stockholm i ett internationellt perspektiv: En handlingsplan mot sexuella trakasserier och brott i transitmiljöer* [Safety on public transport in Stockholm in an international perspective: An action plan against sexual harassment and crime in transit environments]. Kungliga tekniska högskolan. Rerieved February 12, 2024 from http://kth.diva-portal.org/smash/get/diva2:1358136/FULLTEXT01.pdf

Ceccato, V., & Wilhelmsson, M. (2020). Do crime hot spots affect housing prices? *Nordic Journal of Criminology*, *21*(1), 84–102.

Chu, A., Thorne, A., & Guite, H. (2004). The impact on mental well-being of the urban and physical environment: An assessment of the evidence. *Journal of Public Mental Health, 3*(2), 17–32.
Cimellaro, G. P. (2016). *Urban resilience for emergency response and recovery*. Springer.
Colquhoun, I. (2004). Design out crime: Creating safe and sustainable communities. *Crime Prevention and Community Safety, 6*(4), 57–70.
Cozens, P., & Love, T. (2015). A review and current status of Crime Prevention through Environmental Design (CPTED). *Journal of Planning Literature, 30*(4), 393–412.
Crenshaw, K. W. (1994). Mapping the margins: Intersectionality, identity politics, and violence against women of color. In M. A. Fineman (Ed.), *The public nature of private violence* (pp. 93–118). Routledge.
Crowe, T. D., & Fennelly, L. J. (2013). Introduction to CPTED. In T. D. Crowe & L. J. Fennelly (Eds.), *Crime prevention through environmental design* (pp. 3–14). Butterworth-Heinemann.
d'Arbois de Jubainville, H., & Vanier, C. (2017). Women's avoidance behaviours in public transport in the Ile-de-France region. *Crime Prevention and Community Safety, 19*(3–4), 183–198.
da Silva, I. C. M., Payne, V. L. C., Hino, A. A., Varela, A. R., Reis, R. S., Ekelund, U., & Hallal, P. C. (2016). Physical activity and safety from crime among adults: A systematic review. *Journal of Physical Activity and Health, 13*(6), 663–670.
Elfversson, E., & Höglund, K. (2023). Urban growth, resilience, and violence. *Current Opinion in Environmental Sustainability, 64*, 101356. https://doi.org/10.1016/j.cosust.2023.101356
Glaeser, E. L. (2021). Urban resilience. *Urban Studies, 59*(1), 3–35.
Golebiewski, D. (2015). *Roman Catholic traditions and LGBT rights in Poland and France. Rights for all? Sexual orientation, religious traditions, and the challenge of inclusion*. Retrieved February 17, 2024 from http://dx.doi.org/10.2139/ssrn.2640412
Graves, B. S., Hall, M. E., Dias-Karch, C., Haischer, M. H., & Apter, C. (2021). Gender differences in perceived stress and coping among college students. *PLoS One, 16*(8), e0255634. https://doi.org/10.1371/journal.pone.0255634
Greed, C. (2016). Are we there yet? Women and transport revisited. In T. P. Uteng & T. Cresswell (Eds.), *Gendered mobilities* (pp. 243–254). Routledge.
Hale, C. (1996). Fear of crime: A review of the literature. *International Review of Victimology, 4*(2), 79–150.
Hou, F., Bi, F., Jiao, R., Luo, D., & Song, K. (2020). Gender differences of depression and anxiety among social media users during the COVID-19 outbreak in China: A cross-sectional study. *BMC Public Health, 20*(1), 1648. https://doi.org/10.1186/s12889-020-09738-7
Janke, K., Propper, C., & Shields, M. A. (2016). Assaults, murders and walkers: The impact of violent crime on physical activity. *Journal of Health Economics, 47*, 34–49.
Kallus, K. W. (1995). *Der Erholungs-Belastungs-Fragebogen* [The Recovery-Stress Questionnaire]. Swets & Zeitlinger.
Kellmann, M. (2002). Underrecovery and overtraining: Different concepts – similar impact? In M. Kellmann (Ed.), *Enhancing recovery: Preventing underperformance in athletes* (pp. 3–24). Human Kinetics.
Kellmann, M., Jakowski, S., & Beckmann, J. (Eds.). (2023). *The importance of recovery for physical and mental health: Negotiating the effects of underrecovery*. Routledge.
Loukaitou-Sideris, A. (2016). A gendered view of mobility and transport: Next steps and future directions. *Town Planning Review, 87*(5), 547–565.

Loukaitou-Sideris, A. (2020). A gendered view of mobility and transport. In I. Sánchez de Madariaga & M. Neuman (Eds.), *Engendering cities: Designing sustainable urban spaces for all* (pp. 19–37). Routledge.

Massey, D. (2013). *Space, place and gender*. John Wiley & Sons.

Matheson, K., Asokumar, A., & Anisman, H. (2020). Resilience: Safety in the aftermath of traumatic stressor experiences. *Frontiers in Behavioral Neuroscience, 14*, 596919. https://doi.org/10.3389/fnbeh.2020.596919

Meadows, D. H. (2008). *Thinking in systems: A primer*. Chelsea Green Publishing.

Morgan, R., & Smith, M. J. (2012). Crimes against passengers – theft, robbery, assault and indecent assault. In M. J. Smith & D. B. Cornish (Eds.), *Secure and tranquil travel* (pp. 77–102). Routledge.

Mwendwa, M. K. (2020). *Influence of gender mainstreaming on women participation in implementation of county development projects in Kenya: A case of Kilifi county*. University of Nairobi. Retrieved February 17, 2024 from http://erepository.uonbi.ac.ke/bitstream/handle/11295/153295/Mwendwa_Influence%20of%20Gender%20Mainstreaming%20on%20Women%20Participation%20in%20Implementation%20of%20County%20Development%20Projects%20in%20Kenya-%20a%20Case%20of%20Kilifi%20County.pdf?sequence=1&isAllowed=y

Rees-Punia, E., Hathaway, E. D., & Gay, J. L. (2018). Crime, perceived safety, and physical activity: A meta-analysis. *Preventive Medicine, 111*, 307–313.

Roberts, S. (2009). *Infectious fear: Politics, disease, and the health effects of segregation*. The University of North Carolina Press.

Rubio, M. A., Guevara-Aladino, P., Urbano, M., Cabas, S., Mejia-Arbelaez, C., Rodriguez Espinosa, P., Rosas, L. G., King, A. C., Chazdon, S., & Sarmiento, O. L. (2022). Innovative participatory evaluation methodologies to assess and sustain multilevel impacts of two community-based physical activity programs for women in Colombia. *BMC Public Health, 22*(1), 771. https://doi.org/10.1186/s12889-022-13180-2

Sant, A. (2022). *From the ground up: Local efforts to create resilient cities*. Island Press.

Sivak, C. J., Pearson, A. L., & Hurlburt, P. (2021). Effects of vacant lots on human health: A systematic review of the evidence. *Landscape and Urban Planning, 208*, 104020. https://doi.org/10.1016/j.landurbplan.2020.104020

Skogan, W. G. (1992). *Disorder and decline: Crime and the spiral of decay in American neighborhoods*. University of California Press.

Spinks, C. (2001). *A new apartheid? Urban spatiality, (fear of) crime, and segregation in Cape Town, South Africa*. London School of Economics and Political Science, Development Studies Institute.

UNODC. (2020). *Safety governance approach for safe, inclusive, and resilient cities: A practical guide for conducting safety governance assessments in urban environments*. Retrieved February 17, 2024 from https://www.unodc.org/documents/Urban-security/Safety_Governance_Assessment_Guidance_final.pdf

UN Women. (2017). *Safe cities and safe public spaces: Global results report*. Retrieved February 17, 2024 from https://www.unwomen.org/en/digital-library/publications/2017/10/safe-cities-and-safe-public-spaces-global-results-report

van Soomeren, P. (2013). Tackling crime and fear of crime through urban planning and architectural design. In T. D. Crowe & L. J. Fennelly (Eds.), *Crime prevention through environmental design* (pp. 219–272). Butterworth-Heinemann.

Vera-Gray, F. (2018). *The right amount of panic: How women trade freedom for safety*. Policy Press.

Wilhelmsson, M., Ceccato, V., & Gerell, M. (2022). What effect does gun-related violence have on the attractiveness of a residential area? The case of Stockholm, Sweden. *Journal of European Real Estate Research, 15*(1), 39–57.

World Health Organization. (2020). *Gender and health.* Retrieved February 17, 2024 from https://www.who.int/health-topics/gender#tab=tab_1

Yates, A., & Ceccato, V. (2020). Individual and spatial dimensions of women's fear of crime: A Scandinavian study case. *International Journal of Comparative and Applied Criminal Justice, 44*(4), 277–292.

11 Multi-scale urban design and recovery

Strategies, pathways, and implications

Lanqing Gu and Martin Knöll

Introduction

By 2050, 70% of the world population will live in cities. While urban living offers advantages such as access to healthcare and other facilities, individuals in urban areas face higher risks of mental illness compared to those in rural areas. Urbanisation is associated with social and environmental stressors, including poverty and pollution, which contribute to these mental health challenges (Gruebner et al., 2017).

Balancing the negative effects caused by the stressors, also known as recovery, is essential for achieving healthy urban living and requires interdisciplinary efforts. Urban design plays a crucial role in this endeavour by creating high-quality urban public spaces that are integral to residents' daily lives. Effective urban design considers factors such as visual aesthetics, functional needs, environmental qualities, and experience enhancement (Cook, 1980), involving diverse product types in different scales ranging from local monuments to new towns (Lang, 2006).

Human recovery is a multifaceted process encompassing passive, active, and pro-active dimensions, all of which are closely related to situational conditions (Pauleit et al., this volume, Chapter 1). To effectively evoke a recovery process, urban environments should enable individuals to reduce stress, change stress (shift from mental to somatic stress), and take breaks from stress. This implies that urban design should incorporate affordances that protect against environmental stressors, such as the heat island effect, pollution, and noise; facilitate both physical and psychological comfort; and encourage active behaviours and social interactions.

Associations have been built between urban design and recovery benefits, including mood enhancement, as well as mental fatigue and stress reduction (Weber & Trojan, 2018). However, the extensive range of variables involved in research and the lack of a framework for understanding the effects of urban

Gu, L., & Knöll, M. (2025). Multi-scale urban design and recovery: Strategies, pathways, and implications. In S. Pauleit, M. Kellmann, & J. Beckmann (Eds.), *Creating Urban and Workplace Environments for Recovery and Well-being* (pp. 215–230). Routledge.

DOI: 10.4324/9781003435471-14

design on recovery may pose a barrier for designers and policymakers, impeding their ability to translate knowledge into practices and policies aimed at fostering recovery.

Therefore, this chapter will develop a conceptual framework, with the aim to identify multi-scale urban design qualities and strategies that relate to recovery, present pathways linking multi-scale urban design and recovery, and offer implications for future research, practice, and policymaking.

Multi-scale urban design: Qualities and impacts

Based on the scope of design objects, urban design can be categorised into macro and micro scales. These two scales are also referred to as neighbourhood/city scale and street/eye-level scale in research and design practice (Gerike et al., 2023; Roe & McCay, 2021; Zang et al., 2020).

Macro-scale urban design, which operates at the level of urban form, involves design aspects like land use, street network, and density. These design factors play an important role in determining place qualities, such as destination diversity and accessibility (Table 11.1), all of which are related to behaviour-related outcomes, such as mobility patterns and use of a public space (Flowers et al., 2016; Marshall & Garrick, 2010; Nubani & Wineman, 2005). These behavioural outcomes of macro-scale urban design, in turn, exert an influence on psychological perceptions of the environment. For example, a neighbourhood being able to provide more destination diversity and easier access to the destinations can attract more walking activities with potential social interactions, thus influencing perceived fascination and vibrancy of the neighbourhood (Jacobs, 1961). Additionally, macro-scale urban design, including urban street networks planning, can create a resilient urban form, strengthening a city's ability to handle disasters and adverse events (Sharifi, 2019).

Table 11.1 Macro and micro urban design qualities.

	Quality	*Definition*
Macro scale	Diversity	The richness of destination types.
	Accessibility	The possibility to access diverse destinations.
Micro scale	Imageability	How distinct, recognisable, and memorable a place is.
	Enclosure	The degree to which a public space, defined by vertical elements, can be room-like.
	Complexity	The visual richness of a public space.
	Transparency	To which degree one can perceive beyond the edge of a space, such as building facade.
	Human scale	The details of public space design match human size and needs.

Micro-scale urban design plays an essential role in shaping both behaviours and perceptions in an urban space. While macro-scale design factors like street network structure and land-use patterns may not be directly perceived, eye-level design elements, such as building typology, furniture, facilities, and greenery, are immediately noticeable. These design variables contribute to perceived qualities – imageability, enclosure, complexity, transparency, and human scale (Table 11.1) – that are associated with walkability, as well as social, psychological, and physical well-being (Ewing & Handy, 2009; Ewing et al., 2013).

Multi-scale urban design: Qualities and impacts

The conceptual framework linking multi-scale urban design factors and strategies to recovery is presented in Figure 11.1. The framework was developed by synthesising earlier conceptual frameworks (Bornioli & Subiza-Pérez, 2023; Frank et al., 2019) and recent empirical findings.

Recovery includes three essential processes: containment, passive recovery, and active/pro-active recovery. Containment serves as the foundational process, requiring an environment to mitigate stressors, such as air pollution and traffic noise, and ensure safety as well as climate and thermal comfort. While containment itself does not directly promote recovery, it establishes the prerequisite conditions for a recovery experience. Passive recovery, on the other hand, allows individuals to obtain recovery benefits by exposure to environments with inherent recovery potential, without requiring additional efforts. Active recovery involves individuals actively interacting with cultural and social environmental factors to obtain recovery benefits. Such active interactions require spaces to provide resources for activities such as physical exercises and social interactions, as well as for building personal connections, such as place attachment and sense of belonging (Bornioli & Subiza-Pérez, 2023).

Multi-scale urban design can influence recovery processes through pathways in three domains: exposures, behaviours, and personal connections. Exposures contribute by either establishing preconditions for environments to foster recovery (containment) or providing resources conducive to passive recovery. This involves both mitigating negative environmental factors and amplifying positive ones, which are shaped by urban design.

Behaviours have been identified as one crucial pathway through which the built environment influences health (Frank et al., 2019). Active behaviours, including walking, physical activities, and social interactions, are essential strategies for active/pro-active recovery. Therefore, urban design should be able to afford these behaviours by offering adequate resource support.

Personal connections, such as place attachment and sense of belonging, are functional and emotional connections between individuals and places. These connections specially contribute to eudaimonia well-being derived from self-actualisation and meaning (Bornioli & Subiza-Pérez, 2023), as well as memory support and positive emotions (Scannell & Gifford, 2017). Building these connections requires individuals to contribute their own content, including

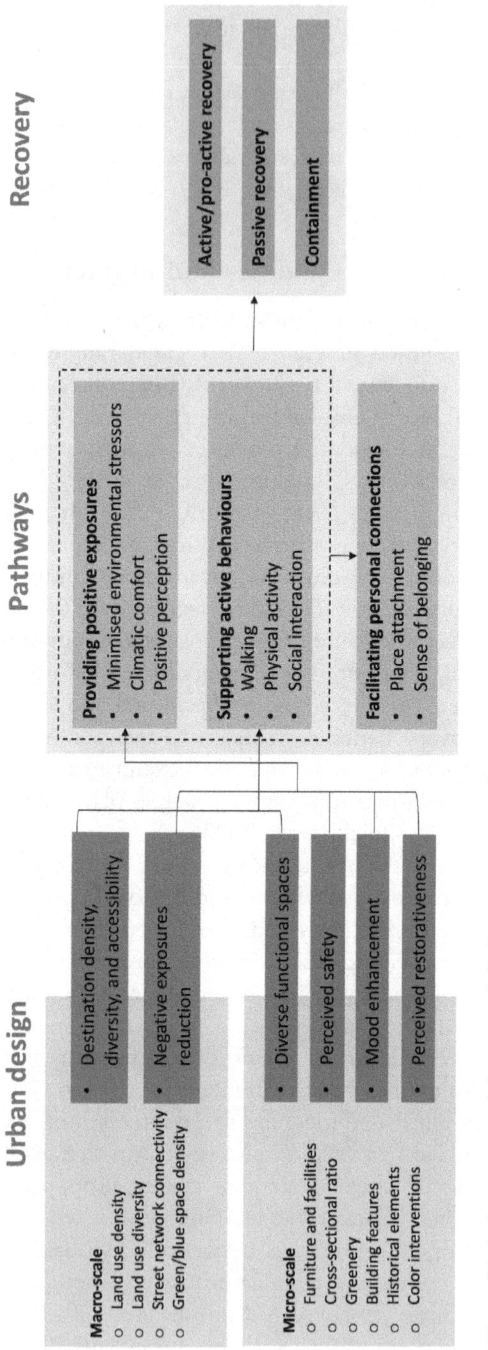

Figure 11.1 A conceptual framework linking macro- and micro-scale urban design to recovery through diverse pathways.

memories and meanings, to the environment (Liu et al., 2020; Ratcliffe & Korpela, 2016). The content itself typically emerges from individuals' interactions with their surroundings, shaped by environmental exposures and behaviours.

Subsequent sections will elucidate the key aspects of multi-scale urban design related to the pathways that are essential to foster recovery processes, grounded in existing empirical evidence.

Macro-scale urban design strategies to support recovery

Urban design at a macro scale encompasses considerations related to urban form, such as land use, street networks, and density, and their consequent impacts on users. To facilitate recovery, macro-scale urban design can focus on two key aspects: enhancing the diversity of destinations within an area and ensuring their accessibility, thereby promoting more active behaviours, and planning urban structures that effectively mitigate the influences of environmental stressors.

Promoting diversity and walking accessibility of destinations

Diverse and accessible destinations can provide diverse 'third spaces' (places separated from home and work) and help individuals connect with local social networks and services, encouraging more social and physical activities (Fonseca et al., 2022; Hajrasouliha & Yin, 2015; Oldenburg, 1999) and reducing social isolation (Kenyon et al., 2002).

Diversity of destinations can be achieved by enhancing land-use mix and the variety of destination types. McConville et al. (2011) measured land-use diversity by counting the number of non-residential land types within a 0.5-mile and 0.25-mile radii of participants' homes, including banks, bus stops, libraries, rail stations, offices, parks, recreation centres, retail stores, schools, and sports facilities. They found a positive correlation between land-use diversity and non-leisure walking. Improving accessibility involves increasing destination density, which reduces travel distance. However, McConville et al. (2011) found that a higher concentration of certain types of destinations, such as bus stops, grocery stores, offices, and retail stores, significantly promote walking. Some research (Yue et al., 2017) argued that destination diversity, a measure reflecting neighbourhood vitality, than density, plays a more essential role in enhancing pedestrian numbers than density.

Street network design is the other aspect to enhance neighbourhood accessibility. A highly connected street network is characterised by a grid pattern, high intersection density, and shorter block lengths. According to *Space Syntax Theory* (Hillier et al., 1993), a street network with high connectivity should have a relatively shallow average topological depth from any street to any other street – in other words, a highly connected street network provides users with easy access to diverse destinations. Such networks encourage behaviours beneficial for recovery, like walking, as they reduce travel distance and offer multiple route options, thereby increasing opportunities and motivations for walking

(Marshall & Garrick, 2010; Wineman et al., 2012). Additionally, highly connected street networks are linked to positive health outcomes, including lower risks of obesity, diabetes, heart disease, and depression (Marshall et al., 2014; Sarkar et al., 2013). These benefits have been explained by active behaviours encouraged by accessible neighbourhood street networks. Recent research also finds that network connectivity is associated with brain activities crucial for stress processing, possibly due to travelling and social behaviours influenced by network design (Dimitrov-Discher et al., 2023).

Reducing negative exposures

Reducing negative environmental exposures, such as pollution, noise, and extreme heat, is crucial for facilitating recovery in urban areas. Green-and-blue space design plays an essential role in mitigating these negative exposures. While macro-scale design characteristics of green and blue spaces, such as density and size, are associated with increased walking, heightened physical activity, and reduced impacts of stressful life events, along with lower risks of depression, anxiety, and mood disorders (Cohen-Cline et al., 2015; Krellenberg et al., 2014; Mytton et al., 2012; Nutsford et al., 2013; van den Berg et al., 2010), these benefits often depend on the micro-scale qualities of these spaces rather than their distribution and size alone. However, a higher amount of green areas reduces impermeable surfaces, mitigates the urban heat island effect, and ensures thermal comfort (Gunawardena et al., 2017). Urban green spaces are also able to purify the air and absorb noise, reducing the negative impacts of these stressors on residents (Gascon et al., 2015; Guo et al., 2019).

Street network design can also contribute to recovery by influencing mobility shares that are related to traffic-related stressors and safety. Neighbourhoods with grid street networks not only encourage more active mobility modes, such as walking and cycling, but are also associated with reduced driving (Marshall & Garrick, 2010, 2011, 2012). This reduction in driving can decrease the negative impacts of traffic-related pollution and noise, as well as lower the incidence of traffic accidents.

Micro-scale urban design strategies to support recovery

Micro-scale urban design closely relates to individuals' experiences in places, involving a wide range of design variables related to all outdoor space interfaces. To promote recovery, the design should provide resources supporting physical activity and social interactions while enhancing perceived qualities related to safety, mood enhancement, and perceived restorativeness.

Creating functional urban public spaces

Public spaces should incorporate diverse functional areas, such as playgrounds, pavilions, sports fields, and health trails, which serve as vital platforms supporting activities beneficial for recovery. The utilization of these spaces is often

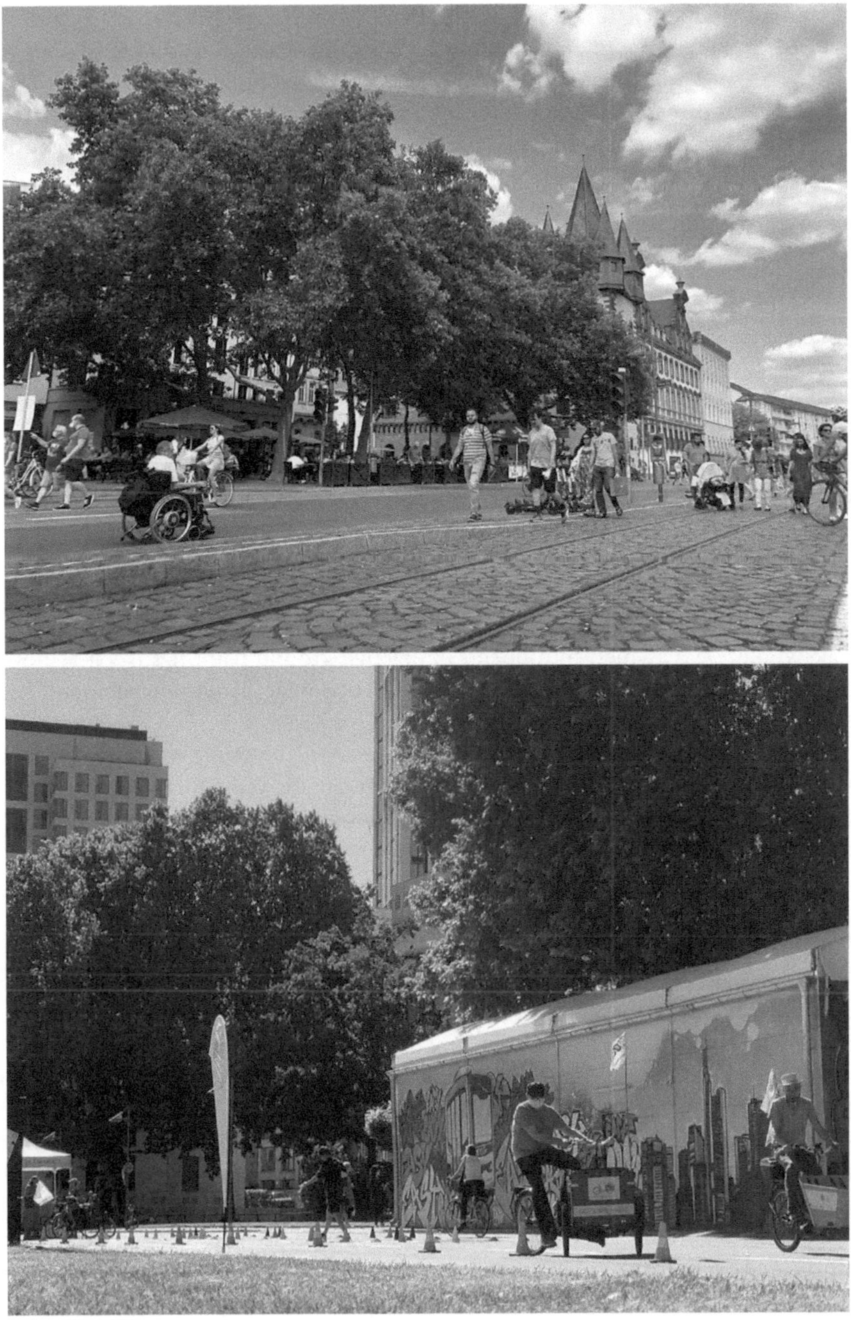

Figure 11.2 Mainkai Street in Frankfurt during the road closure experiment.

driven more by their functional utility than by their aesthetic appeal (Rasidi et al., 2012). Therefore, to enhance functionality, these spaces should be equipped with inclusive, well-maintained, and human-scale amenities that prioritise user comfort and cater to diverse needs. Essential amenities may include seating and secondary seating (e.g., planters, riverbanks, and grass), lighting, and sanitation facilities. These elements not only enhance the physical experience of the space but also contribute to its social and psychological benefits by encouraging prolonged and varied engagement.

For instance, Mainkai Street in Frankfurt (Figure 11.2), along the Main River, is a significant local recreational destination. It offers diverse functional spaces and amenities like outdoor cafés, accessible grass areas, footpaths, riverbanks, and benches, which support plenty of active and stationary activities, including walking, jogging, reading, and social interactions. In 2020, a road closure experiment was carried out, and motorised traffic was excluded from the street. During this time, more benches, movable furniture, club activities, and extended outdoor dining were introduced on the street, resulting in a more pedestrian-friendly scenario: pedestrian volume significantly increased, as well as the types and amount of stationary activities and physical activities (Pandit et al., 2021).

Moreover, interactive design elements like ground murals can also enhance functionality of public spaces, as demonstrated by the 40 West Artline project in Lakewood, USA, which introduced interactive ground paintings, such as hopscotch, along a 4-mile pedestrian path to encourage active engagement and foster a dynamic walking experience.

In addition to all positive behavioural outcomes, the effective usage of urban public spaces also fosters stronger user engagement, providing conditions for developing personal connections with the environment, including place attachment and a sense of belonging.

Improving perceived safety

When individuals feel safe in an urban environment, they are more likely to engage with the space, fostering a sense of comfort and security that supports their recovery process. Conversely, environments perceived as unsafe may provoke stress and anxiety, hindering recovery by discouraging engagement with public spaces. Micro-scale design elements have a stronger impact on perceived safety than macro-scale design (Harvey et al., 2015). Enclosure, the quality that makes urban spaces 'room-like' (Ewing & Handy, 2009), evokes a sense of hereness (Cullen, 2012) and is considered as a quality associated with perceived safety. In urban design, cross-sectional ratio (height-to-width ratio) of a space and vegetation are considered as two essential factors that influence the sense of enclosure (Harvey et al., 2015). While more enclosed streetscapes (having greater cross-sectional ratios and more trees) are perceived as safer (Harvey et al., 2015), excessive enclosure of an urban public space, such as a square or a green space with limited visibility beyond solid vertical interfaces, can hinder

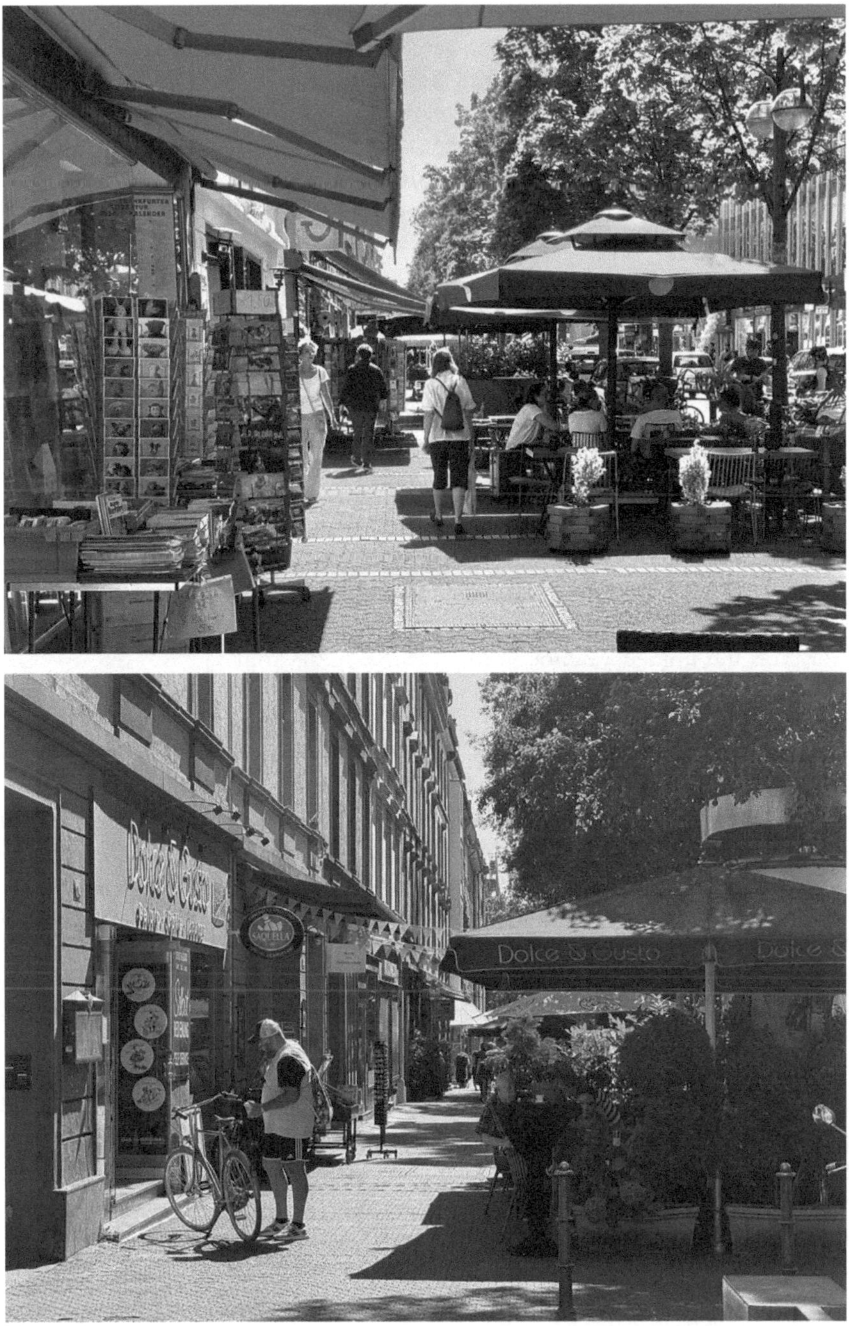

Figure 11.3 Berger Strasse in Frankfurt.

perceived safety. This is because such environments can be related to threats and offenders, indicating a blocked escape and evoking a sense of fear (Herzog & Chernick, 2000; Nasar et al., 1993; Tabrizian et al., 2018). Therefore, urban spaces are suggested to reduce solid wall proportions to enhance perceived safety, such as increasing ground floor facade transparency to increase 'eyes on the street' (Jacobs, 1961; Navarrete-Hernandez et al., 2021).

In addition to enclosure, appropriate lighting in urban public spaces is crucial for night-time safety perception (Zhao & Huang, 2021). The presence of vegetation in urban spaces also directly enhances perceived safety, probably due to the positive association between greenery and a sense of happiness (Seresinhe et al., 2019), given the inner link found between perceived safety and happiness (Mouratidis, 2019).

Improving mood states and perceived restorativeness

Enhanced mood states and perceived restorativeness are key psychological benefits of micro-scale urban design promoting recovery. Perceived restorativeness refers to individuals' evaluations of an environment based on restorative qualities proposed by the *Attention Restoration Theory* (ART; Kaplan, 1992): fascination, being away, extent, and compatibility – these qualities require urban spaces to be engaging and immersive enough to provide a break from daily stress.

Eye-level vegetation plays a crucial role in enhancing mood and perceived restorativeness. The quantity and percentage of greenery in view have been shown to positively influence these psychological outcomes (Jiang et al., 2014; Lindal & Hartig, 2015; Nordh et al., 2009; Zhao et al., 2019). Moreover, vegetation diversity is necessary not only for enhancing space preference but also for creating rich multisensory experiences. These sensory interactions with natural elements, including visual, auditory, and olfactory aspects, are crucial in facilitating passive recovery processes, benefiting individuals both physically and psychologically (He et al., 2022; Michels & Hamers, 2023).

Building facade details, such as silhouette, colour, and ornamentation, contribute to visual complexity in urban spaces and foster effortless attention and involuntary exploration, thereby enhancing perceived restorativeness (Ensari & Akbay, 2018; Lindal & Hartig, 2013; Lyu & Yang, 2023). Ground floor facade design is particularly important for contributing to place fascination, as the transparency of the facades connects indoor and outdoor spaces, generating curiosity (Barros et al., 2021). For example, one crucial aspect contributing to the vibrancy of Berger Strasse in Frankfurt, Germany (Figure 11.3), is the high level of ground floor facade transparency. The large windows of various shops arouse curiosity, allowing people to observe activities inside the buildings. Additionally, the extension of ground floor spaces, such as dining and retail areas, blurs the boundary between indoor and outdoor spaces, facilitating the integration of activities across these spaces.

Cultural and historical elements in urban spaces, such as old buildings and landmarks, enhance place imageability, a quality contributing to fascination.

Interacting with these elements might evoke a sense of being part of history, fostering a sense of being away, as well as personal connections, such as place attachment and belonging (Bornioli et al., 2018).

Colour interventions also have an impact on place perception related to mood and perceived restorativeness. Street art, such as ground murals, increases visual complexity and imageability of a street environment, thereby enhancing the fascination and evoking a sense of being away (Gu et al., 2021, in press). Notable examples include the superblocks in Barcelona and Superkilen in Copenhagen, where colourful ground murals have transformed previously less-appealing urban spaces into vibrant, fascinating areas. The design features of these interventions, such as colour schemes and pattern complexity, have impacts on users' psychological responses. For example, green-coloured murals promote relaxation more effectively than red ones (Gu et al., 2021), and intricate, playful designs elicit greater happiness than simple line designs (Batistatou et al., 2022).

The presence of social landscapes, such as benches, tables, and secondary seating, enriches 'Third Places', increasing perceived complexity, enjoyment, and neighbourhood vitality while triggering a sense of being away (Barros et al., 2021; Hassan et al., 2019; Park et al., 2013). Urban design that supports social interactions not only promotes recovery through user participation but also creates beneficial scenarios for those exposed to them.

Good practice examples

Superblocks, Barcelona, Spain

The superblock project in Barcelona exemplifies the promotion of recovery through multi-scale urban design strategies. The initiative aims to encourage sustainable mobility and create vibrant, healthy neighbourhood life. At a macro scale, the project reconfigured the existing street network to restrict motor vehicle traffic within superblocks, prioritising pedestrians and slow-moving cyclists. The redesign increased green space coverage, as well as public space diversity and density. As a result, these actions significantly reduced air pollution and noise levels within these blocks.

At a micro scale, the project focuses on creating high-quality, functional spaces. Movable planters, colourful ground markings, and furniture were introduced to define areas supporting both active and stationary activities. These spaces, varied in size and layout, offer safe, engaging environments for social interactions and children's play (Figure 11.4a).

Post-implementation, local businesses saw a 30% increase, with over 60% of people reporting significant improvements in walking comfort. Residents and workers within the superblocks noted enhanced perceived well-being, tranquillity, quality of sleep, and social interactions. The city plans to establish over 500 additional superblocks, with the Health Institute BCNecologia predicting an increase in residents' life expectancy by 200 days and a reduction in nitrogen dioxide emissions from 47 mg/m^3 to 36 mg/m^3.

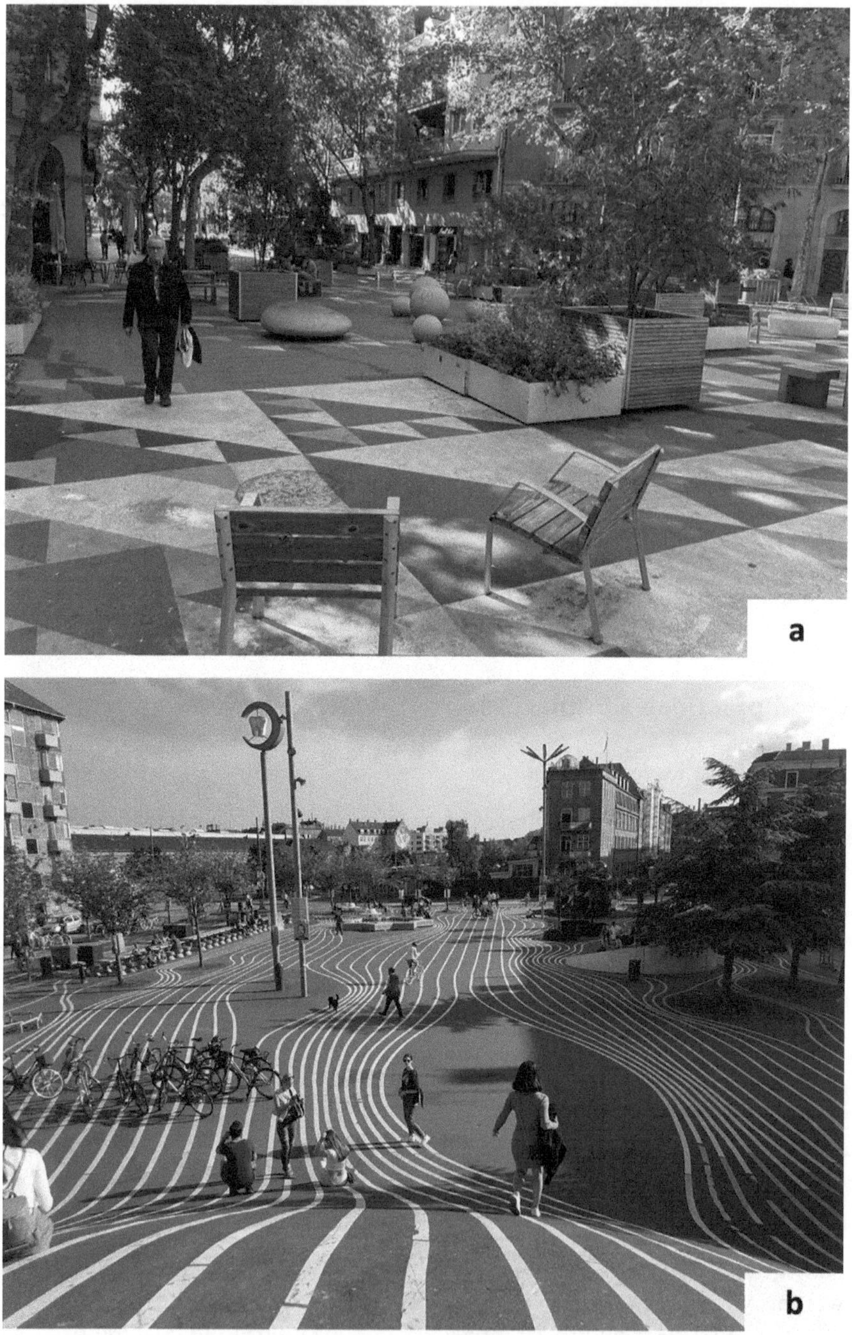

Figure 11.4 a) Application of ground colour interventions, movable furniture, and plants to create liveable and pedestrian-friendly neighbourhood in the superblock project, Barcelona. b) Application of ground painting and objects with diverse culture characteristics for multiculture communication in the Superkilen project, Copenhagen.

Playful City, Copenhagen, Denmark

Promoting active urban living for health is a key development aim of Copenhagen. The city consistently advocates for green mobility, particularly walking and cycling, while also creating playful spaces that support active behaviours.

At a macro scale, the city has followed a transit-oriented development since the 1950s. It enhances its cycling network by considering the total distances and density, as well as introducing unidirectional cycling lanes, improving the accessibility by cycling. Additionally, the city increases the density of recreational facilities, focusing on both new projects and the optimisation of existing public spaces.

At a micro scale, the focus is on human-scale design qualities. The Harbor Bath project, for instance, transforms an industrial dock into a vibrant public space with swimming pools, sunbathing platforms, diving boards, and seating areas, integrating sport and leisure needs. The Superkilen project uses diverse ground paintings, as well as over 60 culturally significant objects and landscapes, to create a lively, multicultural exchange space supporting social interaction and playful experiences for residents and visitors (Figure 11.4b).

Conclusion and implications for research and policies

The chapter proposes a conceptual framework linking multi-scale urban design to recovery with presenting distinctive pathways. The framework is supported by an exploration of existing literature. The framework encourages future research to validate the suggested associations, aiding administrations and planners in implementing policies and strategies for creating cities fostering recovery. Key future research directions include:

- **Empirical validation.** More evidence is needed to validate the pathways – exposures, behaviours, and personal connections – between multi-scale urban design and recovery.
- **Culture differences.** Conduct comparative studies to determine whether certain urban design aspects' impacts on recovery are universal or context-sensitive.
- **Quantifying design factors.** Develop improved methods to capture and quantify multi-scale urban design characteristics.
- **Innovative methodologies.** Integrate virtual reality and physiological measures to study the impact of multi-scale urban design on recovery.

The framework also suggests the following aspects associated with recovery for policymakers to consider:

- **Active city.** Encourage green mobility and active behaviours, especially walking and physical activities. Ensure facility density and accessibility through macro-scale planning, and ensure design quality at a micro scale.

- **Green city.** Enhance urban resilience and create high-quality, accessible, and diverse green spaces for everyday life.
- **Happy city.** Strengthen social coherence by involving the public in conception, design, decision-making, and evaluation processes, and encourage diverse daily activities through public organisation.

This chapter emphasises the role of urban design in fostering recovery. However, achieving urban environments that benefit recovery still calls for transdisciplinary collaboration across multiple sectors, including urban planners, public health officials, architects, environmental psychologists, and community stakeholders. Such collaboration is essential not only during research and conceptualisation but also throughout implementation and maintenance. Integrating diverse perspectives ensures that urban design interventions are holistic, inclusive, and sustainable, creating spaces that are functional, aesthetically pleasing, and beneficial for recovery.

References

Barros, P., Mehta, V., Brindley, P., & Zandieh, R. (2021). The restorative potential of commercial streets. *Landscape Research*, *46*(7), 1017–1037.

Batistatou, A., Vandeville, F., & Delevoye-Turrell, Y. N. (2022). Virtual reality to evaluate the impact of colorful interventions and nature elements on spontaneous walking, gaze, and emotion. *Frontiers in Virtual Reality*, *3*, 81957. https://doi.org/10.3389/frvir.2022.819597

Bornioli, A., Parkhurst, G., & Morgan, P. L. (2018). The psychological wellbeing benefits of place engagement during walking in urban environments: A qualitative photo-elicitation study. *Health & Place*, *53*, 228–236.

Bornioli, A., & Subiza-Pérez, M. (2023). Restorative urban environments for healthy cities: A theoretical model for the study of restorative experiences in urban built settings. *Landscape Research*, *48*(1), 152–163.

Cohen-Cline, H., Turkheimer, E., & Duncan, G. E. (2015). Access to green space, physical activity and mental health: A twin study. *Journal of Epidemiology & Community Health*, *69*(6), 523–529.

Cook, R. S. (1980). *Zoning for downtown urban design: How cities control development*. Lexington Books.

Cullen, G. (2012). *Concise townscape*. Routledge.

Dimitrov-Discher, A., Gu, L., Pandit, L., Veer, I. M., Walter, H., Adli, M., & Knöll, M. (2023). Stress and streets: How the network structure of streets is associated with stress-related brain activation. *Journal of Environmental Psychology*, *91*, 102142. https://doi.org/10.1016/j.jenvp.2023.102142

Ensari, E., & Akbay, S. (2018). *Walkability and colour experience: Façade colours and pedestrian walking preferences on urban streets* [Conference presentation]. AIC Lisboa 2018, Colour & Human Comfort, Lisboa, Portugal.

Ewing, R., & Handy, S. (2009). Measuring the unmeasurable: Urban design qualities related to walkability. *Journal of Urban Design*, *14*(1), 65–84.

Ewing, R. H., Clemente, O., Neckerman, K. M., Purciel-Hill, M., Quinn, J. W., & Rundle, A. (2013). *Measuring urban design: Metrics for livable places* (Vol. 200). Island Press.

Flowers, E. P., Freeman, P., & Gladwell, V. F. (2016). A cross-sectional study examining predictors of visit frequency to local green space and the impact this has on physical activity levels. *BMC Public Health, 16*, 420. https://doi.org/10.1186/s12889-016-3050-9

Fonseca, F., Ribeiro, P. J., Conticelli, E., Jabbari, M., Papageorgiou, G., Tondelli, S., & Ramos, R. A. (2022). Built environment attributes and their influence on walkability. *International Journal of Sustainable Transportation, 16*(7), 660–679.

Frank, L. D., Iroz-Elardo, N., MacLeod, K. E., & Hong, A. (2019). Pathways from built environment to health: A conceptual framework linking behavior and exposure-based impacts. *Journal of Transport & Health, 12*, 319–335.

Gascon, M., Triguero-Mas, M., Martínez, D., Dadvand, P., Forns, J., Plasència, A., & Nieuwenhuijsen, M. J. (2015). Mental health benefits of long-term exposure to residential green and blue spaces: A systematic review. *International Journal of Environmental Research and Public Health, 12*(4), 4354–4379.

Gerike, R., Carlow, V., Görner, H., Hantschel, S., Koszowski, C., Medicus, M., & Krieg, M. (2023). Vibrant streets: Characteristics, success factors and contributions to sustainable development. In R. C. Brears (Ed.), *The circular economy and liveable cities*. Cambridge University Press. https://nbn-resolving.org/urn:nbn:de:bsz:14-qucosa2-872011

Gruebner, O., Rapp, M. A., Adli, M., Kluge, U., Galea, S., & Heinz, A. (2017). Cities and mental health. *Deutsches Ärzteblatt International, 114*(8), 121–127.

Gu, L., Batistatou, A., Delevoye, Y., Roe, J., & Knöll, M. (2021). *Using artificial ground color to promote a restorative sidewalk experience: An experimental study based on manipulated street view images* [Conference presentation]. International Colour Association (AIC) Conference 2021, Milan, Italy.

Gu, L., Dimitrov-Discher, A., Knöll, M., & Roe, J. (in press). Cool colors promote a restorative sidewalk experience: A study on effects of color and pattern design of ground murals on mood states and perceived restorativeness using 2D street view images. *Environment and Planning B: Urban Analytics and City Science*. https://doi.org/10.1177/23998083241272100

Gunawardena, K. R., Wells, M. J., & Kershaw, T. (2017). Utilising green and bluespace to mitigate urban heat island intensity. *Science of The Total Environment, 584–585*, 1040–1055.

Guo, L., Luo, J., Yuan, M., Huang, Y., Shen, H., & Li, T. (2019). The influence of urban planning factors on PM2.5 pollution exposure and implications: A case study in China based on remote sensing, LBS, and GIS data. *Science of The Total Environment, 659*, 1585–1596.

Hajrasouliha, A., & Yin, L. (2015). The impact of street network connectivity on pedestrian volume. *Urban Studies, 52*(13), 2483–2497.

Harvey, C., Aultman-Hall, L., Hurley, S. E., & Troy, A. (2015). Effects of skeletal streetscape design on perceived safety. *Landscape and Urban Planning, 142*, 18–28.

Hassan, D. M., Moustafa, Y. M., & El-Fiki, S. M. (2019). Ground-floor façade design and staying activity patterns on the sidewalk: A case study in the Korba area of Heliopolis, Cairo, Egypt. *Ain Shams Engineering Journal, 10*(3), 453–461.

He, M., Wang, Y., Wang, W. J., & Xie, Z. (2022). Therapeutic plant landscape design of urban forest parks based on the five senses theory: A case study of Stanley Park in Canada. *International Journal of Geoheritage and Parks, 10*(1), 97–112.

Herzog, T. R., & Chernick, K. K. (2000). Tranquility and danger in urban and natural settings. *Journal of Environmental Psychology, 20*(1), 29–39.

Hillier, B., Penn, A., Hanson, J., Grajewski, T., & Xu, J. (1993). Natural movement: Or, configuration and attraction in urban pedestrian movement. *Environment and Planning B: Planning and Design*, *20*(1), 29–66.

Jacobs, J. (1961). *The death and life of great American cities*. Random House.

Jiang, B., Chang, C.-Y., & Sullivan, W. C. (2014). A dose of nature: Tree cover, stress reduction, and gender differences. *Landscape and Urban Planning*, *132*, 26–36.

Kaplan, S. (1992). The restorative environment: Nature and human experience. *The role of horticulture in human well-being and social development* (pp. 134–142). Timber Press.

Kenyon, S., Lyons, G., & Rafferty, J. (2002). Transport and social exclusion: Investigating the possibility of promoting inclusion through virtual mobility. *Journal of Transport Geography*, *10*(3), 207–219.

Krellenberg, K., Welz, J., & Reyes-Päcke, S. (2014). Urban green areas and their potential for social interaction – a case study of a socio-economically mixed neighbourhood in Santiago de Chile. *Habitat International*, *44*, 11–21.

Lang, J. (2006). *Urban design*. Routledge.

Lindal, P. J., & Hartig, T. (2013). Architectural variation, building height, and the restorative quality of urban residential streetscapes. *Journal of Environmental Psychology*, *33*, 26–36.

Lindal, P. J., & Hartig, T. (2015). Effects of urban street vegetation on judgments of restoration likelihood. *Urban Forestry & Urban Greening*, *14*(2), 200–209.

Liu, Q., Wu, Y., Xiao, Y., Fu, W., Zhuo, Z., van den Bosch, C. C. K., Huang, Q., & Lan, S. (2020). More meaningful, more restorative? Linking local landscape characteristics and place attachment to restorative perceptions of urban park visitors. *Landscape and Urban Planning*, *197*, 103763. https://doi.org/10.1016/j.landurbplan.2020.103763

Lyu, C., & Yang, C. (2023). Study on the complexity of urban waterfront interface from the perspective of restorative experience. In A. Hasan, C. Benimana, M. R. Thomson, & M. Tamke (Eds.), *Design for health* (pp. 77–91). Springer.

Marshall, W. E., & Garrick, N. W. (2010). Effect of street network design on walking and biking. *Transportation Research Record*, *2198*(1), 103–115.

Marshall, W. E., & Garrick, N. W. (2011). Does street network design affect traffic safety? *Accident Analysis & Prevention*, *43*(3), 769–781.

Marshall, W. E., & Garrick, N. W. (2012). Community design and how much we drive. *Journal of Transport and Land Use*, *5*(2), 5–20.

Marshall, W. E., Piatkowski, D. P., & Garrick, N. W. (2014). Community design, street networks, and public health. *Journal of Transport & Health*, *1*(4), 326–340.

McConville, M. E., Rodríguez, D. A., Clifton, K., Cho, G., & Fleischhacker, S. (2011). Disaggregate land uses and walking. *American Journal of Preventive Medicine*, *40*(1), 25–32.

Michels, N., & Hamers, P. (2023). Nature sounds for stress recovery and healthy eating: A lab experiment differentiating water and bird sound. *Environment and Behavior*, *55*(3), 175–205.

Mouratidis, K. (2019). Compact city, urban sprawl, and subjective well-being. *Cities*, *92*, 261–272.

Mytton, O. T., Townsend, N., Rutter, H., & Foster, C. (2012). Green space and physical activity: An observational study using health survey for England data. *Health & Place*, *18*(5), 1034–1041.

Nasar, J. L., Fisher, B., & Grannis, M. (1993). Proximate physical cues to fear of crime. *Landscape and Urban Planning*, *26*(1), 161–178.

Navarrete-Hernandez, P., Vetro, A., & Concha, P. (2021). Building safer public spaces: Exploring gender difference in the perception of safety in public space through urban design interventions. *Landscape and Urban Planning*, *214*, 104180. https://doi.org/10.1016/j.landurbplan.2021.104180

Nordh, H., Hartig, T., Hagerhall, C., & Fry, G. (2009). Components of small urban parks that predict the possibility for restoration. *Urban Forestry & Urban Greening*, *8*(4), 225–235.

Nubani, L., & Wineman, J. (2005). The role of space syntax in identifying the relationship between space and crime. *Journal of Chemical Information and Modeling*, *53*, 1689–1699.

Nutsford, D., Pearson, A., & Kingham, S. (2013). An ecological study investigating the association between access to urban green space and mental health. *Public Health*, *127*(11), 1005–1011.

Oldenburg, R. (1999). *The great good place: Cafes, coffee shops, bookstores, bars, hair salons, and other hangouts at the heart of a community*. Da Capo Press.

Pandit, L., Fauggier, G. V., Gu, L., & Knöll, M. (2021). How do people use Frankfurt Mainkai riverfront during a road closure experiment? A snapshot of public space usage during the coronavirus lockdown in May 2020. *Cities & Health*, *5*(Suppl. 1), S243–S262.

Park, S.-H., Kim, J.-H., Choi, Y.-M., & Seo, H.-L. (2013). Design elements to improve pleasantness, vitality, safety, and complexity of the pedestrian environment: Evidence from a Korean neighbourhood walkability case study. *International Journal of Urban Sciences*, *17*(1), 142–160.

Rasidi, M. H., Jamirsah, N., & Said, I. (2012). Urban green space design affects urban residents' social interaction. *Procedia-Social and Behavioral Sciences*, *68*, 464–480.

Ratcliffe, E., & Korpela, K. M. (2016). Memory and place attachment as predictors of imagined restorative perceptions of favourite places. *Journal of Environmental Psychology*, *48*, 120–130.

Roe, J., & McCay, L. (2021). *Restorative cities: Urban design for mental health and wellbeing*. Bloomsbury Publishing.

Sarkar, C., Gallacher, J., & Webster, C. (2013). Urban built environment configuration and psychological distress in older men: Results from the Caerphilly study. *BMC Public Health*, *13*, 695. https://doi.org/10.1186/1471-2458-13-695

Scannell, L., & Gifford, R. (2017). The experienced psychological benefits of place attachment. *Journal of Environmental Psychology*, *51*, 256–269.

Seresinhe, C. I., Preis, T., MacKerron, G., & Moat, H. S. (2019). Happiness is greater in more scenic locations. *Scientific Reports*, *9*(1), 4498. https://doi.org/10.1038/s41598-019-40854-6

Sharifi, A. (2019). Resilient urban forms: A review of literature on streets and street networks. *Building and Environment*, *147*, 171–187.

Tabrizian, P., Baran, P. K., Smith, W. R., & Meentemeyer, R. K. (2018). Exploring perceived restoration potential of urban green enclosure through immersive virtual environments. *Journal of Environmental Psychology*, *55*, 99–109.

van den Berg, A. E., Maas, J., Verheij, R. A., & Groenewegen, P. P. (2010). Green space as a buffer between stressful life events and health. *Social Science & Medicine*, *70*(8), 1203–1210.

Weber, A. M., & Trojan, J. (2018). The restorative value of the urban environment: A systematic review of the existing literature. *Environmental Health Insights*, *12*, 1178630218812805. https://doi.org/10.1177/1178630218812805

Wineman, J. D., Marans, R. W., Schulz, A. J., Van der Westhuizen, D., Mentz, G., & Max, P. (2012). *Neighborhood design and health: Characteristics of the built environment and health-related outcomes for residents of Detroit neighborhoods* [Conference presentation]. Eighth International Space Syntax Symposium, Santiago de Chile, Chile.

Yue, Y., Zhuang, Y., Yeh, A. G., Xie, J.-Y., Ma, C.-L., & Li, Q.-Q. (2017). Measurements of POI-based mixed use and their relationships with neighbourhood vibrancy. *International Journal of Geographical Information Science, 31*(4), 658–675.

Zang, P., Liu, X., Zhao, Y., Guo, H., Lu, Y., & Xue, C. Q. (2020). Eye-level street greenery and walking behaviors of older adults. *International Journal of Environmental Research and Public Health, 17*(17), 6130. https://doi.org/10.3390/ijerph17176130

Zhao, J., & Huang, Y. (2021). Physical characteristics of urban green spaces in relation to perceived safety. *Journal of Urban Planning and Development, 147*(4), 05021032. https://doi.org/10.1061/(ASCE)UP.1943-5444.0000742

Zhao, J., Wu, J., & Wang, H. (2019). Characteristics of urban streets in relation to perceived restorativeness. *Journal of Exposure Science & Environmental Epidemiology, 30*(2), 309–319.

12 Creating urban and workplace environments for recovery and well-being

A concluding summary

Jürgen Beckmann, Michael Kellmann, and Stephan Pauleit

Integrating recovery and resilience: Key insights

The world in the 21st century is facing challenges that require fundamental reorganisation of human societies. The quest for sustainability and climate change adaptation, in conjunction with technological upheavals, is becoming an ever more important factor in current and future urban development. Globalisation affects human health through rapidly spreading pandemics, with consequences for living and working conditions. The way humans live and work is changing due to crisis-like developments.

The concepts of recovery and resilience **are central to meeting these challenges** – both as a personal process and as a systemic response to urban challenges. Urban resilience, as discussed by Pauleit et al. (this volume, Chapter 1), involves not just bouncing back from shocks but also adapting and transforming in the face of adversity. This resilience is intimately tied to the recovery processes that individuals and communities undergo in urban settings. In the Kellmann and Kallus (2001) model, individuals may be high on stress without negative effects on performance, health, and well-being, as long as the stress is balanced by sufficient and appropriate recovery. They may even overcompensate to create a stress buffer. Urban environments should provide resources and affordances that aid the recovery process, such as time, social ties, inclusive communities, well-functioning organisations, and safety. Not least, physical environments for living, working, and commuting need to be planned, designed, and managed to support recovery.

Both recovery and resilience comprise a restorative and a preventive perspective. Urban recovery involves restoration of the infrastructure after natural and human-made disasters, as well as restoration of nature elements, particularly regarding

Beckmann, J., Kellmann, M., & Pauleit, S. (2025). Creating urban and workplace environments for recovery and well-being: A concluding summary. In S. Pauleit, M. Kellmann, & J. Beckmann (Eds.), *Creating Urban and Workplace Environments for Recovery and Well-being* (pp. 231–237). Routledge.

DOI: 10.4324/9781003435471-15

biodiversity. As Egerer and Marselle (this volume, Chapter 8) point out, parallels exist between ecosystem restoration and psychological recovery in urban environments. They consider urban biodiversity as a fundamental link between an ecological and a psychological perspective of resilience. Expanding on Markevych et al. (2017), four pathways between biodiversity and human health can be distinguished: reducing harm, restoring capacities, building capacities, but exposure to nature can also cause harm (Marselle et al., 2021). The latter may comprise pollen allergies or the breeding of mosquitos that transmit malaria. Such aspects should not be neglected in the planning of urban green infrastructure.

Future cities should envisage creating opportunities where ecological resilience can foster psychological resilience, and vice versa (Pauleit et al., this volume, Chapter 1). Notably, urban nature, with its manifold expressions, such as parks, woodlands, gardens, street greenery, surface waters, and wastelands that are recovered by the spontaneous growth of vegetation, seems to moderate the adverse effects of, among others, population density and pollution, directly and indirectly, on people's health and well-being, as several chapters in this volume show (Bengtsson et al., this volume, Chapter 4; de Vries & Chalmin-Pui, this volume, Chapter 7; Egerer & Marselle, this volume, Chapter 8; van den Bosch & Jarvis, this volume, Chapter 6). They provide compelling evidence based on a body of literature that has strongly expanded over the past two decades. Both experimental and population-based studies have confirmed that exposure to nature reduces stress and improves mental health and well-being across various life stages. Theoretical approaches have emphasised nature's role in health promotion through recovery from stress and attention restoration. Recent research addresses resilience as a key pathway to nature's mental health benefits. The *Biopsychosocial Resilience Theory* (White et al., 2023) describes how contact with nature influences resilience across multiple dimensions – biological, psychological, and social – during different phases in the cycle of stress response and recovery (van den Bosch & Jarvis, this volume, Chapter 6). Moreover, the moderation of human heat stress by a strategically developed network of green spaces, also called the urban green infrastructure, is increasingly recognised as a key measure for climate-resilient and healthy cities (Bauer et al., this volume, Chapter 9). In this regard, trees are most effective at cooling the city by casting shade and transpiring water. A biodiverse nature holds particular potential for human recovery. However, as Bengtsson et al. (this volume, Chapter 4) point out, the wider experiential qualities of urban green, such as serenity, shelter, naturalness, and cohesiveness, are important for the recovery of stressed people. There are also people who rather need to seek more stimulating cultural and social experiences to obtain recovery. The authors offer tools to implement these qualities into the purposive design of green spaces and residential areas for human recovery from stress. For the planning of entire urban landscapes, both de Vries and Chalmin-Pui (this volume, Chapter 7) and Egerer and Marselle (this volume, Chapter 8) highlight the important role of nature elements in the immediate vicinity of the residential area, which can be found in residential green spaces, notably home gardens, and in the activity of gardening for human recovery.

Well-connected and multifunctional networks of public green spaces in urban design are very important for human health and well-being. However, they cannot substitute the immediate contact with nature in such residential green spaces. Therefore, the ongoing densification of the built environment in growing cities needs to be questioned. Not only can it threaten the sufficient provision of residential green spaces, but it also can lead to increased crowding of the public green spaces in high-density neighbourhoods (de Vries & Chalmin-Pui, this volume, Chapter 7). This may become particularly problematic during crises, like the Covid-19 pandemic (Poortinga et al., 2021), or when heatwaves strike cities (Pauleit et al., 2020). Setting local targets is essential to ascertain a certain amount of green spaces in each neighbourhood. Yet there is a need to go beyond purely quantitative targets, such as area of green per capita, as various chapters in this book show. Examples are the Accessible Natural Greenspace Standard (Handley et al., 2003) and the 3–30–300 rule that has been recently suggested (Konijnendijk, 2023). The latter requests that one should be able to see three trees from each house, an average tree cover of 30% in each neighbourhood, and a public green space accessible within a 300-metre distance from home. In concurrence, Bauer et al. (this volume, Chapter 9) show that a crown projected tree cover of 25% is needed in densely built inner-city neighbourhoods of central European cities to combat urban heat with its negative effects on human health and well-being in a changing climate. To achieve this goal, a transformation of the streetscape is necessary – away from car streets and towards shared spaces with different purposes. Such streetscapes will also promote active mobility of walking and cycling as a key strategy for healthy cities.

This approach requires interdisciplinary collaboration among urban planners, landscape architects, ecologists, engineers, and not least social scientists and psychologists, to retrofit infrastructures and promote sustainable urban design. Moreover, citizen participation is crucial to align planning efforts with local needs and preferences, ensuring that green spaces are accessible and serve diverse community interests.

Designing work environments for recovery has received little attention so far. The chapter by Koppen et al. (this volume, Chapter 5) presents new perspectives on designing work environments for two specific fields: knowledge workers in offices and health workers in hospitals. For office settings, rediscovering 'Third Places', such as libraries, cafés, and coworking spaces, can enhance employee well-being by offering neutral, leisure-like environments that encourage mobility and interaction. While supporting modern digital work requirements, these spaces can also be integrated within office buildings.

In hospitals, the HEMI architectural concept – (H) *hands on*, (E) *eyes on*, (M_{on}) *mind on*, (M_{off}) *mind off*, (I) *interact* (Koppen et al., this volume, Chapter 5) – offers an innovative approach to improving employee well-being by reorganising work environments based on the nature of patient contact. Environments with direct patient contact should be more private, efficient, and less stimulating, while environments with indirect patient contact can be more open and interactive. Some similarities between this concept and the concept by Bengtsson et al.

(this volume, Chapter 4) of restorative and stimulating perceived sensory dimensions that should be offered in four zones of open spaces can be found.

Gu and Knöll (this volume, Chapter 11) embed the previous suggestions for the planning and design of the built environment with its open spaces into a framework for the multi-scale design of restorative cities. According to these authors, urban planning should, at city scale, primarily enhance the diversity of destinations within an area and ensure their accessibility to promote active behaviours in low-stress environments. Evidence suggests that mixed land use and a variety of destination types, such as banks, bus stops, libraries, railway stations, recreation centres, sports facilities, and parks, accessible through highly connected street networks, are linked to positive health outcomes – provided that environmental stressors, such as excessive levels of air pollution and noise, can be avoided. At the micro-scale, the authors argue for multifunctional public spaces that offer facilities for different uses. A range of design elements, such as cultural heritage, facades, friendly colours, and vegetation, can enhance the quality of open spaces.

Importantly, open space needs to be perceived as safe (Ceccato, this volume, Chapter 10). The latter can be enhanced by physical design, for example, finding the right level of enclosure and lighting, but, as other research has shown, also the management of squares. For instance, vandalism and littering lead to avoidance of public open spaces because they are perceived as unsafe (Maruthaveeran & Konijnendijk van den Bosch, 2014). Safety in public spaces is closely related to inclusivity. Ceccato (this volume, Chapter 10) takes an intersectional perspective as the perception of safety is unequally distributed among urban society and closely linked to personal experiences, such as having been a victim of sexual violence and other crimes. Women, the elderly, ethnic minorities, and members of the LGBTQI+ communities, among others, particularly experience fear of crime and, consequently, may use less and benefit less from open spaces. Strategies for inclusive, gender-sensitive design and policies are outlined in this chapter. Strengthening community involvement is particularly important. Creating liaison units for gender and minority issues, gender-sensitivity training, bystander intervention programmes, and community-led safety audits are promising strategies. Drawing on experience from Global North cities, such as Stockholm, and Global South cities, such as Nairobi and Bogotá, alike makes this chapter distinct in this volume.

Urban environments undergo transformation and demand further planned changes due to a changing environment, particularly climate change, but also developments in the social system. Also, the working environment is changing. The so-called 'New Work' is a new concept fundamentally changing the work environment, replacing traditional structures. The changes are enforced by a structural alteration of the labour market, changing requirements, wishes, and needs of younger generations, as well as the consequences of digitalisation and the corona pandemic. The 'New Work' trend involves decentralisation, a change in the understanding of the workplace and where it is located, and more independent work organisation (Koppen et al., this volume, Chapter 5). Strictly hierarchical leadership styles are increasingly being replaced by a culture of trust and empathy.

Reduced working hours are not only demands made by unions but are also used as means to make a job more attractive, given a shortage of skilled workers. Home office and four-day workweeks have been introduced. Kallus (this volume, Chapter 3) refers to the potential threats to the traditional break and recovery culture in organisations as it becomes more difficult to differentiate between work and leisure time used for recovery. Detachment from work is an essential prerequisite for finding recovery, as several authors point out. Traditionally, commuting between home and the workplace was a potential means of detachment. However, as Kallus highlights, with an increase in working in the home office, this opportunity is lost. Furthermore, Elfering and Huber (this volume, Chapter 2) discuss the potentially stress-aggravating effects of commuting by car. Kallus, as well as Elfering and Huber, point out that the occurring change demands planning and organisation of recovery from work. However, as 'ownership' is a core element in 'New Work', referring to self-determination and taking responsibility for one's work and product, it can be transferred to recovery. With a changing work environment, employees need to increasingly take responsibility for their own recovery. This is particularly important as recovery is highly individuum-specific. What is adequate recovery for one person is not necessarily recovery for another person. Hence, individuals need to learn to recognise their recovery needs and know which kind of recovery suits them best in which situation which involves that recovery requires self-regulation (Beckmann, 2023). In recent years, the concept of health literacy has become popular. Health literacy is defined as the degree to which individuals have the ability to find, understand, and use information and services to inform health-related decisions and actions for themselves and others. Meanwhile, organisational health literacy has been included (Li, 2022). Continuing the considerations from Kallus, given new working conditions that no longer make traditional breaks and recovery culture seem appropriate, employees need to learn a kind of recovery literacy helping them plan recovery activities ahead and know which one is most appropriate in the given time-space context.

A paradigm shift is also required for commuting (Elfering & Huber, this volume, Chapter 2). While flexible work times and places, including working at home, may reduce the overall demand for commuting, it needs to be acknowledged that commuting is and will remain an important part in the life of many. Traditional views of commuting as merely time spent traveling are insufficient; a broader perspective that includes transportation mode, work arrangements, voluntariness, and the potential for personal pursuits during travel is necessary. Conceptualising commuting as both a demand and a potential resource for recovery is essential for identifying factors that can transform it from a stressor into a facilitator of well-being. Active modes of commuting, such as cycling, that promote mental detachment are suggested as a silver bullet to facilitate recovery.

Conclusion: Towards holistic urban futures

The conclusion drawn from these chapters is clear: the future of urban planning must prioritise human recovery and resilience. This entails a paradigm shift towards designing cities that not only withstand environmental and social challenges but also actively support the health and well-being of their residents. Key recommendations refer to:

1. **Integrated strategies for urban resilience and human recovery.** Incorporate human recovery aspects early on, and comprehensively, into urban resilience strategies and integrative urban design at multiple scales, from city and city regions to the design of individual open spaces, homes, and workplaces, ensuring that urban environments facilitate stress reduction, social cohesion, and physical activity. Such strategies should be evidence-based and developed in collaborative and participatory modes to ascertain that they respond to local social and environmental needs and enhance justice.
2. **Environmental quality.** Enhance access to quality green spaces and natural environments that promote mental health and physical well-being. This includes preserving existing green spaces, creating new ones, and ensuring equitable access for all urban dwellers. Employ tools for the design of green spaces to promote perceived sensory dimensions for recovery. Develop targets grounded in scientific evidence for developing multifunctional green infrastructure networks at the city level.
3. **Workplace and commuting.** Redesign work environments to prioritise employee well-being through structured work hours, adequate breaks, and environments that integrate natural elements and opportunities for social interaction. Promote active mobility.
4. **Safety and inclusivity.** Foster urban environments that are safe, inclusive, and supportive of recovery from crime and victimisation. This requires proactive policies and community engagement to address diverse urban experiences and needs.
5. **Biodiversity and ecological resilience.** Integrate biodiversity into urban planning to enhance ecosystem services and promote biopsychosocial resilience through exposure to natural environments.
6. **Climate resilience.** Mitigate the impacts of climate change, notably heat stress and flooding, through green infrastructure, ventilation corridors, passive cooling techniques, and water-sensitive design.
7. **Research and innovation.** Advance inter- and transdisciplinary research to deepen our theoretical understanding of the multifaceted relationships between urban resilience and human recovery. Consolidate more specific concepts related to green space recovery interactions, such as the *Biopsychosocial Resilience Theory* and the pathways model of relationships between biodiversity and human well-being, the HEMI concept for restorative design of healthcare facilities, the potential of break. Develop innovative tools and methodologies to assess and optimise urban environments for human health

and well-being. Identify innovative strategies and governance models for restorative cities. In all this, emphasise the Global South's rapidly expanding cities with their specific challenges of urbanisation.

References

Beckmann, J. (2023). Self-regulation of recovery. In M. Kellmann, S. Jakowski, & J. Beckmann (Eds.), *The importance of recovery for physical and mental health: Negotiating the effects of underrecovery* (pp. 53–69). Routledge.

Handley, J., Pauleit, S., Slinn, P., Barber, A., Baker, M., Jones, C., & Lindley, S. (2003). *Accessible natural greenspace standards in towns and cities: A review and toolkit for their implementation (ENRR526)*. English Nature Research Reports. Retrieved June 17, 2024 from https://publications.naturalengland.org.uk/publication/65021

Kellmann, M., & Kallus, K. W. (2001). *The Recovery-Stress Questionnaire for Athletes: User manual*. Human Kinetics.

Konijnendijk, C. C. (2023). Evidence-based guidelines for greener, healthier, more resilient neighbourhoods: Introducing the 3-30-300 rule. *Journal of Forestry Research, 34*, 821–830.

Li, A. (2022). Individual and organizational health literacies: Moderating psychological distress for individuals with chronic conditions. *Journal of Public Health, 44*(3), 651–662.

Markevych, I., Schoierer, J., Hartig, T., Chudnovsky, A., Hystad, P., Dzhambov, A. M., de Vries, S., Triguero-Mas, M., Brauer, M., Nieuwenhuijsen, M. J., Lupp, G., Richardson, E. A., Astell-Burt, T., Dimitrova, D., Feng, X., Sadeh, M., Standl, M., Heinrich, J., & Fuertes, E. (2017). Exploring pathways linking greenspace to health: Theoretical and methodological guidance. *Environmental Research, 158*, 301–317.

Marselle, M. R., Hartig, T., Cox, D. T. C., de Bell, S., Knapp, S., Lindley, S., Triguero-Mas, M., Böhning-Gaese, K., Braubach, M., Cook, P. A., de Vries, S., Heintz-Buschart, A., Hofmann, M., Irvine, K. N., Kabisch, N., Kolek, F., Kraemer, R., Markevych, I., Martens, D., . . . Bonn, A. (2021). Pathways linking biodiversity to human health: A conceptual framework. *Environment International, 150*, 106420. https://doi.org/10.1016/j.envint.2021.106420

Maruthaveeran, S., & Konijnendijk van den Bosch, C. C. (2014). A socio-ecological exploration of fear of crime in urban green spaces – a systematic review. *Urban Forestry & Urban Greening, 13*, 1–18.

Pauleit, S., Fryd, O., Backhaus, A., & Jensen, M. B. (2020). Green infrastructures to face climate change in an urbanizing world. In R. A. Meyers (Ed.), *Encyclopedia of sustainability science and technology* (pp. 1–29). Springer. https://doi.org/10.1007/978-1-4939-2493-6_212-3

Poortinga, W., Bird, N., Hallingberg, B., Phillips, R., & Williams, D. (2021). The role of perceived public and private green space in subjective health and wellbeing during and after the first peak of the COVID-19 outbreak. *Landscape and Urban Planning, 211*, 104092. https://doi.org/10.1016/j.landurbplan.2021.104092

White, M. P., Hartig, T., Martin, L., Pahl, S., van den Berg, A. E., Wells, N. M., Costongs, C., Dzhambov, A. M., Elliott, L. R., Godfrey, A., Hartl, A., Konijnendijk, C., Litt, J. S., Lovell, R., Lymeus, F., O'Driscoll, C., Pichler, C., Pouso, S., Razani, N., . . . van den Bosch, M. (2023). Nature-based biopsychosocial resilience: An integrative theoretical framework for research on nature and health. *Environment International, 181*, 108234. https://doi.org/10.1016/j.envint.2023.108234

Index

FSC
www.fsc.org
MIX
Papier | Fördert gute Waldnutzung
FSC® C083411

Kolibri 360 GmbH
Ferdinand-Jühlke-Straße 7
99095 Erfurt, Deutschland
produktsicherheit@kolibri360.de